T0145330

Quantitative Methods in Pharmaceutical Research and Development

Olga V. Marchenko • Natallia V. Katenka
Editors

Quantitative Methods in Pharmaceutical Research and Development

Concepts and Applications

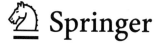 Springer

Editors
Olga V. Marchenko
Statistics and Data Insights Department
Bayer
Whippany, NJ, USA

Natallia V. Katenka
Department of Computer Science
and Statistics
University of Rhode Island
Kingston, RI, USA

ISBN 978-3-030-48557-3   ISBN 978-3-030-48555-9   (eBook)
https://doi.org/10.1007/978-3-030-48555-9

This Springer imprint is published by the registered company Springer Nature Switzerland AG
The registered company address is: Gewerbestrasse 11, 6330 Cham, Switzerland

Preface

The motivation for this book came from a discussion on how to help a young individual interested in quantitative disciplines in school to choose a major for further education and a career. In the old days, if someone were good in quantitative disciplines in school, he or she would go to college to receive a degree in Mathematics or Physics. Nowadays, universities offer a range of different concentration areas that rely on quantitative methods, such as Mathematics, Statistics, Biostatistics, Pharmacometrics, Genetics, Computer Science, Data Science, to name a few. It is not easy to make an educated choice for a future career. We decided to focus on the pharmaceutical industry specifically. There are many books available that describe one specific area, e.g., statistics, or a couple of areas, but we are not aware of books that provide a good overview of different analytics and statistical applications used in the pharmaceutical industry. Additionally, we were trying to understand what quantitative methods different departments at a company use to answer questions in the pharmaceutical industry and how people working at these departments collaborate and build on each other's knowledge.

The book *Quantitative Methods in Pharmaceutical Research and Development* presents an overview of concepts, methods, and applications in different quantitative areas of drug research, development, and marketing. Biostatistics, pharmacometrics, genomics, bioinformatics, pharmacoepidemiology, commercial analytics, and operational analytics—all of these disciplines use quantitative methods and analysis techniques to answer different questions related to drug research, development, and marketing. By bringing theory and applications of these disciplines together in one book, we hope to allow the reader to learn more about different quantitative fields and recognize similarities and differences in theory and applications employed by different disciplines. This book is aimed at people interested in quantitative methods and applications used in the pharmaceutical industry, experts working in these areas, and students looking for applications and career options in quantitative sciences.

Each chapter of this book is self-contained and written by different authors. Chapter 1 provides a brief overview of basic biostatistical principles, selected study designs, and analysis methods used in clinical trials. It also discusses the importance of biostatistics in drug development and highlights some additional considerations for clinical trials, such as defining appropriate estimands, handling outcomes with missing data, applying multiplicity adjustments, analyzing subgroups, planning multiregional clinical trials, and evaluating drug safety. Chapter 2 provides a brief introduction to pharmacometric analysis approaches including pharmacokinetic (PK) models, PK/pharmacodynamics (PD) models, physiologically based pharmacokinetic models, quantitative systems pharmacology models, and model-based meta-analysis. It includes discussions on software, modeling workflow, and major model components, with a focus on population modeling analysis. Chapter 3 gives an overview of bioinformatics and common methods used to address genomics-related questions. In Chapter 4, readers are introduced to common biostatistical methods used in the analysis and interpretation of pharmacoepidemiological data. This chapter also briefly describes how to take into account common issues in observational epidemiology, such as bias, confounding, and interactions, in order to establish a clear causal link between exposure and drug effect.

Chapter 5 provides an overview of the causal inference paradigm, reviewing current methodology and discussing the applications of these concepts to strengthen and improve pharmacoepidemiology. More specifically, this chapter focuses on marginal structural models fitted using inverse probability weights and discusses advanced topics, such as time-varying exposure, instrumental variables, and survival analyses. It also includes a discussion of challenges specific to analyses that employ medical claims and electronic health records. Chapter 6 provides an introduction to the diverse field of data science as viewed from the perspective of a clinical statistician. This chapter discusses data mining and its relationship with machine learning and classical statistics. More specifically, the authors map some common problems occurring in the analysis of clinical data onto general machine learning tasks, such as supervised, unsupervised, and semi-supervised learning, and review key concepts of data mining and machine learning with an emphasis on methods that are most relevant for the analyses of clinical data. Chapter 7 is an introduction to quantitative pharmaceutical market research techniques. It focuses on two types of primary market research: market segmentation and choice modeling. This chapter describes clustering methods that are used to create segments, that is, groups of individuals with unique attitudes and behaviors that allow for more targeted marketing efforts. It also reviews multiple approaches to choice modeling: a family of approaches that aim to deconstruct decisions and identify what attributes drive decision-making. Chapter 8 describes new predictive analytic techniques for efficient modeling and forecasting trial operations, more specifically modeling patient enrollment at different levels and analyzing interim trial performance and risk-based data monitoring using P-values and 2D classification. Chapter 9 provides case studies illustrating the impact of collaboration between biostatisticians, pharmacometricians, clinicians, formulation, and laboratory scientists. It also explains how working as a team and using quantitative modeling and simulation methodologies can result in significant efficiencies and improvements in the drug development process.

This book is a collaborative effort from several authors and based on knowledge and experience gained from working in academia, the pharmaceutical industry, and regulatory agencies. We present material that hopefully will be interesting to a broad and diverse audience. The views expressed in this book are those of the authors and do not necessarily represent the views of organizations with which the authors have been or are presently affiliated.

We would like to acknowledge and thank all authors who contributed to this book and reviewers who helped us review and improve the different chapters. We appreciate the constructive comments provided by José Pinheiro, Michael Hale, Ken Chase, Tony Zagar, Seth Berry, Ilya Lipkovich, and Russell Reeve. From our employers, we thank Torsten Westermeier, Bayer Statistics and Data Insights, and Lisa DiPippo, the University of Rhode Island Department of Computer Science and Statistics, for the encouragement. Additionally, we thank the Springer Publishing Agency for giving us an opportunity to publish this book and the Editor of Mathematics and Statistics, Springer US Christopher Tominich for his patience and helpful tips. Finally, we thank our special friends, Mikhail Benediktovich and Maria Francevna, and our families for encouragement and support.

Whippany, NJ, USA   Olga V. Marchenko
Kingston, RI, USA   Natallia V. Katenka

Contents

Chapter 1
Biostatistics in Clinical Trials

Olga V. Marchenko, Lisa M. LaVange, and Natallia V. Katenka

1.1 Introduction

1.1.1 What Is Biostatistics

Biostatistics is a part of statistics applied in a wide range of areas in the biological sciences. It covers the design of biological experiments, e.g., experiments in medicine, pharmacy, and agriculture; the collection, summarization, and analysis of data from the experiments; and the interpretation of results. A major branch of biostatistics is medical biostatistics that is applied in medicine and health.

As part of drug development, tests are conducted to determine how drugs affect the human body. We can only fully understand these effects—both positive and negative—if they are tested on living organisms. Animal studies are primarily used for testing pharmaceutical compounds in the preclinical development phase, followed by clinical studies with human subjects. In recent years, many new methods have been developed as alternatives to research on animals: in the in vitro method, active ingredients are tested on human cell cultures; in the in silico method, chemical reactions are tested using mathematical and computer-based models. Still, these methods cannot entirely replace tests on animals or humans yet. Clinical studies (clinical trials) are experiments intended to discover or verify the effects of one or more investigational treatments in human subjects, e.g., patients or healthy

O. V. Marchenko (✉)
Statistics and Data Insights Department, Bayer, Whippany, NJ, USA
e-mail: olga.marchenko@bayer.com

L. M. LaVange
Department of Biostatistics, University of North Carolina at Chapel Hill, Chapel Hill, NC, USA

N. V. Katenka
Department of Computer Science and Statistics, University of Rhode Island, Kingston, RI, USA

© Springer Nature Switzerland AG 2020
O. V. Marchenko, N. V. Katenka (eds.), *Quantitative Methods in Pharmaceutical Research and Development*, https://doi.org/10.1007/978-3-030-48555-9_1

volunteers. Biostatistics plays a vital role in the design, conduct, and reporting of clinical trials.

1.1.2 Basic Biostatistics Principals for Clinical Trials

This section briefly describes some important biostatistics principals for designing a clinical trial. There are many statistical books that cover statistical principals and designs of clinical trials in more details (e.g., Snedecor and Cochran 1980; Friedman et al. 2015; Piantadosi 2017). Additional valuable resources include the ICH Guidelines on efficacy and safety. Specifically, ICH Guideline E9 provides succinct information on Statistical Principals for Clinical Trials.

1.1.2.1   Population and Sample

A *population* is an entire group of people we want to understand and make inferences on. The size of the population can vary greatly. For example, the population of patients with diabetes around the world is enormous; the population of people with Pompe disease is quite small. A *sample* is a subgroup of the whole population that can be considered a representative set with respect to the question of interest.

The *study population* (a sample of patients with the disease selected for the study) in a clinical trial is the subset of the population with the condition or characteristics of interest defined by the eligibility criteria, e.g., inclusion and exclusion criteria outlined in a clinical protocol. When reporting a study, it is important to say what patients were studied and how they were selected. Knowledge of the study population helps assess the study's merit and relevance.

If the study population is selected by using very restrictive eligibility criteria, generalizing results from participants in the trial to the study population and then to a population with the condition might be difficult or even impossible. However, if the study includes diverse groups of patients and the treatment is only beneficial to a specific subgroup of patients, the effect of the intervention on a heterogeneous group may be diluted, and the ability to detect a benefit may be reduced. As scientific knowledge advances, the ability to classify improves. Modern trial designs such as platform and basket trial designs allow to include a more diverse group of patients into one trial and treat them with "personalized" treatments, e.g., treatments based on the genotype.

1.1.2.2   Sampling Error and Bias

When a sample is randomly chosen from a population, some variability exists and, therefore, the sample average will not precisely reflect the population average. An error has two components, a random one and a systematic one called bias. *Sampling error* does not necessarily mean that a mistake has been made during the sampling process; it is a fluctuation that remains beyond our ability to attribute it to a specific cause. Because of biologic variations, subject-to-subject differences, measurement error, or other sources of noise, it is impossible to eliminate random error completely. Averaging an increased number of observations and repeating the experiment reduce the magnitude of a random error. As we gain more knowledge, it is possible that some errors that are thought to be random become explainable.

As defined in ICH E9 Guidance (ICH E9 1998), *bias* is "the systematic tendency of any factors associated with the design, conduct, analysis, and interpretation of the results of a clinical trial to estimate a treatment effect deviate from its true value." The presence of bias may compromise the ability to draw valid conclusions. It is important to identify sources of bias in order to eliminate or reduce such bias. In a statistical context (statistical bias), the bias can be quantified. More discussion on the statistical bias is provided in Sect. 1.3 of this chapter. In a clinical context (operational bias), bias can arise from different sources and can rarely be quantified precisely. One type of operational bias is a *selection bias*. For example, if an investigator believes that a particular treatment in a clinical trial works better, he might want to enroll his better patients to this treatment, and therefore, he may affect the validity of the study. By excluding patients from analysis based upon knowledge of their outcomes, one can introduce an *assessment bias* that can enhance or diminish the strength of the actual treatment effect. Such operational biases can be removed or reduced by using an appropriate design, a pre-planned analysis, and a thorough execution of the clinical trial. For example, randomization reduces the selection bias and blinding reduces the assessment bias. Both randomization and blinding are discussed in more details later in this section. Most of the statistical principals and techniques outlined in this chapter deal with the problem of minimizing bias and maximizing the precision of estimation and, therefore, maximizing the validity of conclusions.

1.1.2.3 Choice of Control

Control group is a group of patients that helps understand what would have happened to the patients if they did not receive the experimental treatment or if they received a different treatment known to be effective. Choice of the control group is one of the major elements of the design of a clinical trial. The foundation for the design of controlled experiments was established in agriculture and made its way to the pharmaceutical industry a long time ago.

If the course of disease was uniform or predictable from patient characteristics such that the outcome could be reliably predicted for any given patient or a group of patients, we would not need to have a control group because the results of the treatment could be compared with the known outcome without a treatment. For example, one could assume that without a treatment, the pain would have persisted for a defined time, blood pressure would not change, or tumors would grow following a pre-specified model. If the course of a disease is predictable in a defined population, it may be possible to use previously studied patients as a historical control. In rare diseases, the use of historical control might be the only option. It is also possible to have a very high treatment effect that no comparison group is needed, but successful results of this magnitude are very rare. In most cases, a concurrent control group is needed because it is impossible to predict an outcome with an adequate accuracy or certainty.

The types of control that are mostly used in clinical trials are (1) placebo, (2) active control, or (3) different doses or regimens of the experimental treatment. The experimental treatment and concurrent control groups are sampled from the same population and treated in the same trial over the same period of time. Both groups, including those assigned to the study treatment and the control, should have similar baseline characteristics. Failure to achieve this similarity can introduce a bias into the study.

Study designs that use placebo as the control group are called *placebo-controlled* designs. A placebo is a "dummy" treatment that appears as identical as possible to the experimental treatment with regard to color, shape, weight, taste, and smell but does not contain any active treatment. Such designs almost always use randomization to assign patients to either an experimental treatment or to a placebo for ethical reasons and to eliminate a selection bias. *Active-controlled* (or positive controlled) trials are the trials in which patients are assigned to the experimental treatment and the active control treatment, e.g., the treatment already approved and available on a market. At times even though trials use a placebo arm to make formal comparisons with an experimental treatment arm, an active control arm can be included to validate the study and to help make predictions about a treatment effect of the experimental treatment against the active control. Such designs might be preferable to patients because of the smaller chance of being randomized to the placebo arm. An *add-on study design* is a placebo-controlled design of a new treatment and a placebo, both added to a standard treatment. Such studies are common in oncology, specifically, when the experimental treatment alone does not provide the necessary treatment effect but can improve the clinical outcome of the standard treatment if it is given as a combination treatment. Designs that use several fixed doses of the experimental treatment in addition to placebo allow selection of the most efficacious and safe dose or doses for further development and might help to characterize the dose-response shape.

Sound scientific clinical investigations almost always demand that a control group be a part of a trial to measure and compare a new treatment against a placebo or an active control. ICH E10 Guideline on Choice of Control Group and Related Issues in Clinical Trials (ICH E10, 2001) provides more details on types of a control and how to choose a control group. Randomization is the preferred approach to assign patients to a control group and an experimental group or groups.

1.1.2.4 Randomization and Allocation

Randomization is a process by which each participant has a specific probability (sometimes equal, sometimes not) to be assigned to either a treatment arm(s) or a control arm. Fisher formally suggested the concept of randomization in the 1920s. Amberson et al. in 1931 reported the first clinical trial that used a form of random assignment of participants to study groups. The principal of blinding was also introduced in this trial (Friedman et al. 2015).

Until the new treatment has been proven beneficial, randomization is the most ethical approach. Randomization removes a potential bias (selection bias) in the assignment of patients to study groups. Randomization tends to produce study groups comparable with respect to known and unknown risk factors, measured and unmeasured covariates. Another advantage of randomization is that it helps ensure the validity of statistical tests (Armitage and Berry 1994; Lachin 1988).

Randomization procedures can be fixed or adaptive. *Fixed allocation randomization* assigns participants to different treatment arms with a pre-specified probability, and this allocation probability does not change as the study progresses. The most common types of fixed allocation randomization are complete (simple) randomization, blocked randomization, and stratified randomization. One of the simplest methods of *complete randomization* is to toss an unbiased coin each time a participant is eligible to be randomized. If the coin turns up heads, the participant is assigned to group A; otherwise, the participant is assigned to group B. In practice, a random number generator is used to assign participants to treatment groups. Simple randomization does not take past history into account, as it makes each new treatment assignment regardless of the assignments already made and might create imbalances in the number of patients assigned to treatments. These imbalances become more noticeable when one needs to account for prognostic factors. Even if the number of treatment assignments is balanced, the distribution of patients with different prognostic factors might not be. *Blocked (permuted block) randomization* is used to avoid serious imbalances in the number of participants assigned to each group that might occur if the simple randomization procedure is used. If participants are randomly assigned with equal probability to groups A or B, then for each block of even size (e.g., 4, 6, 8), one-half of the participants is assigned to group A, and the other half is assigned to group B. The number in each group does not differ by more than b/2, where b is a length of the block. Blocks do not need to be the same size. Varying the length of each block randomly can prevent from guessing the treatment assignments in small blocks. One of the objectives of *stratified randomization* in allocating patients to treatments is to achieve between-group balance of certain characteristics known as prognostic or risk factors (e.g., smokers vs. non-smokers). These factors should be available at baseline or at the time of randomization. Within each stratum, the randomization process itself can be a simple randomization, but in practice, most clinical trials use a blocked randomization strategy.

When *adaptive randomization* is used, alterations in the randomization schedule are allowed depending upon the varied or unequal probabilities of treatment

assignments. In contrast to the fixed randomization, the adaptive randomization allows changing the allocation probability as enrollment of participants to a study progresses. Adaptive randomization can be restricted, covariate-adaptive, response-adaptive (outcome-adaptive), or covariate-adjusted response-adaptive. *Restricted randomization* procedures are preferred for many clinical trials because it is often desirable to allocate an equal number of patients to each treatment. This equality is usually achieved by changing the probability of randomization to treatment according to the number of patients that have already been assigned. *Covariate-adaptive randomization* methods are used to ensure the balance between treatments with respect to certain known covariates. These methods are very effective in producing a marginal balance of the treatment groups when many covariates are considered. *Response-adaptive randomization* is used when ethical considerations make it undesirable to have an equal number of patients assigned to each treatment. Adaptive assessment is made sequentially, updating randomization for a next single patient or a cohort of patients using treatment estimates calculated from all available patient data received so far. In this situation, it should be feasible to identify the "better" treatment, and this "better" treatment should not be associated with any potential severe toxicity. A delay in response should be moderate allowing the adaptation to take place. *Covariate-adjusted response-adaptive randomization* combines covariate-adaptive and response-adaptive randomization. These types of adaptive randomization are discussed in details in Rosenberger and Lachin (2002) and Hu and Rosenberger (2006).

Until the new treatment has been proven beneficial, equal allocation to treatments is preferred. This strategy is often the best approach to maximize the efficiency (power) of the primary comparison. At times, an unequal allocation is used to meet important secondary objectives, when the responses have unequal variances or when the costs of treatments differ substantially. Response-adaptive randomization modifies the allocation ratio of patients to treatments during the trial, but as previously mentioned, it should be feasible to identify the "better" treatment before the adaptation.

Large multicenter clinical studies should use blocked randomization stratified by center. A few important risk factors can be used as strata to ensure the balance for these factors. For a large number of prognostic factors, adaptive randomization should be considered and appropriate analyses performed. Stratified analysis can still be performed even if stratified randomization was not done.

The process of implementing the chosen randomization method is fundamental. For fixed randomization, the sequence of assignments can be prepared at the start of the study. However, this is not possible for adaptive randomization because the treatment assignment depends upon the values of the variables for patients already entered the study. To accomplish valid randomization, it is recommended to use an experienced independent center to be responsible for developing and testing the randomization process and monitoring the assignment of patients to the appropriate groups.

1.1.2.5 Blinding

In an unblinded (open-label) trial, both the patient and the investigator know to which study group the patient has been assigned. Some trials can be conducted only in this manner. Such studies include those involving surgical procedures, comparisons of devices, or changes in lifestyle (e.g., eating habits, exercise, smoking). The appeal of such designs is in the simplicity of the trial execution. Additionally, investigators might be more comfortable deciding whether the patient should continue participating in the trial or not if they know the identity of the drug. The main disadvantage of such trials is the possibility of bias. Randomization and blinding are the two techniques usually used to minimize bias and to ensure that the experimental and control groups are similar at the start of the study and are treated similarly in the course of the study (ICH E9 1998).

Blinded studies can be single-blinded, double-blinded, or triple-blinded. In a *single-blinded* study, only patients are unaware of what treatment they receive, but investigators are aware of what treatment each patient is receiving. The advantages of this design are similar to the ones of an unblinded study: it is usually simpler to carry out than a double-blind design, and the knowledge of the intervention may help the investigator exercise their best judgment when caring for patients. It is recognized that bias is partially reduced by keeping patients blinded (especially, if the patient knowledge of the treatment can influence the response variable), but this design is vulnerable to another source of potential bias introduced by investigators. For example, the investigator can influence non-study therapy (concomitant treatment) or the time of their patient's enrollment to the study. In a *double-blinded* study, neither the patients nor the investigators know the treatment assignment of patients whom they treat. A clinical trial should ideally have a double-blinded design to avoid potential problems of bias during data collection and assessment. In studies where such a design is impossible, a single-blinded approach favored and other measures to reduce potential bias are implemented. The *triple-blinded* study design is an extension of the double-blinded design in which the committee monitoring response variables are not aware of the identity of the treatment groups. The Data Monitoring Committee (DMC) receives the study data and analyses with treatment groups as A and B. The actual treatments are revealed only if there is a major safety concern raised by the DMC. In a blinded study (double-, or triple-), blinding to patients and investigator should be preserved during the clinical trial; otherwise, the benefits of randomization can be lost.

1.1.2.6 Sample Size

Questions regarding the quantitative properties of clinical trial designs, specifically, sample size, power, the precision of an estimator, and an optimal study duration, are among the most frequently asked questions by a clinical team to statisticians. Table 1.1 summarizes the quantitative design parameters commonly used in clinical

Table 1.1 Quantitative design parameters commonly used in clinical trials

Parameter	Description
Sample size	Number of patients (subjects) required for the study
Type I error (α)	Concluding that a treatment effect exists when, in reality, it does not
Type II error (β)	Concluding that a treatment effect does not exist when, in reality, it does
Power ($1 - \beta$)	Chance of detecting a difference of a specified size as being statistically significant
Δ	Smallest treatment effect of interest based on clinical consideration (clinically relevant or important difference)
Allocation ratio	Ratio of sample sizes in treatment groups
Accrual rate	Number of patients (subjects) entering a trial per unit of time
Number of events	Number of patients (subjects) achieved an event of interest
Percent censoring	Percent of patients (subjects) left without an event of interest by the end of follow-up
Study duration	Interval from the beginning to the end of the study
Follow-up period	Interval from the end of accrual to the end of follow-up

trials. The *sample size* is the number of patients in a clinical trial. The sample size is a function of different parameters including a significance level (α), a power ($1 - \beta$), and a size of the difference in responses that need to be detected. For trials with a time-to-event endpoint, (e.g., overall survival or disease progression), one must distinguish the sample size from the number of events required by the study design. The actual sample size needed to meet the required number of events depends additionally on the censoring, enrollment, duration of the trial, and its follow-up time.

The underlying theme of sample size considerations in all clinical trials is precision. High precision implies little variation. The precision of estimation is the characteristic of a study that is most directly related to the sample size: the higher the sample size, the better the precision. In contrast, other essential features of the estimates, such as validity, unbiasedness, and reliability, do not necessarily relate to the study sample size. Precision is a consequence of a measurement error, within-person and person-to-person variability, a number of replicates (sample size), experimental design, and methods of analysis. By specifying quantitatively the precision of measurement required, we implicitly outline the sample size and other features of the study. Scientific validity is a consequence of good study design and well-executed study.

There are two widely used frequentist approaches for determining the appropriate sample size for a clinical trial: the first is based on confidence intervals around the effect that we expect to observe, and the second approach is based on the ability of the study to reject the null hypothesis when a specified treatment effect is hypothetically present (based on power). There is a third perspective based on likelihood ratios, a basic biostatistical idea that is appealing theoretically but has not been used widely (Piantadosi 2017). For a more detailed review of fixed sample size calculations, see Donner (1984), Lachin (1981), Chow et al. (2003), Machin et al. (2008), Friedman et al. (2015), and Piantadosi (2017). A good review of group sequential designs and adaptive designs including sample size estimation is given in Jennison and Turnbull (2000), Proschan et al. (2006), Chow and Chang (2007), and Wassmer and Brannath (2016).

It should be noted that the sample size calculations provide only a rough estimate of the needed number of patients for a trial because parameters used to estimate the sample size are estimates and have an element of uncertainty. For example, a study population might be different from a population used to design a trial (sampling error), a control group might have a higher effect than originally assumed, or effect of an experimental drug might be overestimated. Statisticians should use simulations to assess uncertainty, evaluate different scenarios, and understand the quantitative properties and operating characteristics of proposed study designs.

1.1.2.7 Statistical Significance and Clinical Significance

Clinically relevant (important) difference is one of the parameters that are usually used to estimate the sample size for a clinical trial. There are several methods proposed to define the minimal clinically important difference (MCID) including distribution-based methods (use statistical techniques and statistical characteristics of the obtained sample), anchor-based methods (based on comparisons with an external measure which serves as the anchor), and Delphi method (based on the opinion of experts). These methods are described in more details in McGlothlin and Lewis 2014. MCID can be defined from a patient, healthcare professional, or researcher's perspective. Recently, more efforts are made by regulators, researchers, and clinical trial sponsors to include patients' perspective in the design and evaluation of clinical trials.

Once the trial is completed and analyzed, the priority is to see whether the results produced by the data from the trial are statistically significant. The findings can be statistically significant at a pre-specified level (usually, 5%) but unimportant clinically. For example, in a study of overweight people, a weight loss at 12 months on an experimental drug can be only 1 pound more than on a placebo and can produce a statistically significant result if the sample size is very large. However, most likely this degree of weight loss would not be relevant or of interest. Such results would not be clinically significant or even meaningful. Statistical significance does not necessarily mean that the improvements from a trial will be clinically significant (meaningful or relevant to patients). To understand whether the results are clinically significant requires clinical judgment. Even if the MCID was used to design the trial, there is still a possibility that the treatment estimate can be smaller than MCID, for example, if the variability is much smaller than expected. In practice, to minimize the cost of a trial, more substantial treatment effect than MCID is assumed at the trial design, which results in a smaller sample size. If the sample size is underestimated, such a trial might fall short in demonstrating statistical significance even though clinical significance is met. In general, if there is an evidence that the experimental treatment can demonstrate a substantial effect (much larger than MCID), a group sequential design is recommended (Jennison and Turnbull 2000).

1.1.2.8 Role of Biostatistics and Biostatisticians in Clinical Development

Biostatistics is a highly developed information science; it plays a significant role in every stage of drug development. Historically, development of clinical trials has depended mostly on biological and medical advances, as opposed to applied mathematical or statistical developments. Some consider biostatistics to be a useful set of tools that biostatisticians apply when help is needed with the calculation of the study sample size or at the time of the data analysis. Making reasonable, accurate, and reliable inferences from data in the presence of uncertainty is an important intellectual skill that biostatisticians bring to cross-functional teams. In recent years, the recognition and appreciation of biostatistics have considerably improved. Biostatisticians are not only responsible for the quantitative properties of clinical trial designs and for analyzing data from clinical trials, but they are also respected partners of the clinical teams contributing to strategic discussions and helping solve day-to-day issues on studies and clinical programs.

A biostatistician plays an essential role in every stage of clinical research and development, starting from the design and planning stage up to the analysis and interpretation of the results. For example, in pharmaceutical industry, a clinical biostatistician provides statistical expertise to cross-functional teams, leads teams of statisticians and programmers, and ensures the use of appropriate and efficient statistical designs and analysis methods during development, submissions, and life cycle management of drugs, biologics, and devices according to applicable global and regional standards, procedures, and regulatory guidance documents and guidelines.

Biostatisticians drive the development and implementation of the innovative statistical methodology—recent advances in information science and technology enhanced application of innovative statistical designs and methods. High-performing computers and the use of cloud computing facilitated advances in the development of more complex computational algorithms for statistical modeling and simulations. Open-source software and development of handy statistical packages increased the use of advanced methods.

Biostatisticians bring an ability to solve problems efficiently at a level of rigor to data analysis that is a hallmark of our discipline. To have a more significant impact on a clinical program or study design strategy, biostatisticians have to be effective communicators and willing to assume a leadership role in a variety of situations. This is an exciting time in both clinical and statistical research and development, with the promise of personalized medicine and the explosion of computer-intensive statistical tools in development. The job of a biostatistician is exciting, challenging, and rewarding.

1.2 Phases of Clinical Development and Design Types

This section gives a brief overview of clinical development phases and most common design types used in clinical trials: parallel group designs, factorial designs, crossover designs, enrichment designs, group sequential, and adaptive designs. ICH E8 (ICH E8 1997) and ICH E9 (ICH E9 1998) are additional resources that provide information on this topic. ICH E8 guideline on General Considerations for Clinical Trials provides an overview of clinical development phases and gives the classification of clinical trials according to their objectives. This guideline is currently under revision because clinical trial design and conduct have become more complex during the last decade and influenced strategies required to develop drugs. ICH E9 guideline describes statistical principals for clinical trials including a brief description of common design types. The detailed description of clinical trial designs can be found in Chow and Liu (2003), Friedman et al. (2015), Piantadosi (2017), Jennison and Turnbull (2000), and Wassmer and Brannath (2016).

1.2.1 Phases of Clinical Development

Traditionally, a clinical development program consists of four phases: Phase I, Phase II, Phase III, and Phase IV.

Phase I starts with the initial administration of an experimental drug to humans. Phase I clinical trials are designed to evaluate the safety and tolerability of a new drug in a dose range predicted by preclinical research. Such studies are conducted in healthy volunteers or patients with the target disease. Cancer studies are almost always conducted in patients.

Preliminary characterization of a drug's absorption, distribution, metabolism, and excretion is an essential goal of Phase I. Pharmacokinetics (PK) may be assessed in a separate study or as a part of safety and tolerance studies. Pharmacodynamic (PD) studies and studies relating drug blood levels to response (PK/PD studies) may be conducted to provide early estimates of activity and potential efficacy and to guide the dosage and dose regimen in later studies. Preliminary assessment of activity or potential therapeutic benefit is evaluated in Phase I as a secondary objective. For many orally administered drugs, the study of food effects on bioavailability is an important part of Phase I.

The objective of the Phase I trial is to estimate the safe range of doses that can be used in Phase II. Often, the first step is to find how large the dose in a given dose range can be before unacceptable toxicity is experienced by patients. To estimate the maximum tolerated dose (MTD), the process typically begins with the administration of the lowest dose in the dose range and escalates to the next dose until the pre-specified level of toxicity is reached. Dose-escalation designs are typically used in this phase.

Phase II clinical trials are designed to evaluate the level of biological activity of a new agent and continue safety monitoring. Studies in Phase II are typically conducted in a small group of patients selected by relatively narrow criteria. Phase II usually starts with the initiation of studies in which the primary objective is to explore therapeutic efficacy in patients. These studies are often referred to as the proof-of-concept (POC) studies and considered to be Phase IIa studies. An important goal of Phase II is also to determine the dose(s) and regimen for Phase III trial(s). This goal is addressed in Phase IIb studies that are usually dose-ranging trials aimed to estimate the dose-response relationship and choose a dose or doses for Phase III.

Additional objectives of clinical trials conducted in Phase II may include evaluation of multiple study endpoints, therapeutic regimens (including concomitant medications), and different patient subgroups and target populations for further study in Phase II or Phase III. Exploratory analyses can address these objectives, examining subsets of data and by including multiple endpoints in trials. Initial therapeutic exploratory studies may use a variety of study designs. A comparison may consist of a concurrent control group, historical control, or pre-treatment versus post-treatment evaluations. Typically, dose-ranging studies include three to five doses of an experimental agent and a placebo; occasionally, they may include an active control.

Phase III begins with the initiation of studies in which the primary objective is to confirm the therapeutic benefit and the preliminary evidence accumulated in Phase II that a drug is safe and effective for use in the intended indication and population. These studies provide the basis for marketing approval. Studies in Phase III may also further explore the dose-response relationship or evaluate the drug's use in a broader population, in various stages of the disease, or in predefined patients' subgroups. For drugs intended to administer for a long period of time, extension trials or extension phases involving extended exposure to the drug are usually conducted in Phase III. During the last several years, it became more popular to include in Phase III studies conducted not just for marketing approval but also to satisfy payers' requirements. These studies usually use randomized, double-blind, parallel group designs. Group sequential designs and adaptive designs that allow for early stopping, population enrichment, or sample size re-estimation have become more popular in recent years.

Phase IV begins after the initial drug approval. The studies in Phase IV are performed after the drug approval and, usually, are related to the approved indication. They are studies that were not considered necessary for approval but are important for the further evaluation of the drug's use. They may be of any type but should have valid scientific objectives. Commonly conducted studies include additional drug-drug interaction, safety studies, and studies designed to support the use under the approved indication, e.g., mortality/morbidity studies and epidemiological studies. Although some studies in this phase may use randomization, most trials use observational, non-randomized designs. Typical types of observational study designs include cohort and case-control designs. Chapter 4 of this book discusses observational studies and provides more details on the design types used for these studies.

A research goal can overlap with more than one study phase, and some types of studies can be conducted in several phases. Additionally, emerging data can prompt modification of the development strategy. For example, the results of a confirmatory study may suggest a need for an additional human pharmacology study. Recently, seamless trials that combine objectives from two development phases have become more popular in drug development. Seamless designs are used in Phase I/IIa trials, Phase IIa/IIb trials, and Phase IIb/III trials. Such designs aim to reduce the overall sample size, for example, by allowing the patients' data from Phase II to be used in Phase III analysis (inferentially seamless) or by eliminating the time between phases (operationally seamless), which results in a shorter overall drug development time. After the initial approval, drug development may continue with studies of new indications, new dosage regimens, new routes of administration, or additional patient populations. In this case, additional human pharmacology studies may indicate a necessity for a new development plan. Depending on the relevance of the data from the original development plan and therapeutic use, the requirement for some studies may be reduced.

1.2.2   Clinical Trial Designs

1.2.2.1   Parallel Group Designs

A parallel group design is a randomized controlled design in which each patient is randomized to one of two or more treatment arms to receive study treatment. The treatments in this design usually include the investigational product at one or more doses, and one or more control treatments, such as a placebo and/or an active comparator. The assumptions underlying this design are less complicated than for most designs discussed in this section. However, as with other designs, there may be additional features of the trial that complicate the analysis and interpretation (e.g., covariates, repeated measurements over time, protocol violations, intercurrent events, missing data). This design is the most common clinical trial design used for confirmatory trials in Phase III.

1.2.2.2   Factorial Designs

In a factorial design, two or more treatments are evaluated simultaneously to assess the interactions among the treatments. The most straightforward factorial design is 2×2 design in which patients are randomly assigned to four possible combinations of treatments A and B: A alone, B alone, A and B together, and neither A nor B (e.g., a placebo). Factorial designs offer some advantages over conventional parallel group designs. The factorial structure of the design allows for certain comparisons that cannot be achieved by any other designs. When two or more treatments do not interact, factorial designs can test the main effects using smaller sample sizes with greater precision than separate parallel group designs. The precision with which interaction effects are estimated is lower than for main effects, but these designs allow studying the interactions. When there are many treatments or factors, these designs require a large number of treatment groups. In complex designs, if some interactions are not of interest or unimportant, it is possible to omit some treatment groups and reduce the sample size and complexity and, still, estimate the effects of interest. Factorial designs are used mainly in disease prevention studies and to establish the dose response of the combination treatments when the efficacy of each monotherapy has been established.

1.2.2.3 Crossover Designs

The crossover design is a special case of a randomized controlled trial design which allows each participant to serve as his or her control. The simplest crossover design is the two-treatment two-period crossover design (Fig. 1.1). In this type of design, there are two treatment periods, and patients are randomized to the sequence of treatments: either to receive drug A followed by drug B or to receive drug B followed by drug A. Extensions of this design include designs using more than one period for each drug, more than two drugs, or incomplete block design where not all patients receive every studied treatment.

There are some advantages of crossover designs over a parallel group design. For example, because each patient serves as his/her control and because within-subject variability is usually smaller than between-subject variability, the sample size for a crossover design is smaller than for a parallel group design. Another advantage is operational: patient recruitment to the trial might be easier because each patient would have an opportunity to try multiple treatments tested in the trial. A potential problem with crossover designs is the possibility that the treatment effect from one period might continue to the next period. Usually, crossover trials implement a sufficiently long washout interval between the treatment periods to address this problem. Another problem related to the carryover effect is the treatment by period interaction (means that treatment effect is not the same in different treatment periods; it varies over time). This problem is not unique to crossover designs, but carryover

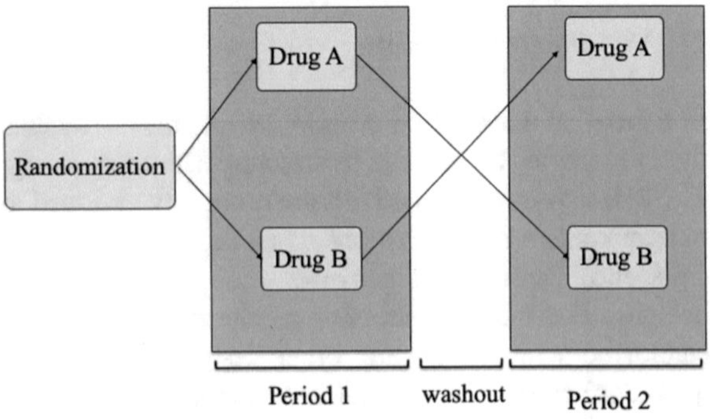

Fig. 1.1 Two-treatment two-period crossover design

effects can cause treatment by period interactions, and for the two-treatment two-period crossover trials, the carryover effect and treatment by period interactions are indistinguishable. Missing data has substantial effects on crossover trials. Usually, the trial duration is longer in crossover trials than in parallel group designs, and the side effects from multiple drugs can increase the chance of patients dropping earlier. ICH E9 guidance suggests restricting crossover designs to trials where loss of subjects and data is expected to be small, and to chronic and stable diseases under study. Crossover designs are commonly used in bioavailability trials.

1.2.2.4 Enrichment Designs

Enrichment designs are the clinical trial designs that aim to enrich the study population by selecting a subset of patients in which the potential effect of a drug can more readily be demonstrated (US Food and Drug Administration 2019a). The FDA guidance on Enrichment Strategies for Clinical Trials identified three broad categories of enrichment strategies: (1) strategies to decrease variability, (2) prognostic enrichment strategies, and (3) predictive enrichment strategies. Many different designs can support each of these strategies. Below, we provide examples of some of them.

Study designs that decrease heterogeneity (nondrug-related variability) and, therefore, increase the study power are widely used in clinical trials. The simplest enrichment design is the placebo lead-in design (Fig. 1.2). In this design, all patients have a run-in period during which they receive a placebo. Patients who respond to placebo are taken off study. Patients who do not respond to placebo are randomized to receive an experimental drug or a placebo. Only randomized patients are included in the final analysis. Placebo lead-in period helps to eliminate patients who improve spontaneously or have large placebo responses. The main advantage of this design is the decreased variability and the increased power to detect the effect in the enriched population.

A slightly more complex and more efficient design is sequential parallel comparison design (SPCD) (Fig. 1.3). This design has a smaller sample size than a traditional two-arm parallel group design because it uses two data points from

Fig. 1.2 Placebo lead-in design

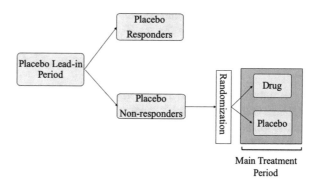

Fig. 1.3 Sequential parallel comparison design

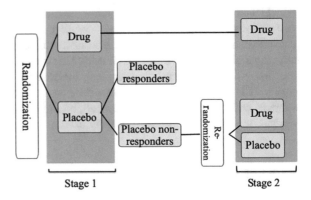

some patients. Compared to the crossover design, the sample size is larger, but there are no concerns about the carryover effect, and we do not need to assume that treatment effects are the same in two periods as they are analyzed separately. More information on these designs can be found in Ivanova et al. (2011) and Baer and Ivanova (2013). Additionally, it is possible to enrich two ways: after Stage 1, one can evaluate both drug and placebo responders and non-responders and then re-randomize placebo non-responders and drug responders to drug and placebo treatment groups (Huang and Tamura 2010). There are other modifications of these designs (Ivanova and Tamura 2015).

Prognostic enrichment strategies mentioned in the FDA guidance on Enrichment Strategies for Clinical Trials (US Food and Drug Administration 2019a) are aimed to identify high-risk patients for the clinical trial before its initiation. For example, type 2 diabetes mellitus therapies have to characterize the cardiovascular (CV) safety profile of the new antidiabetic treatment with a certain level of risk ruled out in the pre-approval stage and a reduced level of risk to be ruled out in the post-approval stage. To meet these requirements, meta-analyses and large cardiovascular outcome trials (CVOTs) are conducted. CVOTs require large sample sizes and, therefore, are very costly studies. Choosing patients at relatively high risk of CV events is critical for these studies to be able to rule out a given level of CV risk with a reasonably feasible study size. Inclusion criteria that are used to identify the high-risk patients for CVOTs include a history of recent myocardial infarction or stroke, the presence of concomitant illness, and certain blood markers. Statistical designs that usually used for these trials are the standard parallel group design, group sequential and adaptive designs that are briefly described in the next subsection. More information on strategies and statistical designs of CVOTs can be found in Marchenko et al. (2015) and Marchenko et al. (2017).

Another type of enrichment designs includes designs focused on a subset of patients with specific genomic patterns that appear to be associated with the response to the therapy. For example, a biomarker-stratified design can be used to prospectively validate the biomarker and compare responses in biomarker-positive and biomarker-negative populations (Fig. 1.4). Exclusion of the marker-negative patients from the trial would be justified when there are evidence based on

Fig. 1.4 Biomarker-stratified design

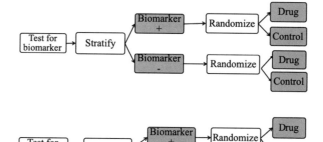

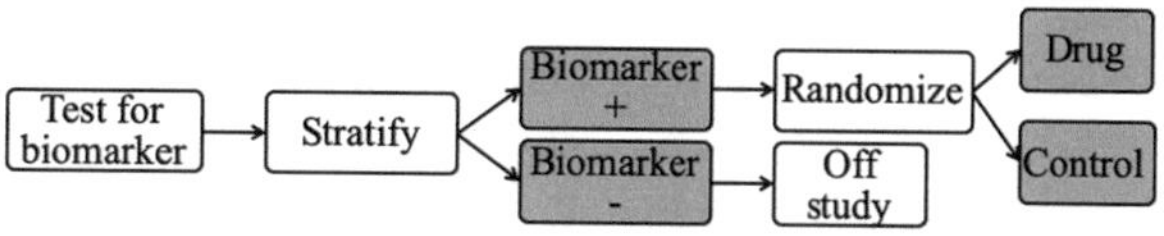

Fig. 1.5 Biomarker enrichment design

mechanistic, nonclinical, or early clinical data that the marker-negative patients would not benefit from the experimental drug or would be exposed to the unreasonable risk. In this case, the biomarker enrichment design that selects only biomarker-positive patients to randomize and study in the trial further will be more appropriate (Fig. 1.5).

If there is uncertainty at the planning stage about the strength of the marker-outcome relationship, a fixed sample enrichment design might not be the best choice. A study design that incorporates planned adaptations with the enrichment strategy, taking advantage of information gained during a clinical trial, could be a better choice.

1.2.2.5 Group Sequential and Adaptive Designs

Designs that allow for prospectively planned adaptations to one or more aspects of the design based on accumulative data from subjects in the trial are called adaptive designs (US Food and Drug Administration 2019b). Some authors consider group sequential designs to be a separate class of designs. Recently released FDA draft guidance on adaptive designs includes group sequential designs as one of the adaptive design types. There are many types of adaptive designs; here we provide some commonly used designs.

Group sequential designs allow stopping a study prematurely due to overwhelming efficacy or futility at a pre-planned interim analysis. The total number of stages (the number of interim analyses plus a final analysis) and the timing and stopping criterion from rejecting or accepting the null hypothesis at each interim analysis are usually pre-planned in advance. The Lan-DeMets alpha-spending approach allows for flexibility in determining the number and timing of interim analyses (Lan and DeMets 1983) if such flexibility is necessary, for example, when the enrollment rate is much slower than anticipated. The timing and number of interim analyses should be evaluated and simulated to navigate the decision process. Although by increasing the number of analyses, the chance of stopping before the end of the trial increases, multiple analyses during the trial might not be practical or even possible due to the fast enrollment or financial constraints. The opportunity to stop a trial early and claim efficacy increases the probability of an erroneous conclusion regarding the new treatment (type I error). For this reason, it is important to choose the method and the significance levels for interim and final analyses carefully so that the overall type I error rate is controlled at a pre-specified level. Usually, stopping rules are based on rejection boundaries, on a conditional power, or on a predictive power. The boundaries determine how conclusions would be drawn following the interim and final analyses, and it is important to pre-specify which type of boundary and spending function (if applicable) would be employed. The conditional power approach is based on an appealing idea of predicting the likelihood of a statistically significant outcome at the end of the trial, given the data observed at the interim and some assumption on the treatment effect. If the conditional power is extremely low, it is wise to stop the trial early for both ethical and financial reasons. Although it is possible to stop the trial and claim the efficacy if the conditional power is exceptionally high, the conditional power is mostly used to stop for futility. The choice of the statistical approach and the type of boundaries should depend on the objective of the trial and the role of the trial in a clinical program. When considering stopping for the overwhelming efficacy, one should keep in mind the implication of stopping early on the secondary endpoints and the safety profile of the drug. Group sequential designs have a reduced minimum and expected sample size but an increased maximum sample size relative to a comparable non-adaptive (fixed sample) parallel group design. In most cases, the increase is not large, and the design is worth considering given the savings from early stopping. The group sequential designs are considered to be more ethical and desirable for patients. More details on sequential designs can be found in Jennison and Turnbull (2000), Proschan et al. (2006), and Wassmer and Brannath (2016).

Adaptive dose-ranging designs allow fuller and more efficient characterization of the dose-response by facilitating iterative learning and decision-making during the trial. Insufficient exploration of a dose-response relationship often leads to a poor choice of the dose selected for the confirmatory trial and may subsequently lead to the failure of the trial and even a clinical program. Understanding of a dose-response relationship with regard to efficacy and safety before entering the confirmatory stage is a necessary step in a drug development. During an early development phase, limited knowledge about a drug opens more opportunities for the adaptive design consideration. Adaptive dose-ranging designs can have several objectives. They can be used to establish an overall dose-response relationship for an efficacy parameter or efficacy and safety parameters, estimate a therapeutic window or regimen, or select a single target dose. The allocation of subjects to the dose currently believed to give best results, or to doses close to the best one, has become very popular in clinical dose-finding studies, specifically, when the intention is to identify the maximum tolerated dose (MTD), the minimum efficacious dose (MED), or the optimal dose. Examples are included in Lai and Robbins (1978); O'Quigley et al. (1990); and Thall and Cook (2004) among others. More rigorous approaches are based on the introduction of utility functions, which quantify the "effectiveness" of a particular dose, and penalty functions, which quantify potential harm due to exposure to toxic or non-efficacious doses. Examples are provided by Li et al. (1995) and Fedorov and Leonov (2013). The FDA draft guidance on adaptive designs (US Food and Drug Administration 2019b) mentions adaptive parallel group designs with multiple dose arms that can be dropped or added at an interim analysis based on the pre-specified algorithm (Bretz et al. 2009; Wassmer and Brannath 2016). A special case of adaptive treatment arm selection occurs in the context of an adaptive platform trial designed to compare more than one experimental treatment against an appropriate control for a disease (Woodcock and LaVange 2017).

Sample size re-estimation designs allow for sample size adjustment or re-estimation based on observed data at an interim time point(s) for which statistical analysis may be conducted in a blinded or unblinded manner. Sample size re-estimation can improve the outcome of a trial if the information used to calculate the original sample size was unreliable, if the change is necessary due to new or additional information from an ongoing or finished trial, or if recent research in the therapeutic area led to new requirements or standards. Although the flexibility to adjust a sample size for a trial during an interim analysis is appealing when information is limited at the design stage, it does not come without a price. When the adjustment is made, it is important to take steps to preserve type I error rate. Sample size re-estimation is an adaptive design feature that mostly used in confirmatory trials to increase the sample size if variability is larger than originally planned. Refer to Chow and Chang (2007) and Bretz et al. (2009) for methods that are commonly used to re-estimate sample size in clinical trials. Similar to adaptive group sequential designs, the timing of a sample size re-estimation requires additional considerations. While it is possible to perform a sample size re-estimation multiple times, it is not recommended to perform it more than once during the trial. Careful consideration must be given to the total sample size utilized for decision-making at the planning stage and the processes that minimize potential bias that may result from knowing an interim-observed treatment effect. In the case of unblinded sample size re-estimation, special considerations should be given to the management of the Data Monitoring Committees (DMC) and the control of the results dissemination.

Adaptive enrichment design allows to decide whether to continue with the overall population or just with the marker-defined subpopulation and re-estimate the study sample size accordantly. Such changes should be prospectively planned and would often need appropriate type I error rate control to account for interim analyses of the accumulating data and subgroup analyses. If the only change were increased sample size based on blinded, pooled results because the prevalence of the marker-defined subgroup was lower than expected, there would be no need for a type I error rate adjustment. Designs that can be used to perform the subgroup search and identifications based on biomarkers are discussed in Lipkovich et al. (2011) and Chap. 6 of this book. Stallard (2010) describes a seamless Phase II/III design based on a selection using a short-term endpoint; Jenkins et al. (2011) present an adaptive seamless Phase II/III design with subpopulation selection using correlated endpoints; and Friede et al. (2012) introduce a conditional error function approach for subgroup selection.

Adaptive seamless designs have become more popular in drug development in recent years. Such designs aim to reduce an overall sample size by allowing the data from one phase to be used in another phase analysis (inferentially seamless) or to reduce the development period by eliminating the time between phases (operationally seamless). For example, an adaptive seamless Phase II/III design is a two-stage design consisting of a so-called learning stage (Phase II) and a confirmatory stage (Phase III). Just as there are a number of Phase II and Phase III designs, there are a number of the corresponding Phase II/III designs. Seamless designs pose many challenges as the time for planning a confirmatory trial is eliminated or rather combined with the planning time of Phase II when the information is limited and the uncertainties of the treatment are more significant. A sufficient benefit should be expected from the combined Phase II/III trial as compared to the strategy with a Phase II trial followed by a separate Phase III trial. To retain the validity, a type I error control is important for the inferentially seamless designs. Approaches based on the combination test principle that combine the stage-wise p-values using a pre-specified combination function or on the conditional error principle which computes the type I error under the null hypothesis conditional on the observed data at interim are usually used to control type I error rate. Bretz et al. (2009) provide a comprehensive review of the methods and offer practical considerations.

The planning stages for an adaptive clinical trial must be completed before finalizing the decision to proceed. Trial simulations that compare different design options, evaluate a range of assumptions, and compare operating characteristics of designs are an essential step in a trial design and planning stage. Simulation tools can also be used to monitor clinical trial outcomes and enrollment during the study to ensure that the study is meeting expectations. Chapter 8 of this book provides more information on the predictive modeling of the clinical trial operations, specifically, predicting patient enrollment at different stages of the study. More information on adaptive design considerations and implementation can be found in He et al. (2014).

1.3   Statistical Methods

Statistical methods in drug development are used for the design and analyses of clinical trials that, in turn, are aimed to determine the effects of particular healthcare treatments, practices, and interventions. While many pharmaceutical studies have utilized mainly randomized trial designs and employed basic inference procedures to assess the efficacy and safety of new interventions and treatments, more recent studies rely on modeling techniques that extend beyond traditional regression-based approaches. Although data in drug development are often collected longitudinally (i.e., data collected repeatedly over time on the same set of subjects), frequently primary and critical secondary analyses rely on a single post-randomization time point (e.g., change from baseline in response at a specific time). While a focus on a single time point may be driven by regulatory requirements in a "confirmatory" setting, longitudinal modeling utilizing the totality of the observed data offers the opportunity to achieve substantial efficiencies in data analysis compared to current prevailing practices at the "learn" stage of drug development. Those efficiencies may translate into faster and more accurate decision-making, increased statistical power and/or estimation precision, and combinations of these, ultimately leading to increased probability of program success, while reducing development costs. For the listed reasons, we decided to dedicate a substantial part of this section to parametric longitudinal modeling methods, the primary goal of which is to characterize the change in response over time and the factors that influence change (Fitzmaurice et al. 2009). In many pharmaceutical studies, the focus is primarily on mortality or survival with a specific interest given to identification of the causes of early death and effectiveness of treatments for delaying death and morbidity. In these types of studies, the survival analysis of time-to-event is utilized (Kleinbaum and Klein 2012a, b).

The rest of this section is organized as follows. We start with a brief overview of the most commonly used probability models and basic principles of parametric estimation and inference in Sect. 1.3.1. Focusing on both categorical and continuous types of response, we continue with the main properties of sampling distributions of estimators commonly used for data analysis. We follow with the concept of regression and generalized linear modeling, thereby unifying the process of model construction for a quantitative and categorical response in Sect. 1.3.2. With this, we lay the ground for longitudinal data analysis described in Sect. 1.3.3 and finish with a brief discussion about inference and modeling techniques for a time-to-event, survival analysis in Sect. 1.3.4. Where appropriate, we include references to available software procedures in R and SAS.

1.3.1 Basic Principals of Probability and Inference

All statistical studies distinguish between response (or dependent, outcome) variables and explanatory (or independent, predictor) variables. Both response and explanatory variables can be qualitative or quantitative.

When a variable takes numerical values in the list or an interval or a set of multiple intervals, this variable is called *quantitative* or *numerical*. Quantitative variables are classified as discrete and continuous. While discrete quantitative variables usually take a few or many values from the list, continuous variables can take a large number of values, in practice, and an infinite number of values, in theory. Examples of continuous response variables in clinical studies include blood pressure, the concentration of white cells, and body temperature.

A *qualitative* (or *categorical*) variable has a measurement scale consisting of a set of categories. Qualitative variables can be of two types of scales: nominal and ordinal. While nominal categorical variables have no inherent natural order in categories (e.g., skin color, sex, personality type, type of side effect), ordinal categorical variables do have ordered categories (e.g., disease stage, patient condition). The choice of statistical analysis depends on the type of distribution of a categorical variable. Agresti presents a comprehensive review of the analysis of categorical data (Agresti 2002).

The first and foremost important step of any statistical analysis is a clear definition of the type and nature of the response and explanatory variables. This step helps to determine an appropriate set of descriptive and inferential methods for analysis and, if needed, leads to a proper choice of class of models. While descriptive analysis relies only on the assumption of the randomness of the data, inferential data analyses also rely on assumptions of the specific distribution of the variables under consideration. For instance, for linear regression models with continuous responses, the assumption of normality is essential; for logistic regression, the distribution of responses is assumed to be binomial.

1.3.1.1 Probability Distributions

Many statistical inference procedures rely on the assumption of a particular distribution. For example, the assumption of normal distribution is required for statistical procedures such as t-tests, linear regression analysis, discriminant analysis, and analysis of variance, and when violated, interpretation and inferences may not be reliable or valid. Here, we provide an overview of the probability distributions most commonly used in pharmaceutical data analyses. Specifically, we focus on normal, multivariate normal, binomial, hypergeometric, multinomial, Poisson, and negative binomial distributions.

Normal Distribution

Normal random variable, Y, is the most frequently used and most studied univariate continuous random variable in theory of statistics and probability that is completely characterized by its *expected value (mean)* μ and the *standard deviation* σ. Most of the inferential and modeling procedures for continuous response (e.g., regression, one- and two-sample inference for population mean) rely on an assumption of normality of some sort, as well as large sample procedure for categorical response (e.g., one- and two-sample inference for population proportion). Similarly, studies with a multivariate continuous response (e.g., repeated measurement over time and/or conditions, clustered data) rely on assumption of multivariate normality. *Multivariate normal distribution* of random vector $Y = (Y_1, Y_2, \ldots, Y_k)$ is fully defined by a mean vector μ and a covariance matrix Σ. Table 1.2 contains a summary for univariate and multivariate normal distribution.

Table 1.2 Distributions of the most commonly used categorical variables

Distribution	Probability density/mass function	Mean	Variance/covariance
Normal	$f(y) = \frac{1}{\sqrt{2\pi\sigma^2}} e^{-\frac{(y-\mu)^2}{2\sigma^2}}$	$E(Y) = \mu$	$var(Y) = \sigma^2$
Multivariate normal	$f(y) = \frac{1}{|2\pi\Sigma|^{\frac{1}{2}}} e^{-(y-\mu)'\Sigma^{-1}(y-\mu)}$	$E(\boldsymbol{Y}) = \boldsymbol{\mu}$	$Cov(\boldsymbol{Y}) = \Sigma$
Binomial	$\Pr(Y = y) = \binom{n}{y} p^y (1-p)^{n-y}$	$E(Y) = np$	$var(Y) = np(1-p)$
Hypergeometric	$\Pr(Y = y) = \frac{\binom{A}{y}\binom{N-K}{n-y}}{\binom{N}{n}}$	$E(Y) = \frac{nA}{N}$	$var(Y) = \frac{nA}{N}\left(1 - \frac{A}{N}\right)\left(\frac{N-n}{N-1}\right)$
Multinomial	$\Pr(Y_1 = y, \ldots, Y_k = y_k) = \frac{n!}{(y_1! \ldots y_k!)} p_1^{y_1} \cdots p_k^{y_k}$	$E(Y_i) = p\pi_i$	$var(Y_i) = np_i(1 - p_i)$ cov $(Y_i, Y_j) = -np_ip_j, \; i \neq j$
Poisson	$\Pr(Y = y) = \frac{e^{-\lambda}\lambda^y}{y!}$	$E(Y) = \lambda$	$var(Y) = \lambda$
Negative binomial	$\Pr(Y = y) = \binom{y+r-1}{y} p^y (1-p)^r$	$E(Y) = \frac{pr}{1-p}$	$var(Y) = \frac{pr}{(1-p)^2}$

In R software, density/mass distribution function, cumulative distribution function, quintile function, and random variable generation for many standard probability distributions available in the **stats** package and named in the form of dxxx, pxxx, qxxx, and rxxx, where xxx stands for the name of the distribution (e.g., dhyper, phorm, qpois, rbinom). Similar functions are available for multivariate normal distribution in mvtnorm package

Binomial Distribution

Many pharmaceutical applications use a binary response to report, for example, presence or absence of a certain disease, side effect, effectiveness of a drug, etc. Let $y_1, y_2, \ldots, y_n$ denote binary responses for n independent individuals related to n independent random variables $Y_1, Y_2, \ldots, Y_n$. For a binomial model, we assume that each person's response is an independent and identical Bernoulli experiments with $P(Y_i = 1) = p$ and $P(Y_i = 0) = 1 - p$, where outcomes 1 and 0 are labeled as "success" and "failure" and p is the same across all responders. The total number of successes, $Y = \sum_{i=1}^{n} Y_i$, is a binomial random variable with a *fixed* number of experiments, n, and a probability of success, p. Table 1.2 provides the binomial probability mass function with a corresponding mean and variance. As a number of experiments grows and p remains fixed, the distribution of Y converges to normal. In some cases when there is no guarantee that successive response experiments are independent or identical, one can use the *hypergeometric distribution* that samples n binary outcomes without replacement from a finite population of size N with A successes (Agresti 2002).

Multinomial Distribution

In some sense, it represents an extension of binomial distribution when each person's response is exactly one of k possible categories. Consider, for example, a blood type where each person can be either of O, A, B, or AB type. In this case, response of person i is a k-dimensional vector $y_i = (y_{i1}, y_{i2}, \ldots, y_{ik})$ with only a single non-zero value 1 (e.g., a person with AB blood type has a multinomial outcome vector (0,0,0,1)). The total sum of responses is a random vector $Y = (Y_1, Y_2, \ldots, Y_k)$, where each entry Y_j is the sum of all responses for category j. The sum of all responses across all categories, $\sum_{j=1}^{k} Y_i$, always equals to the number of responses, n. The probability of success in category k on each experiment is fixed, p_i, and $\sum_{i=1}^{k} p_i = 1$. The probability mass function of $Y = (Y_1, Y_2, \ldots, Y_k) \sim Multinomial(n, p_1, p_2, \ldots, p_k)$ along with the means and variances for each category as well as covariances between categories is summarized in Table 1.2.

Poisson and Negative Binomial Distribution

Poisson random variable is a discrete random variable that is used for counts of events that occur randomly over a continuum (time or space), when outcomes in disjoint segments (periods or regions) are independent. In theory, a Poisson random variable can take discrete values from an infinite list of possible values, though in practice only some values can happen with non-trivial probability. The distribution of a Poisson random variable, Y, depends on a single parameter λ, which defines both its mean and variance. Moreover, the variance equals to the mean of Poisson distribution (see Table 1.2). In practice, this means that sample counts vary more when their mean is higher. Often, however, sample count observations exhibit variability exceeding expected by the Poisson distribution, phenomena is known as overdispersion. In these cases, assumption of a Poisson distribution for count data is too simplistic and the *negative binomial* distribution can serve as an alternative model for count data that permits the variance to exceed the mean. *Negative binomial distribution* is a discrete probability distribution that counts the number of successes, y, in a sequence of independent and identically distributed Bernoulli experiments until a pre-specified (fixed in advance) number of failures, r, occurs. Analogously to binomial, each Bernoulli experiments results in one of the outcomes, success or failure, with probabilities p and $(1 - p)$, respectively.

1.3.1.2   Statistical Estimation

In general, the choice of the distribution for a response variable is one of the essential steps. Each distribution is defined by one parameter or a set of parameters that in practice are unknown and need to be estimated using sample data. In this chapter, we follow the approach described by Agresti (2002), and we first focus on *maximum likelihood* (ML) estimators that under weak regularity conditions possess important properties for large samples: such as for approximate normality of sampling distributions, asymptotical consistency (converging to the parameter as sample size increases), and efficiency (producing standard errors no higher than those using other methods).

Suppose response variables Y_1, Y_2, Y_3, ..., Y_n have the following joint density function (for continuous variables) or the probability mass distribution function (for discrete random variables) $f(y_1, y_2, ..., y_n | \theta)$, where θ can be a single parameter (e.g., $\theta = p$) or a vector of parameters (e.g., $\theta = (\mu, \sigma)$, $\theta = (\beta_0, \beta_1, \beta_2, ..., \beta_q)$). Given observed values $Y_1 = y_1$, $Y_2 = y_2$, ..., $Y_n = y_n$, the likelihood of θ is the probability of observing the given data as a function of θ, $L(\theta) = f(y_1, y_2, ..., y_n | \theta)$. The value of $\widehat{\theta}$ that maximizes $L(\theta)$, $\widehat{\theta} = arg\ max_\theta\ L(\theta)$, is called the *maximum likelihood estimate* (MLE) of parameter θ. The MLE is also a value of the parameter that maximizes $l(\theta) = \log L(\theta) = \sum_i \log f(y_i | \theta) = \sum_i l_i(\theta)$ and guarantees that observed data have the highest probability of occurrence.

The standard error of $\widehat{\theta}$, in general, can be obtained from the asymptotic covariance matrix of $\widehat{\theta}$, which under certain regularity conditions equals to the inverse of information matrix $I(\theta)^{-1}$ (Rao 1973), where the information matrix is defined as $I\left(\widehat{\theta}\right) = -E\left[\frac{\partial^2 l(\theta)}{\partial \theta \partial \theta'}\right]$. The standard errors of each parameter of interest are the square roots of diagonal elements of the inverse of information matrix evaluated at the maximum likelihood estimator, $\widehat{\theta}$. A number of other variance/covariance estimators include negative Hessian variance estimator $\left(-\sum_i \frac{\partial^2 l_i(\theta)}{\partial \theta \partial \theta'}\right)^{-1}$, outer product of gradient $\left(-\sum_i \frac{\partial l_i(\theta)}{\partial \theta} \frac{\partial l_i(\theta)}{\partial \theta}'\right)^{-1}$, and the result of M-estimation

$\left(\sum_i \frac{\partial^2 l_i(\theta)}{\partial \theta \partial \theta'}\right)^{-1} \left(\sum_i \frac{\partial l_i(\theta)}{\partial \theta} \frac{\partial l_i(\theta)}{\partial \theta}'\right) \left(-\sum_i \frac{\partial^2 l_i(\theta)}{\partial \theta \partial \theta'}\right)^{-1}$, also known as the empirical or

"sandwich" estimator. M-estimators and their asymptotic properties were initially introduced by Huber (Huber 1964, 1967). In the biostatistics literature, M-estimators were brought under the name of generalizes estimation equations (GEE) by Liang and Zeger (Liang and Zeger 1986, 1995). Serving as an alternative to maximum likelihood estimation, the GEE approach provides a more general methodology for analyzing correlated responses that can be discrete or continuous (Fitzmaurice et al. 1993). The well-known generalized least squares (GLS) approach used in regression model can be considered a special case of the GEE approach. The key idea behind the GEE is to extend the usual likelihood equations by incorporating the covariance matrix of the vector responses.

In practice, it is more informative to construct confidence intervals than to report estimates and their corresponding standard errors. Based on the asymptotical consistency and normality of the MLE of $\widehat{\theta}$ and using both the values of the estimates and standard errors, one can construct $100(1 - \alpha)\%$ Wald confidence interval. The Wald confidence interval (Wald 1943) for univariate parameter is a set of θ values between $\widehat{\theta} - z_{\frac{\alpha}{2}} SE\left(\widehat{\theta}\right)$ and $\widehat{\theta} + z_{\frac{\alpha}{2}} SE\left(\widehat{\theta}\right)$, where $z_{\frac{\alpha}{2}}$ denotes the $100(1 - \alpha)$ percentile of the standard normal distribution. For categorical data and data with a small sample size, the likelihood-ratio-based confidence interval is more preferable. The likelihood-ratio-based confidence interval is based on the $100(1 - \alpha)$ percentile of the chi-square distribution, $X_{df}^2(\alpha)$, with q degrees of freedom (with one degree of freedom for a single parameter). In general, this interval represents a q-dimensional confidence region space for multivariate parameter θ: $-2\left[L(\theta) - L\left(\widehat{\theta}\right)\right] < X_{df}^2(\alpha)$.

The likelihood-ratio-based approach to construction of a confidence region (interval) remains reliable when the assumption of normality of $\widehat{\theta}$ is violated (Pierce and Peters 1992). See Kauermann and Carroll (2001) for a more recent discussion of the properties of the "sandwich" estimator and corresponding coverage probability of confidence intervals (Kauermann and Carroll 2001).

1.3.1.3 Statistical Inference

Here we focus on two standard approaches to perform large sample inference of a parameter of interest: one using the reported maximum likelihood estimates and corresponding standard errors and another based on the likelihood-ratio test. Consider a significance test of a null hypothesis $H_0 : \theta = \theta_0$. Using the first approach, the Wald test statistic $z = \left(\widehat{\theta} - \theta_0\right)/SE\left(\widehat{\theta}\right)$ has an approximate standard normal distribution when $\theta = \theta_0$. Depending on the alternative hypothesis H_1 (one- or two-sided), one can follow with the computation of p-value or reference the standard normal table for appropriate critical values.

A second method uses maximization of the likelihood function under two conditions: (1) when H_0 is true and $\theta = \theta_0$ and (2) permitting H_0 or H_1 to be true. The likelihood maximized under the second condition L_1 will always be as large as or larger than the likelihood maximized under the first condition L_0 due to maximization of an unrestricted set of parameters. The likelihood-ratio test statistics $-2 \log [L_0/L_1]$ under H_0 converges to chi-square distribution with the degrees of freedom equal to the difference between the dimension of the full parameter space and the dimension of the parameter space restricted by H_0 (Willks 1938). For large samples, both approaches provide the estimates asymptotically equivalent; for small to moderate samples sizes, the likelihood-ratio test is usually more reliable (Cox 1970). Overall, the traditional approach to statistical inference focuses on hypothesis testing of a single test or a number of multiple test with some chosen multiplicity adjustment strategy (see Alosh et al. 2014; Dmitrienko and D'Agostino 2013; and Tamhane and Gou 2017).

Evidently, knowledge of a sampling distribution or at least the expected value and the standard error of a sample statistics significantly simplify the process of statistical inference that is based on the probability distribution of a statistic, rather than on the likelihood function built on all sample values. A sampling distribution is the probability distribution of a given sample statistic, or more specifically, if a large number of random samples of size n was drawn from the same population of interest, and each sample was used to produce one value of a sample statistic (e.g., the sample mean), then the probability distribution of the values that the statistic takes on is called the sampling distribution. Many sampling distributions are not observed in practice but instead derived in theory via various versions of the Central Limit Theorem. For example, when a random sample is drawn from a normal population or the sample size n that is relatively large (roughly 30 or more), the sample mean follows normal or approximately normal distribution with the same mean as the population mean μ and the standard error as a ratio of the population standard deviation and a square root on the sample size, $\frac{\sigma}{\sqrt{n}}$. In cases, when the population standard deviation is unknown and is estimated using a sample standard deviation, the same statement applies except the sampling distribution is the Student's t-distribution, rather than normal. The exact sampling distribution of a sample proportion of successes in n Bernoulli trials $\widehat{p}$ is $n\widehat{p}Binomial(n, p)$ that can be also approximated by a normal distribution, $\widehat{p} \sim N\left(p, \sqrt{\frac{p(1-p)}{n}}\right)$. There are other sampling distributions derived for many sample statistics that are out of the scope of this Section.

1.3.2   Linear Regression and Generalized Linear Models

The objective of statistical modeling is usually twofold: (1) the interpretability and the prediction power of the model and (2) the inference about the effect of individual predictors on the response. For example, in many pharmaceutical studies, one of the objectives is (1) to test a statistically significant effect of some treatment (e.g., new analgesic vs. placebo) on a response variable (e.g., pain relief score) and (2) to estimate the magnitude of the treatment effect. Consistently with these two objectives, statistical modeling approaches often rely on certain assumptions regarding the relationship between the response and predictors and the distribution of the response. By fitting a simple regression model with the treatment represented as one of the independent variables (categorical), one can perform a test of statistical significance essentially equivalent to t-test for the difference in population means. Using the regression approach, it is also possible to adjust the model for other independent (pre-treatment) variables, such as baseline patient characteristics.

1.3.2.1   Linear Regression Model

Classical regression model focuses on a continuous dependent variable, or response, and has the general form of:

$$Y = E(Y|X) + \varepsilon,$$

where X denotes a set of independent predictor variables (with the first column assumed to be one) and ε represents a random error induced by some source of uncertainty (e.g., random sampling). While the expected value of the response Y is considered to be a linear combination of predictors $E(Y|X) = X'\beta$, error term ε is assumed to follow a normal distribution with the expected value of zero and the variance of σ^2 and to be independent of X.

   More specifically, let's consider N independent observations of a single response variable, Y, that can be either continuous, binary, or count. Let Y_i ($i = 1, 2, \ldots, N$) denote the response variable for the ith subject and assume a p-dimensional vector of covariates, $X_i = (X_{i1}, \ldots, X_{ip})$ associated with each outcome Y_i, where X_{ik} denotes the kth covariate for the ith subject. The classical linear regression model for Y_i can be written as:

$$Y_i = \beta_1 X_{i1} + \beta_2 X_{i2} + \ldots + \beta_p X_{ip} + e_i,$$

where $X_{i1} = 1$ for all individuals and β_1 is the regression intercept. According to this model, the expected value of Y_i is the average for all individuals with the pre-specified covariate values that vary linearly with the values of the covariates,

$$E\left(Y_i|X_{i1}, \ldots, X_{ip}\right) = \mu_{\left(Y_i|X_{i1},\ldots,X_{ip}\right)} = \beta_1 X_{i1} + \beta_2 X_{i2} + \ldots + \beta_p X_{ip}.$$

Vector of coefficients $\boldsymbol{\beta} = (\beta_1, \beta_2, \ldots, \beta_p)$ is estimated using the least squares (LS) approach of the maximum likelihood (ML) method and has the following interpretation. The population intercept (for $X_1 = 1$), β_1, is the mean value of the response when all of the covariates equal zero. In turn, the population slope, say β_k, has interpretation in terms of the expected change in the mean response for a single-unit change in X_k given that all of the other covariates remain constant.

The basic idea behind the least squares (LS) estimation is to choose the estimates of $\beta_1, \ldots, \beta_p$ $(\widehat{\beta}_1, \ldots, \widehat{\beta}_p)$ such that the fitted regression model "deviates" the least from the observed data or minimizes the residual sums of squares defined as:

$$\sum_{i=1}^{N} \left(Y_i - \widehat{Y}_i\right)^2 = \sum_{i=1}^{N} \widehat{e}_i^2,$$

where $\widehat{e}_i$ is an estimated residual, Y_i is an observed value of the response, and $\widehat{Y}_i$ a fitted value of the response of the ith subject:

$$\widehat{Y}_i = \widehat{\beta}_1 X_{i1} + \widehat{\beta}_2 X_{i2} + \ldots + \widehat{\beta}_p X_{ip}.$$

Recall that according to ML approach, the estimates of $\beta_1, \ldots, \beta_p$ $(\widehat{\beta}_1, \ldots, \widehat{\beta}_p)$, and $\sigma^2(\widehat{\sigma}^2)$ are the values that are most "likely" for the observed data that can be found as the values that maximize the log-likelihood:

$$\begin{aligned}
l\left(\beta_1, \ldots, \beta_p, \sigma^2\right) &= \ln L\left(\beta_1, \ldots, \beta_p, \sigma^2 | Y_i, X_i, i = 1, \ldots, N\right) \\
&= -\frac{N}{2} \ln\left(2\pi\sigma^2\right) \\
&\quad - 1/\left(2\sigma^2\right) \sum_{i=1}^{N} \left(Y_i - \beta_1 X_{i1} + \beta_2 X_{i2} + \ldots + \beta_p X_{ip}\right)^2.
\end{aligned}$$

It turns out that the estimates found by ML and LS approaches are equivalent and in the vector/matrix notation form can be written as:

$$\widehat{\boldsymbol{\beta}} = \left(\widehat{\beta}_1, \ldots, \widehat{\beta}_p\right) = \left[\sum_{i=1}^{N} \left(X_i X_i'\right)\right]^{-1} \sum_{i=1}^{N} \left(X_i Y_i\right).$$

This value of the estimate is the one usually produced by any statistical software for linear regression. In SAS, one can use PROG GLM or PROC REG and the "lm" function (as a part of standard 'stats' package) in R.

Provided that the main linear regression model assumptions are satisfied, the ML (LS) estimator of regression coefficients possesses the following important properties. The estimator of β is unbiased that is $E\left(\widehat{\beta}\right) = \beta$; and the sampling distribution of $\widehat{\beta}$ is asymptotically normal,

$$\widehat{\beta} \sim N\left(\beta, \sigma^2 \left[\sum_{i=1}^{N} \left(X_i X_i'\right)\right]^{-1}\right).$$

Note that in this chapter, we do not provide a detailed description of classical methodology of the analysis of variance (ANOVA) and the analysis of covariances (ANCOVA). Both of these concepts can be formulated and interpreted in term of the general linear models. See Rutherford (2011) for a comprehensive review and detailed explanation of how ANOVA and ANCOVA are incorporated in GLMs. In his book, Rutherford (2011) also discusses corresponding different multiple comparisons procedures and the power analysis in relation to the sample size computation.

1.3.2.2 Generalized Linear Models

In many pharmaceutical and biomedical applications, the response is not continuous, for example, presence or absence of some particular side effect or counts of the number of epileptic seizures over some period of time or the number of acne pimples over a certain body area or the type of response to cancer treatment (e.g., complete response, partial response, stable disease, progression). When the response variable is discrete (e.g., binary, ordinal, or a count), the linear regression models are no longer appropriate. Instead, generalized linear models can serve as an alternative for relating changes in the expected response to covariates. Generalized linear models extend the class of linear regression models to settings where the outcome variable can be categorical, continuous, or count using the distribution models appropriate for each type of response.

First, we consider methods for analyzing cross-sectional data and then we extend them to longitudinal and clustered data settings. Assume N independent observations of a single response variable, Y, that can be either continuous, binary, or count. As before, we let Y_i ($i = 1, 2, \ldots, N$) denote the response variable for the ith subject and assume a p-dimensional vector of covariates, $X_i = (X_{i1}, \ldots, X_{ip})$ associated with each outcome Y_i, where X_{ik} denotes the kth covariate for the ith subject with $X_{i1} = 1$ for all subjects. The primary goal of a generalized linear model is to relate the mean of Y_i, $\mu_i = E(Y_i | X_{i1}, \ldots, X_{ip})$, to the covariates X_i in some linear form through the specification of (1) a distribution for Y_i, (2) a systematics component, and (3) a link function.

The distribution of the response is assumed to belong to the exponential family of distributions, the density function of which can be expressed in a form:

Table 1.3 Scale factor, variance functions, and canonical link for normal, Bernoulli, and Poisson distributions

Distribution	Scale factor	Variance function	Location parameter/canonical link function
Normal	$\phi = \sigma^2$	$v(\mu) = 1$	Identity: $\theta = g(\mu) = \mu$
Bernoulli	$\phi = 1$	$v(\mu) = \mu(1 - \mu)$	Logit: $\theta = g(\mu) = \log\left(\frac{\mu}{1-\mu}\right)$
Poisson	$\phi = 1$	$v(\mu) = \mu$	Identity: $\theta = g(\mu) = \log(\mu)$

$$f(y_i; \theta_i, \phi) = \exp\left[\frac{\{y_i\theta_i - a(\theta_i)\}}{\phi} + b(y_i, \phi)\right],$$

where $a(\cdot)$ and $b(\cdot)$ are specifically defined for each particular distribution. All exponential family distributions share some common statistical properties. Focusing on the mean and the variance of exponential family distributions, it can be shown that the mean of Y_i can be computed as a derivative of the function $a(\theta_i)$, that is $E(Y_i) = \mu_i = \frac{\partial a(\theta_i)}{\partial \theta}$, and the variance of the response can be computed using a second derivative of $a(\theta_i)$ and expressed in terms of the product of a positive dispersion parameter, $\phi > 0$, and a variance function of mean, $v(\mu_i)$, that is $Var(Y_i) = \phi\frac{\partial^2 a(\theta_i)}{\partial \theta^2} = \phi v(\mu_i)$. In fact, the normal, Bernoulli, binomial, and Poisson distributions all belong to the exponential family distributions. For instance, by re-arranging terms in the normal density function, $f(y_i; \mu_i, \sigma^2)$, one can represent it in a general form of exponential density with canonical location parameter $\theta_i = \mu_i$, scale parameter $\phi = 1$, $a(\theta_i) = \mu_i^2/2$, and $b(y_i, \phi) = -1/2 \{y_i^2/\sigma^2 + \log(2\pi\sigma^2)\}$. Scale factors and variance functions for normal, Bernoulli, and Poisson distributions are summarized in Table 1.3.

The systematic component of a generalized linear model specifies the effect of the covariates, X_i, on the mean of Y_i that can be expressed in a linear combination of the unknown regression coefficient and covariates (or even transformed coefficients), denoted by η_i,

$$\eta_i = \beta_1 X_{i1} + \beta_2 X_{i2} + \ldots + \beta_p X_{ip}.$$

By taking a suitable transformation of the mean response, μ_i, and relating the transformed response to the covariates through an appropriate link function, $g(\mu_i)$, the specification of a generalized linear model becomes

$$g(\mu_i) = \eta_i = \beta_1 X_{i1} + \beta_2 X_{i2} + \ldots + \beta_p X_{ip}.$$

The link function, $g(\mu_i)$, is some known function. For example, for the normal distribution of the responses, the link function is an identity function, $g(\mu_i) = \mu_i$; for count data following the Poisson distribution, the link function is a natural logarithm $g(\mu_i) = \log(\mu_i)$. Table 1.3 contains canonical link functions for three most used distributions that are normal, Bernoulli, and Poisson.

In general, the estimation of the regression coefficients in a generalized linear model is based on the maximum likelihood approach that requires an iterative procedure that has been implemented in many statistical packages. In SAS, one can use PROC GENMOD and the "glm" function in R.

Logistic Regression for Binary Responses

In situations when the response for each subject is binary (i.e., can be mapped to $1 = $ "success" and $0 = $ "failure"), $Y_i \in \{0, 1\}$, the mean of the binary response variable, denoted as p, is the proportion of successes or the probability that the response takes on the value one, $p_i = E(Y_i|X_i) = \Pr(Y_i = 1|X_i)$. Estimation of p_i and relating this to a set of covariates X is usually done using logistic regression:

$$\ln\left(\frac{p_i}{1 - p_i}\right) = X_i'\beta = \beta_1 X_{i1} + \beta_2 X_{i2} + \ldots + \beta_p X_{ip},$$

where $\ln\left(\frac{p_i}{1-p_i}\right)$ defines the logarithm of the odds of success and replaces the mean of the continuous response used in linear regression model, hence imposing a nonlinear relationship between p and the covariates. Under the assumption that the binary responses $(Y_1, Y_2, \ldots, Y_n)$ are binomial (Bernoulli) random variables, one can use ML estimation to obtain estimates of the logistic regression parameters and adopt the interpretation similar to linear regression coefficients but in terms of log odds of success. Specifically, the population intercept, β_1, is the log odds of success when all of the covariates equal zero; and the population slope, β_k, is the change in log odds of success for a single-unit change in X_{ik} given that all of the other covariates remain constant.

Log-Linear Regression for Counts

In Poisson regression, the response variable Y_i is a count (e.g., number of specific symptoms of a disease in a given period of time) assumed to follow the Poisson distribution with the expected count or number of events $E(Y_i|X_i) = \lambda_i$. This provides the basis for model likelihood-based inference. As a basis for direct comparison, counts are often expressed as rates; the corresponding expected rate is given by λ_i/t, where t is a relevant baseline measure. Poisson regression relates the expected counts or rates to a set of covariates:

$$\ln(\lambda_i) = X_i'\beta = \beta_1 X_{i1} + \beta_2 X_{i2} + \ldots + \beta_p X_{ip},$$

or the expected rates to a set of covariates:

$$\ln(\lambda_i) = \ln(t) + X_i'\beta = \ln(t) + \beta_1 X_{i1} + \beta_2 X_{i2} + \ldots + \beta_p X_{ip},$$

where $\ln(t)$ is an adjustment term known as an "offset."

Thus, modeling λ_i (or λ_i/t) with a logarithm function can be considered equivalent to a linear regression model but replacing the mean of Y_i by the logarithm of the expected count (or rate). The coefficients of the model are interpreted in terms of the logarithm of the expected count (or rate), respectively.

Both logistic and Poisson regression models as well as linear regression models fall within generalized linear models. Note that when a Poisson regression model is applied to data consisting of very small rates (e.g., applicable to studies with rare events), then the rate is approximately equal to corresponding probability, p_i, and $\ln\frac{\lambda_i}{t} \approx \ln\frac{p_i}{1-p_i}$, hence making the estimates of the regression coefficients for Poisson regression and logistic regression models approximately equal and the results of the inference not discernibly different. See Agresti (2002) for comprehensive description of regression models for ordinal model and Hilbe (2007) for negative binomial regression.

Overdispersion

One of the important properties of Poisson random variable is an equality of the expected value and variance. However, in practice count data variable often has variability far exceeding the expected value. This phenomenon is referred to in statistics as overdispersion. Although overdispersion has negligible effect on the estimated model coefficients, failure to account for overdispersion results in underestimated standard errors that lead to potentially misleading inferences such as too narrow confidence intervals and too small p-values. There are several options to address the issue of overdispersion. First option is to make the adjustment to nominal standard errors by including a scale factor ϕ in specification of the Poisson variance, $Var(Y) = \phi E(Y)$. This option makes an assumption of variance increasing linearly as a function of mean; seemingly simplified, in practice, it tends to work well. Second option to handle overdispersion is to include in the log-linear model an additional source of random variability, say some additional random error e that arises due to unmeasured individual factors:

$$\ln(E(Y_i|X_i; e_i)) = \ln(t_i) + \beta_1 X_{i1} + \beta_2 X_{i2} + \ldots + \beta_p X_{ip} + e_i.$$

The inclusion of random errors with normal distribution with zero mean and variance σ_e^2 implies a more complicated dependence of the variance of Y from the mean: $Var(Y) = E(Y) + (\exp(\sigma_e^2) - 1)E^2(Y)$. However, the model with additional normal errors does not have a closed form of the likelihood and requires computationally demanding integration techniques. At the same time, assuming a gamma distribution for the exponentiated errors, $\exp(e)$, with mean of 1 and variance γ results in the model that has a closed-form likelihood corresponding to a negative binomial distribution, leading to a more straightforward estimation of the model parameters. This approach of adjusting for overdispersion also allows for the quadratic dependence of the variance of the counts: $Var(Y) = E(Y) + \gamma E^2(Y)$.

We finish our discussion on overdispersion with a final note about situations when overdispersion arises with a discernably large number of zero counts in the data. This prevalence of zeros often leads to the inflation of the count variability compared to the mean value of Poisson distribution. Using, for example, a scale factor or inclusion of the additional variation in these situations can solve only partially the problem of overdispersion and explain the excess of zeros. One way to account for zeros is to explicitly incorporate them in the regression-like models. So-called "zero-inflated Poisson" (ZIP) models have been developed specifically to account for excess of zeros (Lambert 1992). These models assume two unobserved groups "always-zero group" and "sometimes-zero group." For example, it may be of interest to model the average number of times patients refill their prescriptions for opioids. In this example, patients can be thought as belonging to one of two groups: those who never refill a prescription for opioids (the "always-zero group") and those who refill a prescription whenever they feel pain that is severe (the "sometimes-zero group"). Observed zero counts are realized from the first group (those who never refill their opioid prescriptions) and a proportion of patients from the second group (those who would refill but not during the period of the study). Zero-inflated models are available for binomial and negative binomial types of distributions (Hall 2001). See Yang et al. (2016) for a more detailed review and comparison of different methods for zero-inflated data with application to health surveys. Similar extensions have been made to incorporate inflations other than zero for multinomial or ordinal outcomes (see Sweeney and Parnell 2018). Package "pscl" with function "zeroinfl" has been developed in R for zero-inflated count data (see also R help manual for more details).

Model Selection

Performance assessment is an essential step that guides the selection process of the best model. In order to select a model, one can distinguish between two situations when (a) competing models are nested and (b) competing models are not nested. Nested models can be compared using the likelihood-ratio test. Two models are nested if a set of the parameters in a simpler (or reduced) model is a subset of the parameters of a more complex (or full) model or, alternatively, if the full model can be transformed into the reduced model by putting constraints on a subset of the parameters. The likelihood-ratio test statistics $-2 \log \left[L_{reduced} / L_{full} \right] = 2 \left(\widehat{l_{full}} - \widehat{l_{red}} \right)$ under H_0 (no significant difference between full and reduced models) converges to chi-square distribution with the degrees of freedom equal to the difference between the dimension of the full model and the reduced model. This approach can be used in backward or forward variable subset selection approaches. In R, one can use ANOVA (model1, model2) function to implement a comparison.

When one compares non-nested models, other statistics may be used to assess the quality of each model. These statistics include Mallow's C_p, Akaike information criterion (AIC), Bayesian information criterion (BIC), and adjusted R^2.

1.3.3   Applied Longitudinal Analysis

Longitudinal studies allow direct evaluation of change in response over time and the factors that influence this change. While many of the longitudinal studies are observational, more and more recent longitudinal studies are designed as randomized experiments. In this Section, we summarize the main concepts described in Fitzmaurice et al. (2011).

In a longitudinal study, participants (subjects or patients) are measured repeatedly at different occasions or times. When the number and the timing of occasions are the same for each participant in the study, then the design of the study is called balanced. Generally, both the number of occasions and the timing can vary from one participant to another, which can happen due to the nature of the study design or due to the incompleteness of the data collection. In order to obtain valid inferences, longitudinal data analysis methods must account for correlation (dependence), which is usually present between repeated measures on the same individual, and variability, which is often heterogeneous across measurement occasions. Both correlation between observations and heterogeneity violate the fundamental assumptions of independence and homoscedasticity in the linear regression modeling. Failure to account for correlation and heterogeneity often results in large standard errors, increasing the risk of type II error.

Let Y_{ij} denote the response variable for the ith individual ($i = 1, \ldots, N$) at the jth occasion ($j = 1, \ldots, n_i$). The expected average and the variance for each occasion among N individuals are denoted as $\mu_j = E(Y_{ij})$ and $\sigma_j^2 = E\left[Y_{ij} - E(Y_{ij})\right]^2 = E\left(Y_{ij} - \mu_j\right),^2$ respectively. The covariance is a measure of the linear dependence between two variables Y_{ij} and Y_{ik}, denoted by $\sigma_{jk} = E[(Y_{ij} - \mu_j)(Y_{ik} - \mu_k)]$. The correlation between Y_{ij} and Y_{ij} is denoted by $\rho_{ik} = \frac{E\left[(Y_{ij}-\mu_j)(Y_{ik}-\mu_k)\right]}{\sigma_j \sigma_k}$, where σ_j and σ_k are the standard deviations of Y_{ij} and Y_{ik}. For the vector of repeated measures, $Y_i = (Y_{i1}, Y_{i2}, \ldots, Y_{in})'$, we define the symmetric variance-covariance matrix, Σ_i.

The independence assumption between observations measured on the same individual and homoscedasticity of observations at different occasions would lead to (incorrect) estimates of the variance of change in the mean over time. As a result the estimated standard errors and the corresponding p-values would be under- or overestimated, leading to misleading statistical inference. Thus, longitudinal data modeling would require proper modeling of both mean responses over time and modeling of covariance among repeated measures. When proposing the final longitudinal model, one must jointly specify models for the mean and covariance.

Analogously to classical regression models, longitudinal models adopt the general form of the relationship between a dependent variable and a set of covariates:

$Y_i = X_i'\beta + \varepsilon_i, E\left(Y_{ij}|X_{ij1}, \ldots, X_{ijp}\right) = \mu_{ij} = \beta_1 X_{ij1} + \beta_2 X_{ij2} + \ldots + \beta_p X_{ijp}$, but unlike classical models with a univariate response, longitudinal models focus on a multivariate response and assume multivariate normal distribution for random errors. In this case, the values of response Y_i follow a multivariate normal distribution, and in order to find maximum likelihood estimates of a vector of coefficients β, we must maximize the log-likelihood based on the product of multivariate normal densities. Assuming known and constant (across all individuals) covariance matrix Σ, the log-likelihood of interest has a form:

$$l(\beta) = \ln\left\{(2\pi)^{-\frac{Nn}{2}}|\Sigma|^{-\frac{N}{2}}\exp\left[-\frac{\sum_{i=1}^{N}(Y_i - X_i\beta)'\Sigma^{-1}(Y_i - X_i\beta)}{2}\right]\right\}.$$

The solution to this optimization problem has a closed form expression for the vector of regression coefficients β, the corresponding ML estimate, also known in the literature as the generalized least squares (GLS) estimate:

$$\widehat{\beta} = \left[\sum_{i=1}^{N}\left(X_i'\Sigma^{-1}X_i\right)\right]^{-1}\sum_{i=1}^{N}\left(X_i'\Sigma^{-1}Y_i\right).$$

The GLS estimate of β is an unbiased and consistent estimate that follows asymptotically multivariate normal distribution, $\widehat{\beta} \sim N\left(\beta, \left[\sum_{i=1}^{N}\left(X_i'\Sigma^{-1}X_i\right)\right]^{-1}\right)$. In the beginning of this section, we assumed a known covariance matrix, Σ; in practice, however, Σ must be estimated from the data. Unfortunately, no closed form ML expression is available from the multivariate normal log-likelihood. One can obtain the ML estimate of Σ via numerical approximation and then substitute the corresponding $\widehat{\Sigma}$ in the ML expression for a vector of coefficient $\widehat{\beta}$, which, in turn, for sufficiently large samples holds the same properties as the estimator $\widehat{\beta}$ when Σ is known. When Σ is unknown and the sample size is small, the ML can potentially underestimate diagonal elements of Σ (i.e., variances). As an alternative to MLE, one can utilize the method of residual or restricted maximum likelihood estimation (REML). The key idea behind REML is to utilize the likelihood for the residuals after estimating β:

$$l(\beta) = \ln\left\{(2\pi)^{-\frac{Nn}{2}}|\Sigma|^{-\frac{N}{2}}\exp\left[-\frac{\sum_{i=1}^{N}(Y_i - X_i\beta)'\Sigma^{-1}(Y_i - X_i\beta)}{2}\right]\left|\sum_{i=1}^{N}\left(X_i'\Sigma^{-1}X_i\right)\right|^{-\frac{1}{2}}\right\}.$$

Maximizing the residual log-likelihood, we obtain less biased estimate of Σ and the same GLS estimator of β but with modified covariance:

$$Cov\left(\widehat{\boldsymbol{\beta}}\right) = \left[\sum_{i=1}^{N} \left(X_i'\widehat{\Sigma}^{-1}X_i\right)\right]^{-1} \sum_{i=1}^{N} \left(X_i'\widehat{\Sigma}^{-1}Cov(Y_i)\widehat{\Sigma}^{-1}X_i\right) \left[\sum_{i=1}^{N} \left(X_i'\widehat{\Sigma}^{-1}X_i\right)\right]^{-1},$$

where $Cov(Y_i)$ can estimated as $\widehat{V}_i = \left(Y_i - X_i\widehat{\beta}\right)\left(Y_i - X_i\widehat{\beta}\right)'.$

In practice it is important to note that the REML can be used to compare different models for the covariance structure, but the standard ML should be used to compare different regression models for the mean. Also, if the covariance $Cov\,(\boldsymbol{Y}_i)$ has been misspecified, an empirical, so-called sandwich, or robust variance estimate of $Cov\left(\widehat{\boldsymbol{\beta}}\right)$ is obtained by using M-estimator approach (see Fitzmaurice et al. (2011) for details).

1.3.3.1 Mean Response Profiles for Continuous Longitudinal Data

When the purpose of the study is to characterize change patterns in the mean response over time in groups and to determine whether and how the shapes of profiles differ among groups, one can compare groups of subjects in terms of mean response profiles over time. Given any level of some group effect, we refer to the mean response profile as the sequence of means over time computed for a given group. Although this approach is particularly useful in situations when the study design is balanced and there is only one of a few categorical covariates are at the consideration, the analysis of response profiles can be extended to handle more than a single group factor and missing data.

Consider the following example of a randomized trial with two treatment groups (new treatment vs. placebo or control treatment) and three time measurements that are the same for each study participant. This study design is a simple example of a balanced longitudinal randomized experiment, for which the mean response profiles analysis is the most straightforward. The main focus of the analysis is on the testing of the null hypothesis that the difference in the mean response profiles in two groups is not significant (i.e., the mean response profiles are parallel). To test such hypotheses, it is usually assumed that both treatment group and time are categorical variables. In this regard, the analysis of the mean response profiles is similar to two-way analysis of variances, but unlike classical ANOVA, the mean response profile approach must account for dependencies and variability in repeated measurements on the same individuals.

Referring back to the two-treatment example, we use a constant and a set of three indicator variables as covariates to formulate a simple response profile model:

$$Y_{ij} = \beta_1 X_{ij1} + \beta_2 X_{ij2} + \beta_3 X_{ij3} + \beta_4 X_{ij4} + \beta_5 X_{ij2}X_{ij3} + \beta_6 X_{ij2}X_{ij4} + e_{ij}$$

where $X_{ij1} = 1$, $X_{ij2} = I$(patient i randomized to new drug), $X_{ij3} = I(j = 2)$, $X_{ij4} = I$ $(j = 3)$.

For many longitudinal studies, especially longitudinal clinical trials, the main interest is on the time × treatment (or similarly, time × group) interaction effect. Thus, the null hypothesis of interest in the hypothetical trial above can be reformulated in terms of the group and time interaction effect or using the regression coefficients: $H_0 : \beta_5 = \beta_6 = 0$. To test this null hypothesis of no time × treatment interaction effect, one can use a multivariate Wald statistics that under certain regularity conditions follows chi-square distribution with $(n - 1)$ degrees of freedom. When the number of treatments (groups) exceeds two, the same type of test can be applied with $(n - k + 1)$ degrees of freedom, where k is a number of treatments. In general, the Wald test requires the estimation of regression coefficients and the corresponding standard errors. At the same time, the analysis that is based on the repeated measure on the same patients must account for the correlation structure among these measurements. In our example, the analysis of response profiles requires the estimates of three (generally n) variances for each occasion and three (generally $n(n - 1)/2$) pairwise correlations. When no additional assumption is made on the covariance/correlation structure among repeated measurements and all values are estimated separately, the structure of the covariance matrix is called unrestricted.

Note that a significant test based on a multivariate Wald statistics only indicates that groups differ but does not tell us how they differ. The two single contrasts (each based on a univariate test in a general linear model) for time × treatment interaction have direct interpretations in terms of treatment comparisons of changes from baseline. In longitudinal clinical trials, a natural baseline for a group variable is a control, often a placebo, or an existing standard treatment. A natural baseline level for a categorical time variable is "time zero" that can be referred to a pre-treatment visit. The baseline response measurement, or the response at "time zero," is often analyzed within a vector of post-treatment outcomes, but alternatively it can be used to transform post-treatment outcomes to a vector of differences from the baseline; and sometimes when there are no missing values at "time zero," the baseline response can be effectively incorporated in a set of covariates.

It is also worth to mention that if the Wald test is not significant, the secondary hypotheses concerning the mean response profiles could be formulated as follows. Assuming the mean response profiles are parallel ($\beta_5 = \beta_6 = 0$), one can test (1) if the means are also constant over time, $H_0 : \beta_3 = \beta_4 = 0$, or (2) if the mean response profiles for the groups coincide, $H_0 : \beta_2 = 0$

There are some obvious advantages of using the analysis of mean response profiles when a longitudinal study design is balanced with time measurements common for all individuals and no mistimed measurements. The analysis is fairly straightforward and allows for arbitrary patterns in the change of mean response over time as well as in the covariance/correlation structure. In addition, the response profiles can be adjusted for missing response data, and essentially there is no potential risk of bias that often arises due to misspecification of the model.

Despite outlined advantages, the analysis of response profiles does have a number of disadvantages and restrictions that make it infeasible for many longitudinal studies. The method cannot be applied when repeated measurements are obtained from participants with different measurement schedules. Disregarding the time ordering, the response profiles approach tends to fail to recognize time trends of the repeated measures in a longitudinal study. And finally, it becomes computationally inefficient rapidly when the number of time occasions and groups grows. To analyze the longitudinal data using the mean response profiles approach, one can adopt PROC MIXED in SAS and "gls" function with "nlme" package in R, respectively.

1.3.3.2   Parametric Curve Models for Continuous Response

As mentioned earlier, the analysis of response profiles may be infeasible for many longitudinal studies due to its numerous restrictions. Unlike response profile models, fitting parametric or semi-parametric curves to longitudinal data allows to describe the patterns of change in the mean response over time in terms of simple polynomial trends, model means as an explicit function of time, handle highly unbalanced designs in a relatively seamless way, and incorporate mistimed measurements. For example, to compare treatment and control in a two-group clinical trial, where changes in mean response are approximately linear and measurements are not necessarily taken on the same schedule, one can use the following simple linear model:

$$E\left(Y_{ij}\right) = \mu_{ij} = \beta_1 + \beta_2 time_{ij} + \beta_3 group_i + \beta_4 time_{ij} group_i,$$

where $time_{ij}$ refers to the actual value of jth time measurement on i^{th} individual and as $group_i$ is a time invariant group indicator which equals one for treatment and zero for control. Then intercept β_1 refers to average baseline response for the control group, $(\beta_1 + \beta_3)$ refers to the average baseline response for the treatment group, and the slopes β_2 and $(\beta_2 + \beta_4)$ have a direct interpretation in terms of a constant rate of change in mean response for a single unit change in time for control and treatment groups, respectively. The null hypothesis of interest would be here $H_0 : \beta_4 = 0$, and if it is not rejected, then the two groups do not defer in terms of change in the mean response over time.

When changes in the mean response over time are not linear, one can consider fitting a model with a quadratic or higher-order polynomial trend. In a quadratic trend model, for example, the rate of change depends on time and must be represented in terms of two parameters for each treatment group. When fitting polynomial trends, one must include a sufficient number of terms to account for model complexity and test higher-order terms before lower-order terms. Also, it is advisable to replace time observations by their deviations from the mean (i.e., center variable by a time step) to avoid problems of collinearity.

If change over time represents a sequence of joined linear or higher-order segments that produce a piecewise polynomial pattern, one can extend a simpler polynomial model to a spline model to accommodate trends that cannot be approximated by just fitting a polynomial in time. The basic idea behind the spline models is to divide time axis into a sequence of segments and consider piecewise polynomial trends on each segment with different sets of parameters but joined at fixed times (known as "knots"). The simplest possible spline model has only one knot. For two-group example, linear spline model with knot at $t*$:

$$E(Y_{ij}) = \mu_{ij}$$
$$= \beta_1 + \beta_2 time_{ij} + \beta_3 (time_{ij} - t^*)_+ + \beta_4 group_i + \beta_5 time_{ij} \ group_i$$
$$+ \beta_6 (time_{ij} - t^*)_+ group_i,$$

where $(x)_+$ is a truncated line function that takes the value of x, if $x > 0$, and zero, otherwise.

To analyze the longitudinal data using the polynomial curves or spline modeling, one can adopt PROC MIXED in SAS and "gls" function with "nlme" package in R, respectively. These are the same functions that are used for the mean response profiles approach with one important difference. For the polynomial curves or spline modeling, time is considered to be continuous, not categorical like in the mean response profiles. In SAS, however, one needs to create an additional copy of the time variable, say t, and include it in the CLASS statement and repeated statement of the PROC MIXED; time is included in the MODEL statement as a continuous predictor and in REPEATED statement. For a spline model, one must create one additional variable for each knot t^* corresponding to $time^* = (time - t^*)_+$ function and include all of them in the MODEL statement in SAS or as a set of continues variables in the "glm" formula in R.

1.3.3.3   Modeling the Covariance

Choice of models for mean response for longitudinal observations often interrelated with the choice of covariance model. In turn, a model for the covariance must be selected based on the chosen model for the mean response, because the covariance between residuals depends on the model for the mean and therefore depends on β.

When the longitudinal design is balanced (i.e., with the same schedule and the number of occasions for each patient) and the number of occasions is relatively small, unstructured covariance, which does not require any explicit structure assumption except homogeneity of covariance across different individuals, may be appropriate. With n measurement occasions, unstructured covariance matrix has n variance and $n \times (n - 1)/2$ pairwise covariance parameters. The total number of parameters grows rapidly with an increasing number of occasions/assessment times. This design of covariance structure can be used in the combination with the mean response profiles model; other covariance (pattern) models that impose some structure on covariance have often been used in combination with the parametric curve models. In what follows, we briefly discuss several covariance models to choose from when fitting parametric models for mean response.

Compound symmetry covariance model assumes constant variance across all occasions, and the constant pairwise correlations, $Corr(Y_{ij}, Y_{ik}) = \rho$ for all j and k. Despite its simplicity and a minimal number of parameters (i.e., two) that does not depend on the number of occasions, this covariance model may not be valid for most of longitudinal datasets. *Toeplitz* covariance model assumes constant variance across occasions and $Corr(Y_{ij}, Y_{i,j+k}) = \rho_k$ for all j and k, i.e., a constant correlation among responses at adjacent measurement occasions. This model has a total of n parameters and is more flexibility in terms of the correlation structure than compound symmetry but still restrictive and applicable when measurements are taken at equal intervals in time. A special case of the Toeplitz covariance models is the (first-order) *autoregressive* covariance, where $\rho_k = \rho^k$ for all j and k. Relaxing assumption of constant variance across time, one can fit heterogeneous versions of the Toeplitz (and also autoregressive) covariance models that would require additional $(n - 1)$ parameters. When time measurements are not equally spaced over time, then, for example, the parsimonious (heterogeneous or homogeneous) *autoregressive* model can be extended by fitting correlation between any pair of repeated measures by a function which decreases exponentially with the time separations between them, $Corr\left(Y_{ij}, Y_{ik}\right) = \rho^{|t_{ij}-t_{ik}|}$ for all i and k.

Choice of models for covariance and mean are interdependent, and choice of model for covariance should be based on a "maximal" model for the mean response (e.g., based on AIC, BIC). For nested covariance pattern models, a log-likelihood ratio test statistic built on REML can be constructed (e.g., compound symmetry model is nested within the Toeplitz model). For comparing non-nested covariance models, AIC or BIC can be used.

We conclude that the covariance models attempt to characterize and model the covariance between longitudinal time measurements with a relatively small number of parameters. While parametric models permit patients to be measured on different number of occasions and at different times, not many covariance models (except unrestricted) can handle data from inherently unbalanced longitudinal designs. Moreover, because the models for the mean and covariance are interdependent, the best choice of each can be difficult.

To analyze the longitudinal data using the polynomial curves or splines with a chosen covariance model, one can use PROC MIXED in SAS and "gls" function with "nlme" package in R, respectively. In PROC MIXED, a covariance mode is identified under REPEATED …/TYPE = [covariance type] statement. In "gls" function, a type of covariance is included in a set of parameters under "corr= [corSymm, corAR, corExp]" statement specified for a compound symmetry, autoregressive, or exponential models, respectively.

1.3.3.4 Linear Mixed Effects Models

As an alternative to the described models, one can use linear mixed effects models to account for sources of natural heterogeneity in the population over time. These models are the regression-based models. The term mixed effects comes from the fact that the mean response is modeled as a combination of population parameters, shared by all individuals and referred as fixed effects, and subject-specific parameters, referred as random effects, which vary randomly from one individual to another, and assumed to be unique to a particular individual. In these settings, individuals in the population are allowed to have their own subject-specific mean response trajectories over time. Also, the introduction of random effects self-induces subject-specific covariance (among individual's responses) that has a distinctive random effects structure and that can be expressed as a function of time with relatively few parameters, regardless of the number and the timing of measurements.

Linear mixed effects models allow (a) estimation of parameters describing the mean response changes in the population of interest and (b) prediction of individual response trajectories over time. In the context of clinical trials, for instance, these predictions can help to identify those participants who do not respond well or somewhat very different from expected.

One of the main advantages of linear mixed effects models, in comparison to the models described in the previous subsections, is their flexibility in accommodating unbalanced data that is when subjects have a different number of observations and measurements taken at different times.

A simple example of linear mixed effects models is a model with an intercept and a slope that vary randomly among individuals. In this model, each subject has its own baseline level of response and the level of change in the response over time. This model can be generalized to incorporate additional randomly varying regression parameters related to time changing covariates. The effects of covariates (e.g., due to treatments, exposures) are included by allowing mean of intercepts and slopes to depend on covariates. In general settings, the linear effects model can be expressed as

$$Y_{ij} = X'_{ij} \beta + Z'_{ij} b_i + \epsilon_{ij},$$

where β is p-dimensional vector of fixed effects, b_i is q-dimensional vector of random effects, $X_i = \left\{ X'_{ij}, j = 1, \ldots, n_i \right\}$ is a matrix of covariates with n_i rows (matching the number of measurement occasions for subject i) and p columns, $Z'_{ij} = \left\{ Z_{ij}, j = 1, \ldots, n_i \right\}$ is a matrix of time-varying covariates with n_i rows and q columns, with $q \leq p$, and $\epsilon_i = \{ e_{ij}, j = 1, \ldots, n_i \}$ is a n_i-dimensional vector of errors assumed to be independent of b_i with a multivariate normal distribution with mean zero and covariance diagonal matrix $R_i = \sigma^2 I_{n_i}$. Often, the columns of the matrix of time-varying covariates Z_i are a subset of the matrix X_i, and the random effects, b_i, are assumed to be independent of X_i and to have a multivariate normal distribution with mean zero $(E(b_i) = 0)$ and covariance matrix G. The latter assumption is essential for the prediction of the random effects as well as the interpretation of conditional or subject-specific mean. Combining fixed effects and random effects, conditional mean describes the mean response profile for the ith individual:

$$E(Y_{ij}|X_{ij}, b_i) = X'_{ij}\beta + Z'_{ij}b_i.$$

In this model, the response for the ith subject at jth occasion is assumed to differ from the population mean $E\left(Y_{ij}|X'_{ij}\right)$, by a subject effect, $Z'_{ij}b_i$. That is the marginal population-averaged mean of Y_i, $E(Y_{ij}|X_{ij}) = X'_{ij}\beta$.

The introduction of a random subject effect induces correlation among the repeated measures. The conditional and marginal covariances can be distinguished in a similar way as conditional and marginal means. Using a vector-matrix notation, the conditional covariance of Y_i, given b_i, is

$$Cov(Y_i|X_i, b_i) = Cov(\epsilon_i) = R_i = \sigma^2 I_{n_i},$$

and the marginal (population-averaged) covariance of Y_i, averaged over the distribution of random effects b_i, is $Cov(Y_i) = Z_i G Z'_i + R_i$.

If the mixed effect model includes only a random intercept, then the covariance matrix of the repeated measurements has the form of the compound symmetry. To allow variance heterogeneity among variances of time measurements, a model with a random intercept and a slope serves as a yet simple alternative. In this random intercept and slope model and more complex mixed effect models for longitudinal data, the variances and covariances are individual and do not require any additional specification (self-induced) with the terms expressed as explicit functions of time thereby accounting for inherently unbalanced designs with a different number of time occasions per subject.

In many pharmaceutical- and health outcome-related studies, the primary focus is on estimation and inference of fixed effects, $\beta_1, \beta_2, \ldots, \beta_p$. When the researchers also desire to estimate subject-specific random effects, b_i, they can do it using maximum likelihood or restricted maximum likelihood approach and construct so-called best linear unbiased predictor (BLUP) for each individual subject in a form of $\widehat{b}_i = E\left(b_i|Y_i; \widehat{\beta}, \widehat{G}, \widehat{\sigma}^2\right)$. To predict subject-specific response trajectories over time, one can simply plug in the estimated values of fixed effects and predicted values of random effects in a definition of conditional mean, $\widehat{Y}_{ij} = X'_{ij}\widehat{\beta} + Z'_{ij}\widehat{b}_i$.

To analyze the longitudinal data using the mixed effect models, one can adopt PROC MIXED in SAS and "lme" function with "nlme" package in R, respectively. In PROC MIXED, for example, a mixed effects model with a random intercept and a slope for time is identified under REPEATED INTERCEPT time/statement. In "lme" function, the same model is included in a set of parameters under "random = ~ time| id" statement. One can also obtain BLUPs in SAS and R, using outlined functions.

When the response variable in a longitudinal study is categorical (e.g., binary and count data), previously discussed generalized linear models can be extended to handle the correlated outcomes. There are two different analytic approaches: generalized marginal models and mixed effects models (see Chapters 12–15, Fitzmaurice et al. 2011). Note also that both linear and generalized mixed effects models can be used to analyze multilevel data (see Chapter 22, Fitzmaurice et al. 2011). Multilevel models are especially effective in studies where the primary goal is on the assessment of health services and/or outcomes with information obtained from patients who are nested within different sites and clinics. Such data can be regarded as hierarchical or multilevel data.

1.3.4 Analysis of Time-to-Event Outcome

The theoretical background represented in this subsection is mainly based on the book of Kleinbaum and Klein (2012a, b). Analysis of time-to-event outcome, or survival analysis, is a collection of statistical procedures for data analysis for which the outcome variable of interest is time until an event occurs. An event, in survival analysis also referred as a failure, is usually related to (but not limited to) some negative experience, for example, death in patients with heart transplant or relapse in remission in cancer patients. It could also be a positive experience such as recovery from obstructive pulmonary disease or any experience or event of interest that can happen to an individual. Time, in the survival analysis referred as survival time, can be counted in years, months, weeks, or any other suitable units characterizing period from the beginning of follow-up of an individual until an occurrence of an event. In this section, we focus on traditional survival analysis settings when only one event of interest is analyzed. In case, when more than one event of interest needs to be analyzed, we refer our reader to the read about recurrent event survival analysis and competing risks survival analysis described in Kleinbaum and Klein (2012a, b); Austin et al. (2016); De Glas et al. (2016); and references therein.

Censoring is a common problem related to survival analysis. Censoring occurs when we have some information about individual survival time, but the exact survival time is unavailable. This can happen due to the following reasons. A patient does not experience the event of interest before the trial ends, or a patient withdraws from the trial earlier due to a specific reason or fails to follow-up during the trial period. In these examples, the survival time of a patient becomes incomplete or cut off at the right side of the observed survival time interval. These observations are further marked as right-censored. Less frequently than right-censored, survival times can also be left-censored or interval-censored. A patient's survival time is marked as left-censored if a patient's true survival time is less than or equal to the pre-specified observed survival time. For example, in an observational study, some women had babies before the pre-specified 250-day mark. If a procedure is administered multiple times during the study period and a patient's true survival time falls within a known time interval but the actual time is unknown, such event will be considered as interval-censored. In what follows we focus on the analysis of right-censored observations that are more common in clinical trials.

Formally, let T be a random variable for a person's survival time. By construction, T can take only non-negative values less than or equal to the length of the study period. A specific realization of T is denoted by t. Together with the random variable for survival time, we define a binary (dichotomous) random variable d indicating event occurrence or censorship. That is $d = 1$, if the event of interest occurs during the study, and $d = 0$, if and only if one of the following happens: a patient does not experience an event of interest until the end of the study and a patient is lost to follow-up or withdraws from the study.

Given the above notation, we now can define two critical functions of survival time, namely, the survival function $S(t)$ and the hazard function $h(t)$. The survival function $S(t)$ provides the probability that a patient survives longer than some specified time t, $S(t) = P(T > t)$. In theory, $S(t)$ is a non-increasing function of t with $S(0) = 1$, indicating no event occurrences for any patients at the beginning of the study, and $S(\infty) = 0$, indicating all patients are experiencing an event occurrence at the end of the study. In practice, however, when using actual observations and the fixed study period (not infinite), the survival function $S(t)$ may not approach zero at the end of the study. The hazard function, $h(t)$, provides the instantaneous potential per unit time for event occurrence, given that the individual has survived (has not experienced an event) up to time t. Formally, $h(t)$ equals the limit of conditional probability $P(t \leq T < t + \Delta t \mid T \geq t)$ as Δt approaches zero, and in this formulation is also called a conditional failure rate. While $h(t)$ is not limited to start at one and go down to zero like $S(t)$, for any fixed value of t, the hazard function is always non-negative and has no upper bound.

Both the survival function and the hazard function are equally important in practice. The survival function directly describes the survival from the observations; the hazard function is used for modeling by taking a specific form with a known distribution. Knowing the form of $h(t)$, one can derive the corresponding S(t), and vice versa. The relationship between the two can be expressed as follows:

$$S(t) = \exp\left[-\int_0^t h(u)du\right], h(t) = -\left[\frac{dS(t)/dt}{S(t)}\right].$$

Given the time-to-event outcome, one can pursue the following steps in the survival analysis. The analysis starts with the first step that includes estimation and the interpretation of the survival and/or hazards functions from observed survival data. In clinical studies with the time-to-event outcome, this step could be used to compare survival trends and/or hazard rates over time for patients in a treatment group and a placebo group. The two survival curves are estimated, for example, using the Kaplan-Meier method, and then graphed on the same axis to aid the further visual comparison. A formal comparison of two or more survival curves estimating a common curve can be performed via the log-rank test. Before the comparison over time, one can compute simple descriptive measures including the average survival time, $\overline{T} = \sum_{i=1}^{n} t_i/n$, and the average hazard rate, $\overline{h} = \#events / \sum_{i=1}^{n} t_i$, to provide overall preliminary comparison. Since the average survival time includes censored data (if present) in the computation, it may significantly underestimate the true average survival time. As an alternative, median survival time can provide a better measure to compare. If the study also collects additional variables, one can also look at the survival curves considering the possible confounding effect of any available variables or proceed with the second step of survival analysis that may include the statistical modeling with the purpose to assess the relationship between the survival time and the explanatory variables. The most commonly used model for this step is the Cox proportional hazards model, which is described later in this chapter.

1.3.4.1 Kaplan-Meier Survival Curves and the Log-Rank Test

Descriptive statistics of survival times provide overall comparisons but do not compare two or more groups at different times of follow-up. In this subsection, we discuss how to estimate a survival curve $S(t)$ using the Kaplan-Meier (KM) method and how to decide whether or not two or more survival curves are equivalent using the log-rank test or similar tests of hypotheses. We also provide equations for computing 95% confidence intervals for KM curves and for the median survival time.

The general theoretical formula for an estimate of a survival curve $\widehat{S}(t_{(f)})$ at time-to-event $t_{(f)}$ using KM method can be expressed as the probability of surviving past the previous time-to-event $t_{(f-1)}$, multiplied by the conditional probability of surviving past time $t_{(f)}$, given survival to at least time $t_{(f)}$:

$$\widehat{S}(t_{(f)}) = \widehat{S}(t_{(f-1)}) \times \widehat{Pr}(T > t_{(f)}|T \geq t_{(f)}).$$

Equivalently, KM curve $\widehat{S}(t_{(f)})$ can be written as a product of all fractions that estimate the conditional probabilities for time-to-event and earlier:

$$\widehat{S}(t_{(f)}) = \prod_{i=1}^{f} \widehat{Pr}(T > t_{(f)}|T \geq t_{(f)}).$$

In practice, KM curves can be constructed as follows. For convenience, the collected survival data should be organized in a form of the tables with at least three columns for each group or treatment: ordered survival times from smallest to largest; frequency counts of failures (events) at each distinct failure time; and frequency counts of those subjects censored in time interval $[t_{(f)}, t_{(f+1)})$. To estimate the survival probability at a given time, one can use the information in these columns. If there are no censored cases in a group, one can compute the survival probabilities $\widehat{S}(t_{(f)})$ as the number of subjects surviving past the specified time being considered and divided by the number of subjects at the start of the follow-up, $\widehat{S}(t_{(f)}) = \frac{\#surviving\ at\ or\ past\ time\ t_{(f)}}{\#group\ sample\ size}$. If a group contains any censored subjects, the Kaplan-Meier approach that utilizes a product-limit formula can be used. The first survival estimate $\widehat{S}(0)$ in both cases, with and without censored subjects, is always one as the probability of surviving past time zero. The following survival estimates are calculated by multiplying the preceding survival estimate $\widehat{S}(t_{(f-1)})$ by a fraction of subjects surviving past time $t_{(f)}$ out of subjects at risk at time $t_{(f)}$ or $\widehat{Pr}\left(T > t_{(f)} | T \geq t_{(f)}\right)$.

To better understand the behavior of the estimated KM survival curves, the appropriate confidence bounds for $\widehat{S}_{KM}(t)$ can be also estimated:

$$\widehat{S}_{KM}(t) \pm Z_{\frac{\alpha}{2}} \sqrt{\widehat{Var}\left[\widehat{S}_{KM}(t)\right]},$$

using the Greenwood's formula for computation of the standard error:

$$\widehat{Var}\left[\widehat{S}_{KM}(t)\right] = \left(\widehat{S}_{KM}(t)\right)^2 \times \sum_{f:t_{(f)} \leq t} \left[\frac{m_f}{n_f(n_f - m_f)}\right],$$

where m_f is the total observed number of failures and n_f is the total number of subjects at risk in all groups at time $t_{(f)}$ for a given group. At this point, we resume the estimation of survival curves and continue with the overview of the hypothesis testing using the log-rank approach and later with the modeling using the Cox proportional hazard model.

To evaluate whether or not KM curves for two or more groups ($G \geq 2$) are significantly different, and test $H_0 : S_1(t) = S_2(t) = \ldots = S_G(t)$, one can use the log-rank test. The log-rank test is a large-sample chi-squared test that is based on the idea of comparing observed and expected counts in different categories over failure times. Thus, for each ordered failure time, $t_{(f)}$ ($f = 1, 2, \ldots, k$), in the entire data and for each group i, ($i = 1, 2, \ldots, G$), one needs to obtain the number of subjects at risk in group i, n_{if}, the observed number of failures in group i, m_{if}, and the expected number of failures in group i, e_{if}. While values of n_{if} and m_{if} for each failure time can be derived directly from the data, the expected counts e_{if} are computed as

$$e_{if} = n_{if} \frac{m_f}{n_f},$$

where $m_f = \sum_{i=1}^{G} m_{if}$ is the total observed number of failures and $n_f = \sum_{i=1}^{G} n_{if}$ is the total number of subjects at risk in all groups at time $t_{(f)}$. Given the observed and expected counts, the next step is to compute a set of the differences aggregated over time and their corresponding variances and covariances:

$$O_i - E_i = \sum_{f=1}^{k} \left(m_{if} - e_{if}\right), \; Var(O_i - E_i) = \sum_{f=1}^{k} \left(\frac{n_{if}\left(n_f - n_{if}\right)m_f\left(n_f - m_f\right)}{n_f^2\left(n_f - 1\right)}\right),$$

$$Cov(O_i - E_i, O_l - E_l) = \sum_{f=1}^{k} \left(\frac{-n_{if}n_{lf}m_f\left(n_f - m_f\right)}{n_f^2\left(n_f - 1\right)}\right).$$

By letting $D = (O_1 - E_1,\ O_2 - E_2, \ldots, O_{G-1} - E_{G-1})$ be the vector of difference between observed and expected failure counts, and V be the matrix containing variances and covariances of D, one can compute the log-rank test statistics, which in the matrix notation has a form, $D'C^{-1}D$, and for a large sample size under the null hypothesis follows a chi-squared distribution with $(G-1)$ degrees of freedom. In practice, for large samples, an approximation of the log-rank statistic that does not require computation of variances and covariances can be used to compare two or more survival curves. The approximate formula includes the sum over all groups of the square of the observed minus expected values divided by the expected value, $\sum_{i=1}^{G} \frac{(O_i - E_i)^2}{E_i} \sim \chi^2_{df=G-1}$. When survival curves are being compared for two groups, the log-rank test is formed using the difference and its variance for one of the two groups without using any covariance information.

There are several variations of the log-rank test approach that are designed to test the equivalence of two or more survival curves. The most commonly used variations include the methods that incorporate the weights for different failure times such as the Wilcoxon, the Tarone-Ware, the Peto, and the Flemington-Harrington tests. Although all of these tests should provide similar results and lead to the same clinical conclusions, one needs to make a priori decision which test to use and why. The decision should be based on both considerations of the power of the test and the possible violations of assumptions behind the null hypothesis. Another extension of the log-rank test is a stratified log-rank test that allows controlling the comparison for the stratified explanatory variable. For more details, see Kleinbaum and Klein (2012a, b).

1.3.4.2 The Cox Proportional Hazards Model and Its Characteristics

The Cox proportional hazards model is the most common model used for the analysis of time-to-event or survival data. This model provides an expression for the hazard at time t for an individual with a given specification of a set of p explanatory variables $X = (X_1, X_2, \ldots, X_p)$ and can be represented in a form of a product of the baseline function, $h_0(t)$, and the exponential expression depending on a linear combination of explanatory variables and parameters, $X'\beta$:

$$h(t, X) = h_0(t)e^{X'\beta}.$$

In general, it is possible to consider explanatory variables that are time-dependent (i.e., depending on t). In this case, one can use the extended Cox model. The focus of this section is on the time-invariant X variables that do not change their values over time (e.g., sex, race, family history). When all covariates X are equal to zero, the Cox model reduces to the baseline hazard $h_0(t)$, which does not have to be specified. This property among others makes the Cox model a widely used semiparametric model. It does not require specification of the baseline hazard but allows obtaining estimates of the regression coefficients, hazard ratios, and adjusted survival curves. At the same, if the correct form of a parametric hazard function is known (typically not), a corresponding parametric model may be preferred (e.g., Weibull, Exponential, Log-Normal). When in doubt, one can choose the Cox model as a reasonable choice of a robust model.

To obtain the estimates for the parameter coefficients β of the Cox model, the Cox model uses so-called "partial" maximum likelihood approach, which consists of probabilities for subjects that fail (or experience event), but does not include probabilities for censored subjects. However, the process of construction of the partial likelihood as a product of likelihoods at all failure times incorporates the censored data implicitly.

Once the estimates coefficients are obtained, one can fit the model and compare two individuals with different values of the predictors, say $X_a = (X_{1a}, X_{2a}, \ldots, X_{pa})$ and $X_b = (X_{1b}, X_{2b}, \ldots, X_{pb})$. For example, the goal could be to compare hazard rates of two patients with similar baseline characteristics assigned to placebo and treatment. Using general notation above, the estimated hazard ratio is:

$$\widehat{HR} = \exp\left[\sum_{i=1}^{p} \widehat{\beta}_i (X_{ia} - X_{ib})\right].$$

As one can notice, the formula for $\widehat{HR}$ does not depend on time, or equivalently, it implies that the hazard for one individual is proportional to the hazard for any other individual and the proportionality is constant. This statement briefly explains the concept of the proportional hazard assumption, which usually requires being formally tested using, for instance, so-called Schoenfeld residuals (see Chapter 4 of Kleinbaum and Klein 2012a, b for more details).

Maximum likelihood approach can be also used to compute the corresponding standard error and the confidence interval of the HR. If the confidence interval contains one (i.e., $H_0 : HR = 1$), this would indicate no significant difference (statistically speaking) in terms of the hazard ratio for two subjects. Similarly, one can use the confidence intervals (and standard errors) of the estimated parameters to make inference about the effect of the predictors on individual hazard rates or HR (i.e., in terms of $H_0 : \beta = 0$).

Additionally, the estimated coefficients $\widehat{\beta}$ from the Cox model can be used to produce the adjusted survival curves, the survival curves that are adjusted for the explanatory variables:

$$\widehat{S}(t, X) = \left[\widehat{S}_0(t)\right]^{\exp X'\widehat{\beta}},$$

where the estimate of $\widehat{S}_0(t)$ is also produced by fitting the Cox model; the values of X should be specified by the investigator. The obtained adjusted survival curves can be produced for two or more groups analogously to the KM curves that are fitted without any model assumption.

To analyze the time-to-event outcome data in SAS, one can use PROC LEFETEST, PROC PHREG, and PROC LIFEREG. PROC LEFETEST is used to construct Kaplan-Meier survival estimates and plots. In addition, it produces output for life table estimates, the log rank, and Wilcoxon test statistics. PROC PHREG can be used to fit the traditional Cox proportional hazard model, a stratified Cox model, and a Cox model with time-varying covariates. For a comprehensive graphical output PROC PHREG can be used in a combination with PROC GPLOT. PROC LIFEREG is used to obtain the output for parametric accelerated failure time (ATF) models, survival models that are less restrictive than proportional hazard models (see Chapter 7 of Kleinbaum and Klein 2012a, b for more details).

In R, the following functions are available for analysis of the time-to-event outcome data within "survival" package. Function "surv" serves as an essential first step to create a survival object. This object is used as input variable for other survival functions including "survfit," a function that produces Kaplan-Meier survival estimates; "survdiff," a function that tests the equality of survival functions; "coxph," a function that fits the Cox proportional hazard model, a stratified Cox model, and an extended Cox model; and "survereg," a function that fits ATF and other parametric survival models.

1.4 Important Considerations in Clinical Trials

There are many points to consider when designing and analyzing clinical trials. Estimation of the clinical trial sample size depends on the choice of statistical methods and pre-defined set of parameters that depend on our knowledge about disease under the study, study population, study drugs and actions, tolerability of the drug and other safety issues, acceptability of endpoints, enrollment rate, participating countries, drop-out mechanism, etc. To account for different scenarios and uncertainties in our knowledge, in addition to pre-defined primary analysis of the clinical trial endpoints, sensitivity analyses are usually planned and conducted. This section focuses on some common statistical considerations that affect the design, execution, and analysis of clinical trials including missing data issues and prevention, defining an appropriate estimand, handling multiple objectives, analyzing subgroups, planning multiregional clinical trials, and evaluating drug safety.

1.4.1 Missing Data and Patient Retention

Missing data is a common problem in clinical trials. There are many reasons why data can be missing, including patient dropout due to adverse events, lack of efficacy, or any other reasons either related or unrelated to the study treatment or the primary objective. Loss to follow-up is generally considered to be one of the most important and preventable reasons for missing data. Even if a patient completes the study, one may still have elements of incomplete data due to different aspects of study conduct. For example, patients can complete a trial but discontinue the study treatment early, requiring careful consideration about the appropriate use of the data collected, or have missed measurements at one or more visits. Missing data can lead to loss of power and biased results that affect the quality and validity of clinical trials. There are three common types of missing data defined by the reason the data are missing: missing completely at random (MCAR), missing at random (MAR), and missing not at random (MNAR). There are many statistical methods available to handle incomplete data, but different methods require different assumptions and can lead to different conclusions in extreme cases of missing data. The detailed description of the various methods with applications can be found in the literature including Little and Rubin (2002), O'Kelly and Ratitch (2014), and Mallinckrodt and Lipkovich (2017).

In 2010, the National Research Council (NRC) published the report *The Prevention and Treatment of Missing Data in Clinical Trials* (National Research Council 2010). The NRC report advocated preventing missing data through increased follow-up efforts for patients who discontinue treatment or otherwise violate the study protocol. The report provided a review of available methods for handling missing data during the data analysis stage, but rather than recommending any one method as best, it stressed the importance of clearly defining the estimand at the design stage of a trial. The term "estimand" as used here refers to the treatment effect—the quantity to be estimated with study data. The report argued against the use of single-value imputation methods, such as last observation carried forward or baseline carried forward, due to potential underestimation of the variability of the resulting treatment effect estimates.

At the time of the NRC report publication, drug development clinical trials with continuous outcomes (e.g., blood pressure, lung function, blood glucose levels, or patient reported symptom scores) often relied on mixed models for repeated measurements (MMRM) as the primary analysis strategy for estimating and testing hypotheses about treatment effects. Implicit in the use of these methods is the assumption that dropouts would behave similarly to other patients in the same treatment group, and possibly with similar covariate values, had they not dropped out. Such an assumption, however, may not be reasonable if a patient discontinues therapy for intolerability. Focusing on the appropriate estimand at the design stage can help bring considerations such as these to the forefront, ultimately resulting in the most appropriate treatment effect definition and analysis strategy for a particular setting.

The International Council for Harmonisation (ICH) published a first revision of the E9 Statistical Principles in Clinical Trials guideline in 2017 (ICH E9 R1 2017). This draft guideline ICH E9 (R1) sets forth basic principles for defining estimands or treatment effects, taking into consideration the target population, the outcome variable or trial endpoint, the method to account for intercurrent events (e.g., dropouts or use of rescue medications), and the population summary measure that provides the basis for comparing treatments (e.g., differences in means or risk ratios). The guidance suggests some potential strategies for constructing estimands, including the following:

- *Treatment policy estimand*—the actual value of the outcome variable is obtained and used in the analysis, regardless of any post-randomization events that occurred (e.g., taking rescue medication). There are no statistical issues with this estimand, as it preserves the advantages of randomization and may come closest to mimicking medical practice, but prescribers and patients often find it less desirable, being too far removed from a pharmacologic effect. An additional benefit is that retrieved data on dropouts can be used to impute outcomes for dropouts whose data were unable to be retrieved.
- *Composite estimand*—the post-randomization event becomes the outcome of interest for patients experiencing the event, and treatment effects are defined using composite endpoints combining measured values for some patients and events for others. This approach is particularly useful when a measurement following an event is not meaningful but the fact that the event occurred is. Other approaches, such as trimmed means (Permutt and Li 2016), may also be useful in these settings.
- *Principal stratification*—the treatment effect is defined in patients able to tolerate the test drug, even if the patient was assigned to control. Note this is not a completer's analysis but is what clinicians are often most interested in—what is the effect of the drug among those able to take it? It is, however, difficult to implement, requiring identification of patients in the control group who would have tolerated the drug, had they been assigned to it.
- *Hypothetical effect*—the treatment effect is defined under alternative conditions (e.g., if adherence had been perfect or if rescue medications were withheld). Analyses that involve estimating the effect that would have been observed had all patients tolerated treatment and completed the trial are not generally acceptable from a regulatory standpoint. The effect if rescue medications are withheld may be of interest, but a trial that allows direct estimation of this effect is usually unethical to conduct.
- *Effect while on treatment*—the treatment effect is defined based on measurements obtained while each patient remained on treatment. Because every patient has a measured value to contribute to the analysis, there are no statistical issues with this strategy. Note, however, that although measurements were taken when treatment stops, regardless of when that occurs, and are available for all patients, the treatment effect based on those measurements will not usually provide a valid estimate of the effect at the planned end of the trial and could, therefore, raise problems when labeling the drug. The relevance of this estimand will usually be a clinical decision.

Sensitivity analyses are often performed to assess the impact of assumptions, required for a particular analysis strategy but unable to be verified, on a study's findings. ICH E9 (R1) addresses the need to plan for sensitivity analyses to assess the impact of missing data on a trial's results. In this application, conducting additional analyses that make the same missing data assumptions as the primary analysis will rarely be useful. For example, if a primary analysis involves fitting an MMRM that assumes data are missing at random, then sensitivity analyses based on multiple imputations that make the same missing-at-random assumption will be less informative than sensitivity analyses that vary the reasons the data are missing and include missing not-at-random scenarios. When planning sensitivity analyses to assess the impact of missing data on study results, the number of different analyses to be conducted is usually less important than how the missing data assumptions are varied.

Tipping point analyses are mentioned in Permutt et al. (2016b) as being particularly useful for regulatory purposes. With these analyses, unverifiable assumptions about missing data are varied in such a way as to identify the scenarios under which the analysis results are tipped away from success, followed by an assessment of how likely those scenarios would be. As discussed in LaVange (2019), a useful example of a pharmaceutical sponsor's use of tipping point analysis can be found in the briefing materials for the June 20, 2017 meeting of the Endocrinologic and Metabolic Drugs Advisory Committee (US Food and Drug Administration 2017a). During this meeting, a tipping point analysis used to address missing data in a large cardiovascular outcome trial of liraglutide to treat type 2 diabetes was discussed. The sponsor presented sensitivity analyses that identified (1) the number of liraglutide patients with missing outcomes who would need to experience an event and (2) the number of placebo patients with missing outcomes who would need to not experience any events before superiority of the hazard ratio would be reversed. The argument was made that the resulting tipping point scenario was unlikely to occur, thereby supporting the trial's finding of superiority.

The US FDA and some sponsor organizations are becoming increasingly concerned with the misuse of sensitivity analyses during regulatory reviews and the impact of those analyses on approval decisions. An example illustrating this problem is included in LaVange (2013) based on a 2012 meeting of the Gastrointestinal Drugs Advisory Committee. Additional manuscripts describing the agency's thinking on missing data, estimands, and sensitivity analysis appeared in recent years (LaVange and Permutt 2016; Permutt et al. 2016a, b). FDA advises sponsors on the adequacy of their proposed approach to missing data and sensitivity analyses through protocol reviews of new trial designs and statistical reviews of submitted trial data for nearly every application submitted, and although the ICH E9 (R1) guidance provides a framework for addressing missing data problems, application of some of the approaches described therein can pose challenges (LaVange 2019).

As mentioned previously, prevention of missing data through the development of strategies to increase patient retention is an essential component of study planning, especially in long-term studies where challenges with patient retention are the most notable. Statisticians can help with missing data prevention at the study design stage by quantifying the amount of missing data in similar studies and illustrating its effect, translating finding into information to inform future subject care, educating the clinical study team, and participating in the creation of missing data prevention plans (Hughes 2014).

1.4.2   Multiple Objectives and Multiplicity Adjustments

Efficacy endpoints in a clinical trial are measures intended to reflect the effect of a drug or drugs (treatment effect) on patients or healthy volunteers. Clinical trials are often designed to examine the treatment effect on more than one endpoint. Endpoints in clinical trials are usually classified into three families: primary, secondary, and exploratory. Endpoints are frequently ordered by clinical importance, with the most important being a primary endpoint or co-primary endpoints. Alternatively, endpoints can be ordered by the likelihood of demonstrating an effect. For example, time-to-disease progression is often selected as the primary endpoint in oncology trials even though survival is the most important endpoint. The reasons are that an effect on disease progression can be detected earlier and is often larger than the observed effect on survival, because the latter can be diluted by subsequent post-progression treatment. Determination of which endpoints are primary, secondary, or exploratory should always be made prospectively.

The statistical approach commonly used to evaluate a treatment effect on a chosen clinical endpoint is based on the test of hypothesis. The rejection of the null hypothesis supports the study conclusion that there is a difference between treatment groups but does not constitute absolute proof that the null hypothesis is false. There is always some possibility of mistakenly rejecting the null hypothesis when it is true, making a type I error. An essential element of type I error rate control is the prospective specification of all endpoints to be tested and all data analyses to be performed to test hypotheses for the pre-specified endpoints. The statistical analysis plan should describe how the endpoints are tested, including the order of testing and the alpha level applied to each specific test (US Food and Drug Administration 2017b).

Multiplicity issues are encountered in clinical trials with multiple testing due to multiple objectives multiple endpoints (primary or secondary), multiple treatment groups, multiple dose levels, evaluation of multiple subgroups, analyses at multiple time points, or some combination thereof. Testing multiple hypotheses without any adjustments for multiplicity can increase the probability of erroneously rejecting at least one true null hypothesis, the error known as the familywise error rate (FWER). In confirmatory clinical trials, strong control of the FWER across the primary trial objectives (endpoints) is mandated by some regulatory authorities (e.g., EMA 2017; US Food and Drug Administration 2017b). As mentioned previously, a multiplicity adjustment procedure must be pre-defined to preserve the FWER across the null hypotheses associated with the individual tests.

The most basic multiplicity adjustment, e.g., a Bonferroni adjustment, examines each null hypothesis independently of the other null hypotheses and then adjusts alpha accordingly. This procedure is known as a single-step test. More efficient tests that result in a higher overall probability of success for the trial while also controlling for multiplicity are stepwise tests; these tests are applied in a pre-defined sequential order thought to maximize the chance of detecting a treatment effect under the alternative hypothesis. The fixed-sequence and fallback procedures are examples of stepwise tests. Alternatively, the null hypotheses can be tested in the order determined by the significance of the hypothesis test statistics. Such testing is more flexible than fixed-sequence testing. The Holm and Hochberg procedures are examples of the stepwise tests.

When selecting the method for handling multiplicity, it is recommended to utilize the available information on the joint distribution of the hypothesis test statistics associated with the hypotheses of interest. Nonparametric procedures (or p-value based procedures) such as Bonferroni, Holm, and fixed-sequence procedures do not make any assumptions on the joint distribution of the test statistics, and they are uniformly less powerful than semiparametric procedures such as a Hochberg test or parametric procedures such as Dunnett's test. Nonparametric procedures tend to perform poorly when the testing problem involves a large number of hypotheses or the test statistics are strongly correlated. Semiparametric procedures control the overall type I error rate under the assumption that the test statistics follow a multivariate normal distribution with non-negative pairwise correlations. Parametric procedures require full specification of the joint test statistics distribution. Another class of multiple testing procedures includes resampling-based procedures. The critical feature of these procedures is that they estimate the joint distribution directly rather than making assumptions about that distribution. The estimates are obtained by applying bootstrap or permutation methods.

Many multiplicity adjustment methods have been developed and are discussed in the literature. For example, books by Hochberg and Tamhane (1987), Hsu (1996), Dmitrienko et al. (2010), and Bretz et al. (2011) provide a detailed description of multiple testing methods and analysis techniques; some include SAS and R code for illustration. The paper by Dmitrienko and D'Agostino (2013) provides a comprehensive tutorial summarizing traditional multiplicity adjustment methods used in clinical trials, including comparisons of methods and recommendations on the choice of the procedures to use. The tutorial by Alosh et al. (2014) describes more advanced multiplicity adjustment procedures that allow recycling of significance levels of hypotheses to address complex multiplicity problems. Both tutorials are aimed to help statisticians working in clinical trials to select an appropriate method for their applications and calculate critical values, adjusted p-values, and, in more simple scenarios, adjusted confidence intervals.

In January 2017, the US FDA released draft guidance on Multiple Endpoints in Clinical Trials (US Food and Drug Administration 2017b). The focus of the draft guidance is on methods to manage multiplicity due to multiple endpoints in demonstrating the effectiveness of a drug to support its approval. Although the guidance addresses only one source of multiplicity, the principles described therein may apply to others (e.g., multiple doses, multiple analyses, multiple analysis populations, and multiple subgroups). The guidance explains the agency's use of co-primary and composite endpoints in some disease areas and also touches on situations where multiplicity adjustments may not be needed, such as the use of additional analyses to better characterize the effects of a drug, following a positive finding that the drug is effective based on the primary hypothesis test with appropriate multiplicity control.

In LaVange (2019), an interesting example is provided to illustrate the need for additional guidance on multiple endpoints. During the May 12, 2015 meeting of the Pulmonary-Allergy Drugs Advisory Committee (US Food and Drug Administration 2015a), an application for a combination product to treat cystic fibrosis was discussed. Results from two Phase III trials were presented (Wainwright et al. 2015) during the meeting. Both trials relied on a testing hierarchy to manage multiplicity due to multiple secondary endpoints following success on the primary endpoint in each trial. A non-significant result occurred in both trials for an endpoint early in the hierarchy, precluding the availability of any evidence to support findings for endpoints further down the list. A pre-specified analysis of a key secondary clinical endpoint, pulmonary exacerbation, was carried out using data combined from the two trials to increase the power available for testing, but this analysis was outside of the testing hierarchy of either trial. It was clear from the discussion at the meeting that Advisory Committee members were impressed with the significant results of the combined analysis on exacerbations, but it was not clear how the carefully followed approach for managing multiplicity in these trials applied in interpreting this analysis. As the agency and industry gain more experience with complex cases such as this, these and other questions regarding multiplicity in clinical trials will be addressed and hopefully clarified in the final FDA guidance on Multiple Endpoints in Clinical Trials.

1.4.3   Subgroup Analysis

Subgroups of the study population are defined for most clinical trials, and while they serve different purposes, their consideration in the planning of statistical analyses is essential. LaVange (2019) categorized subgroups of interest for drug development clinical trials into three broad types:

- Demographic subgroups (e.g., age, sex, race/ethnicity) defined for reporting purposes. Although the subgroup-specific effects are of interest, differences among groups are usually not expected.
- Regional subgroups defined for global trials (e.g., the USA vs. Europe). Differences are often expected due to intrinsic factors (e.g., patient characteristics) or extrinsic factors (e.g., medical practice).
- Biomarker subgroups defined based on a valid assay, typically reflecting an expectation that one or more of the groups will experience more benefit or less harm than others.

The primary results of a clinical trial relating to treatment effects are usually based on the estimation and testing of average effects across all patients, even though we know that not all treatments will affect all patients the same. Some variability in the way a particular treatment affects different patients and different subgroups of patients is almost always expected. To investigate this variability, subgroup-specific treatment effects may also be estimated, and tests of hypotheses about differences between subgroups assessed. The challenge is to be able to differentiate true subgroup differences from those due to random variability. Further, it is often the case that the sample sizes of some subgroups are small and the confidence intervals about them are wide, making inference about subgroup effects difficult. Estimating the treatment effect for the overall study population requires an assumption that the effect is the same for all patients, and although this approach increases the precision of the estimate, it may be systematically wrong for some particular subgroups. In planning for subgroup analyses, therefore, the analyst has three options: (1) compute subgroup-specific estimates to report for subgroups of interest, (2) assume that overall estimates of effects based on the entire study population apply to each subgroup, or (3) use shrinkage estimators to produce subgroup-specific estimates that rely on some borrowing of information across subgroups to reduce variability and increase the precision of the subgroup estimates. The advantages and disadvantages of each approach will depend in part on the type of subgroup and purpose of subgroup reporting and should be carefully considered during the trial planning stage.

Representing an internal FDA working group on subgroup analysis, Alosh et al. (2015) described several subgroup analysis problems commonly faced by FDA reviewers and offered solutions for different trial scenarios and subgrouping schema. An example is the problem of how to interpret significant findings in the overall study population, when a trial is designed to show an effect primarily in a biomarker-positive subgroup. If the drug is not expected to work in the biomarker-negative subgroup, but a reasonable number of biomarker-negative patients are enrolled in the trial, how should positive overall study results be interpreted for those patients? This is not an easy question to address but one that impacts product labeling, if the drug is approved for marketing. The working group manuscript emphasizes the importance of planning for subgroup analyses and the difficulty of trying to explain surprising subgroup results after a trial is completed. The use of data visualization methods is advocated, and a variety of statistical methods are described, including Bayesian subgroup estimators that can be used in some settings to reduce the number of random highs expected with the use of more traditional subgroup estimators and to provide greater precision of subgroup-specific estimates. The working group manuscript offers some suggestions to sponsors when planning for subgroup analyses, but to date, formal FDA guidance on this topic has not yet been issued.

The European Medicines Agency (EMA) guideline on the investigation of subgroups in confirmatory clinical trials (EMA 2014) recommends proceeding with caution when performing exploratory subgroup analyses, taking into consideration all available evidence, not only the point estimates for individual subgroups. Data visualization methods, when appropriately applied, can greatly facilitate the interpretation of results from any data analysis, and subgroup analyses are no exception. Many clinicians and statisticians favor forest plots as a convenient and concise way to describe subgroup estimates in a clinical trial. Clinical trial subgroups defined by baseline characteristics (e.g., age, sex, baseline disease status, geographic region), however, are not independent (the same patients appear in more than one subgroup) and, consistency among subgroups, therefore, should not be over-interpreted as providing independent verification of results. Caution is also advised in over-interpreting what appears to be extreme effects in a forest plot depicting subgroup effects, as some random variation among subgroups is expected.

In some cases, a subgroup effect is observed that requires further exploration of underlying factors to explain the differential effects. In LaVange (2019), the Platelet Inhibition and Patient Outcomes (PLATO) trial (Wellentin et al. 2009) is described as an example where a regional difference apparent in the subgroup forest plot for the trial prompted an examination of confounding factors and low-dose aspirin use was identified as a likely candidate (US Food and Drug Administration 2011; Carroll and Fleming 2013). Another example of regional subgroup differences is provided by the Advisory Committee discussion of the cardiovascular safety trial mentioned above to illustrate tipping point analyses (US Food and Drug Administration 2017a). Based on a forest plot presented by the sponsor , increased benefit in the Asian region and decreased benefit in the USA were apparent. The sample size for the Asian subgroup was small compared to other regions, and the variability in the USA estimate was such that it was difficult to determine whether the true effect was likely to be different from that observed for the overall population. The decision was ultimately made to approve this drug for the USA.

Progress in precision medicine produces yet another interesting subgroup analysis problem, as increasingly specific drug targets translate to smaller and smaller subgroups of patients that can benefit from treatment. In LaVange (2019), the ivacaftor story was used to illustrate the problem. Ivacaftor received FDA approval in 2012 as the first genetic medicine for cystic fibrosis, but it targeted a small subset (4%) of the approximately 30,000 cystic fibrosis patients in the USA. The sponsor identified additional genetic mutations that might benefit from treatment, based on the mechanism of action of the drug, for subsequent clinical trials. A 2014 Advisory Committee was convened to discuss expansion of the indication to another mutation, and the FDA statistical reviewer raised the issue during that meeting of how to determine the set of patients a drug benefits once it has been shown to work in some (US Food and Drug Administration 2014b). The statistical reviewer pointed out that simple pre-specification of a primary analysis cannot control the different errors possible in this scenario, and alternative statistical approaches were needed. As smaller and smaller genetic subgroups are studied, the issue of error control is compounded with the issue of insufficient subgroup sample sizes to support inference. Even when a clinical trial of rare mutations in a rare disease shows overall benefit, sample sizes will usually be insufficient to make attribution of benefit to specific mutations possible. The most recent ivacaftor approval expanded the number of genetic mutations from 10 to 33 (US Food and Drug Administration 2017c), but approval was made under the accelerated approval pathway and based mainly on laboratory data. Draft guidance on rare subsets of diseases was issued to clarify the agency's expectations in this scenario (US Food and Drug Administration 2017d), and a companion publication provides additional details on the agency's thinking in developing the guidance (Schuck et al. 2018).

Subgroup analyses are frequently performed for both efficacy and safety endpoints. Subgroup analyses are beneficial because they can inform clinicians on the potential for differential treatment response within important demographic, genetic, disease, environmental, behavioral, or regional subgroups, which furthers our understanding of the benefit-risk of the drug or even a class of drugs. Subgroup analyses, however, have numerous statistical challenges; some of them have been mentioned already. The analysis and interpretation of subgroups should be approached cautiously to reduce the potential for over-interpretation and erroneous conclusions. One can find a detailed explanation of the issues, case studies, and recommendations in a tutorial on statistical considerations on subgroup analysis in confirmatory clinical trials published by Alosh et al. (2017) and a tutorial on data-driven subgroup identification and analysis in clinical trials by Lipkovich et al. (2017). Some additional information on exploratory subgroup analyses can be found in Chap. 6 of this book.

1.4.4 Multiregional Trials

Drug development has been globalized, and many multiregional clinical trials (MRCTs) have been conducted by pharmaceutical companies to expedite global clinical development and facilitate simultaneous registration in multiple regions around the world. MRCTs provide pharmaceutical sponsors with a larger and more diverse pool of patients and give an opportunity to local scientific and medical communities to use advanced technologies and try new medical treatments. Although MRCTs can provide many benefits, they also bring challenges. Differences among various geographic regions and countries may lead to difficulties with planning and execution of the study and later with interpreting the study results. The differences might include patient demographics and disease characteristics; local practices and standards of care; availability of a control arm medication or concomitant medications (e.g., drugs can be approved in certain countries but not in others, and medical practices may also differ); availability of therapeutic procedures, imaging modalities, and specialized laboratory tests; differences in clinical trial operations and costs among regions; regional targets or objectives of treatment with choice of efficacy variables; methods of assessment of safety; duration of the trial; and similarity of dose and dosing regimens. The ICH E5 guideline was adopted in 1998 with the purpose of facilitating the registration of medicinal products among different ICH regions by recommending a framework for evaluating the impact of ethnic factors upon the efficacy or safety of a product (ICH E5 1998). ICH E5 states that if the data developed in one region satisfy the requirements for evidence in a new region, but there is a concern about possible differences in ethnic factors, both intrinsic and extrinsic, between the two regions, then it might be possible to extrapolate the data to the new region with a single bridging study. The bridging study could be a pharmacodynamic study or a full clinical trial, possibly a dose-response study.

Defining the treatment effect in a multi-regional trial is discussed in the recently finalized ICH E17 guideline on Principles for Designing and Planning a Multi-

Regional Clinical Trial (ICH E17 2017). The guidance does not make explicit recommendations about statistical methods most suitable for an MRCT, but it provides general recommendations on subject selection, choice of endpoints, selection of doses, sample size planning, pooling strategies, examination of consistency across regions, subgroup analysis, and other aspects of MRCT planning and analysis. At the planning stage, regional variability should be carefully considered in determining the role MRCTs can play in a drug development program. MRCTs are typically designed to address treatment effects in the entire study population; they are usually not powered to assess the country- or region-specific treatment effects. The key consideration for sample size calculation is ensuring a sufficient number of patients to be able to evaluate the overall treatment effect under the assumption that the treatment effect applies to the entire target population, specifically to the population in regions included in the trial. The MRCT should be planned to also include an evaluation of the consistency of treatment effects among regions. When results appear inconsistent across regions, regulatory authorities may question the validity of the results in their countries. In this case a structured exploration of these differences should be planned. Additional references on this topic include Quan et al. (2010), Chen et al. (2010), Binkowitz and Ibia (2011), and Chen and Quan (2016).

1.4.5 Safety Evaluation

Safety evaluation is fundamental to medical product development. It takes a long time and a large amount of data to fully understand the safety profile of a medical product. Randomized clinical trials are the gold standard for evaluating the efficacy of new treatments. Clinical trials are sized and powered to identify differences among treatment groups for a small number of efficacy endpoints, usually for a primary endpoint or co-primary endpoints. At times, key secondary endpoints are taken into consideration when the trial sample size is calculated. The available sample size results in treatment comparisons for safety that is often underpowered.

In practice, there are numerous safety endpoints to consider in a trial and even more as a medical product proceeds through clinical development. Adverse events (AEs), death, laboratory values, vital signs, physical examinations, hospitalizations, and electrocardiograms (ECGs) are examples of safety parameters collected in a clinical trial. In addition, efficacy outcomes that fail to improve or worsen over time can contribute to the safety of the new treatment. Safety outcomes have important characteristics to consider including duration, severity, and investigator's assessment of causal relationship to drug, resulting in numerous sensitivity analyses. Not all safety endpoints and analyses can be pre-specified. Safety issues may occur spontaneously at any time during the trial and often occur between study visits. Clinical trials are often not big or long enough to capture all the risks. For indications requiring chronic treatment, such as diabetes, clinical trials may be of short duration even though real-world use may for many years, and a safety concern may only be evident with long-term exposure to a product. Often the inclusion/exclusion criteria fail to reflect the population that uses the product once approved or licensed. Many safety signals are not identified until after a product is on the market and a large number of patients with more varied conditions are exposed. Zink et al. (2018) discussed the limitations of evaluating safety solely using clinical trial data. Despite these challenges, it is essential to proactively plan for a comprehensive safety evaluation and signal detection at the start of any development program, considering the underlying challenges of the disease and the unique features of treatment and patient management.

The goal of a development program is to identify safety signals as early as possible, to prevent further safety issues where feasible, and to highlight areas requiring greater focus during post-approval safety monitoring if the new treatment has a benefit-risk profile allowing for the market authorization. Initial information on a medical product's toxicity is investigated in basic research, discovery, and nonclinical animal models. With data accumulating from different phases of clinical trials, the safety profile is gradually established. At the time of filing a product to a regulatory authority, safety data collected from clinical trials are analyzed and summarized to provide sufficient evidence for a benefit-risk assessment.

Given the volume and complexity of the data available for safety outcomes, efficient and informative reporting is crucial. Traditionally, safety analyses have been descriptive in nature; AEs are usually summarized by number and percent of patients with events coded by Preferred Term and grouped by System Organ Class in order of decreasing frequency of occurrence. Binary outcomes, such as whether a patient experienced a particular AE or not, are often reported using a risk difference, risk ratio, or odds ratio (Chuang-Stein et al. 2014; Zhou et al. 2015). Pros and cons for the various measures are discussed in Zhou et al. (2015). Given a large number of potential treatment group comparisons for adverse events, Crowe and co-authors suggested a three-tier approach for the analysis of adverse events (Crowe et al. 2009). The approach provides a reasonable balance between committing to type I error rate control without overly sacrificing the power to detect potential safety signals. In the analysis of AEs, type II errors are equally if not more important, because failing to flag a real drug-AE interaction is probably a higher public health risk than falsely identifying such an interaction. Another approach is based on the false discovery rate (FDR) method. It provides a good balance between type I error and power (Benjamini and Hochberg 1995; Benjamini and Yekutieli 2005). Bayesian methods such as hierarchical modeling can help correct for multiplicity arising in the analysis of safety data and capture the biological relationship among various AEs (Berry and Berry 2004; Berry et al. 2011). Given the amount of data and their complexity, visualization of safety is important. Visual tools play a significant role in understanding the data and in interpreting results from data analyses. Forest plots and dot plots are often used to visualize results from the analysis of AEs (Amit et al. 2018). A volcano plot can be used to effectively summarize the incidence of adverse events (Zink et al. 2013). A shift plot and a waterfall plot are used to show the change from baseline in laboratory parameters (Chuang-Stein et al. 2001; Ivanova et al. 2019). Additional references on graphical presentations of safety data include

Krause and O'Connell (2012), Duke et al. (2005), Matange (2016), and Zink et al. (2018).

There has been increased interest in the systematic monitoring of safety for a compound throughout the drug development life cycle. While some methods are available to monitor the safety of novel therapies, many challenges remain. For example, it is often challenging to assess the causality of AEs in relation to the investigational drug due to the severity of symptoms of the underlying disease, the toxicity from other concurrent therapies, and the frequent use of non-randomized study designs. Further, in randomized Phase II and Phase III studies, safety is considered to be one of the components of the benefit-risk trade-off, a complex and comprehensive process that often requires an independent group of experts such as a Data Monitoring Committee (DMC) to evaluate the well-being of patients in ongoing trials. *Data and safety monitoring* in clinical trials is defined as a planned, ongoing process of reviewing the data collected in a clinical trial with the primary purpose of protecting the safety of trial participants, the credibility of the trial, and the validity of trial results (Ellenberg et al. 2002). In the FDA guidance on Establishment and Operation of Clinical Trial Data Monitoring Committees, a *DMC* is defined as a group of individuals with pertinent expertise that reviews regularly accumulating data from one or more ongoing clinical trials (US Food and Drug Administration 2006). An independent DMC is usually responsible for the data and safety monitoring of randomized Phase II and Phase III studies. Though it is possible to have an independent DMC for Phase I trials, it is not a common practice. In the FDA draft guidance on Safety Assessment for IND Safety Reporting, the FDA recommends that sponsors consider the use of a *Safety Assessment Committee* (SAC) (US Food and Drug Administration 2015b). The SAC would oversee the evolving safety profile of the investigational drug by evaluating the cumulative serious adverse events from all of the trials in the development program, as well as other available important safety information. The SAC is distinct from a DMC, in that a DMC is typically responsible for a single study, while an SAC oversees safety for an entire development program. If both are used, then consideration is required to ensure their respective roles and responsibilities are clearly defined.

The European Medicines Agency and the US FDA allow sponsors to file for accelerated and conditional approvals of severe conditions (US Food and Drug Administration 2014a; EMA 2016). There are some concerns that accelerated development might result in a simplified and shortened process of the development of a new drug. In this case, interim analyses pose an ethical dilemma of safeguarding the interests of patients enrolled in clinical trials, while simultaneously protecting society from premature claims of treatment benefit. Trials stopped early because of safety or futility tend to result in prompt discontinuation of useless or potentially harmful interventions. In contrast, trials stopped early for benefit may result in the fast approval and dissemination of promising new treatments. Given the severe and life-threatening nature of cancer and patients' expectations for promising treatments, quicker clinical drug development is required. This may, however, lead to a poorly defined benefit-risk profile of a new therapy. Of particular concern is the potential for early stopping of trials based on surrogate efficacy endpoints such as disease-free survival or time to recurrence, when delayed toxicity of the therapy might be observed with longer follow-up. Further, not observing a full benefit of a new treatment might result in rejection or just the partial reimbursement of the treatment by payers that could also lead to a new drug being not at all or hardly adopted by the medical community. Due to limitations of pre-marketing clinical trials and clinical development programs stopped early for success, ongoing safety monitoring and assessment are critical in post-marketing to fully establish the medical product's safety profile and understand the impact on patient populations. Discussions on sources of safety data outside of traditional randomized clinical trials and statistical strategies can be found in Izem et al. (2018) and Marchenko et al. (2018). Additional references on safety monitoring and analysis include books by Jiang and Xia (2014) and Gould (2015).

1.5   Concluding Remarks

Biostatistics is a highly developed information science, and it plays a significant role in every stage of drug development. Biostatisticians provide statistical expertise to cross-functional teams and ensure the use of appropriate and efficient statistical designs and analysis methods during development, submissions, and life cycle management of drugs. Making reasonable, accurate, and reliable inference from data in the presence of uncertainty is an important responsibilities of biostatisticians. This is an exciting time in both clinical and statistical research and development, with the promise of personalized medicine and the explosion of computer-intensive statistical tools in development. Many new advanced and efficient designs and analysis methods have become available and increased in use in pharmaceutical industry because of biostatisticians. Today the job of a biostatistician is exciting, challenging, and rewarding.

In this chapter, we briefly covered some basic biostatistical principles, some designs, and some selected analysis methods used in clinical trials. Where appropriate, references to available software procedures in R and SAS were provided. Additionally, we briefly highlighted some important considerations for clinical trials, such as defining appropriate estimands, handling outcomes with missing data, applying multiplicity adjustments, analyzing subgroups, planning multiregional clinical trials, and evaluating drug safety. There are many other topics not covered in this chapter, including the use of Bayesian statistical methods to design trials and analyze data. Bayesian methods in clinical trial design have become more popular in recent years, particularly for monitoring efficacy and toxicity simultaneously, and in data analysis due to their flexibility of use and the corresponding ease of interpretation of results. High-performance computers have facilitated widespread advances in the development of computational algorithms that have enhanced the use of Bayesian and hybrid designs in clinical trials, specifically in early phase trial development. We refer readers interested in Bayesian methods to Spiegelhalter et al. (2004), Berry et al. (2011), and Yuan et al. (2016).

References

Agresti A (2002). Categorical Data Analysis. Second Edition. Wiley Series in Probability and Statistics.

Alosh M, Bretz F, Huque M (2014). Advanced multiplicity adjustment methods in clinical trials. Statistics in Medicine 33(4).

Alosh M, Fritsch K, Huque M, Mahjoob K, Pennello G, Rothmann M, Russek-Cohen E, Smith F, Wilson S & Yue L (2015). Statistical considerations on subgroup analysis in clinical trials. Statistics in Biopharmaceutical Research 7: 286-303.

Alosh M, Huque MF, Bretz F, D'Agostino R (2017). Tutorial on statistical considerations on subgroup analysis in confirmatory clinical trials. Statistics in Medicine, 36 (8): 1334-1360.

Amit O, Heiberger RM, and Lane PW (2018). Graphical approaches to the analysis of safety data from clinical trials. Pharmaceutical Statistics 7: 20–35.

Armitage P, Berry G (1994). Statistical Methods in Medical Research, 3rd ed. Oxford: Blackwell.

Austin PC, Lee DS, Fine JP. (2016). Introduction to the Analysis of Survival Data in the Presence of Competing Risks. *Circulation*. 6133(6):601–609.

Baer L, Ivanova A (2013). When should the sequential parallel comparison design be used in clinical trials? Clinical Investigation 3:832–833.

Benjamini Y, Hochberg Y (1995). Controlling the false discovery rate: a practical and powerful approach to multiple testing. Journal of the Royal Statistical Society, 57: 289–300.

Benjamini Y, Yekutieli D (2005). False discovery rate-adjusted multiple confidence intervals for selected parameters. Journal of the American Statistical Association 100: 71-81.

Berry SM & Berry DA (2004). Accounting for multiplicities in assessing drug safety: A three-level hierarchical mixture model. Biometrics 60: 418-426.

Berry SM, Carlin BP, Lee JJ, and Muller P (2011). Bayesian Adaptive Methods for Clinical Trials. CRC Press, Taylor and Francis Group, Boca Raton, FL.

Binkowitz B, Ibia E (2011). Multiregional clinical trials: An introduction from an industry perspective. Ther Innov Regul Sci., 45:569–73.

Bretz F, Koenig F, Brannath W, Glimm E, Posch M (2009). Adaptive designs for confirmatory clinical trials. Statistics in Medicine, 28:1181-1217.

Bretz F, Horthorn T, and Westfall P (2011). Multiple Comparisons Using R. CRC Press, Taylor and Francis Group, Boca Raton, FL.

Carroll KJ, Fleming TJ (2013). Statistical Evaluation and Analysis of Regional Interactions: The PLATO Trial Case Study. Statistics in Biopharmaceutical Research, 5(2): 91-101.

Chen, J, Quan, H, Binkowitz, B (2010). Assessing consistent treatment effect in a multi-regional clinical trial: A systematic review. Pharm Stat., 9:242–253.

Chen J, Quan H (2016). Multiregional Clinical Trials for Simultaneous Global New Drug Development. Boca Raton, FL: Chapman and Hall/CRC.

Chow SC, Shao J, Wang H (2003). Sample Size Calculation in Clinical Research. Marcel Dekker, New York.

Chow SC and Chang M (2007). Adaptive Design Methods in Clinical Trials. Chapman & Hall/CRC.

Chow SC and Liu JP (2003). Design and Analysis of Clinical Trials, 2nd edition. John Wiley and Sons, New York.

Chuang-Stein C, Le V, & Chen W (2001). Recent advancements in the analysis and presentation of safety data. Drug Information Journal 35: 377-397.

Chuang-Stein C, Li Y, Kawai N, Komiyama O and Kuribayashi K (2014). Detecting safety signals in subgroups. In: Jiang Q & Xia HA, eds. Quantitative Evaluation of Safety in Drug Development: Design, Analysis and Reporting. Boca Raton, Florida: CRC Press.

Crowe BJ, Xia HA, Berlin JA, et al. (2009). Recommendations for safety planning, data collection, evaluation and reporting during drug, biologic and vaccine development: a report of the safety planning, evaluation, and reporting team. Clinical Trials 6: 430-440.

Cox DR (1970). Analysis of Binary Data, 1st ed. New York: Chapman and Hall/CRC Press.

Dmitrienko A, Tamhane AC, and Bretz F (2010). Multiple Testing Problems in Pharmaceutical Statistics. CRC Press, Taylor and Francis Group, Boca Raton, FL.

Dmitrienko A and D'Agostino R (2013). Traditional multiplicity adjustment methods in clinical trials. Statistics in Medicine 32(29).

Donner A (1984). Approaches to sample size estimation in the design of clinical trials—A review. Stat. Med. 3: 199–214.

Duke SP, Bancken F, Crowe B, Soukup M, Botsis T and Forshee R (2005). Seeing is believing: good graphic design principles for medical research. Statistics in Medicine 34: 3040-3059.

Ellenberg SS, Fleming TR & DeMets DL (2002). Data monitoring committees in clinical trials: a practical perspective. John Wiley & Sons.

EMA (2014). European Medicines Agency. Guideline on the investigation of subgroups in confirmatory clinical trials (Draft). Available at https://www.ema.europa.eu/en/documents/scientific-guideline/draft-guideline-investigation-subgroups-confirmatory-clinical-trials_en.pdf

EMA (2016). European Medicines Agency. Guideline on the scientific application and the practical arrangements necessary to implement Commission Regulation (EC) No 507/2006 on the conditional marketing authorisation for medicinal products for human use falling within the scope of Regulation (EC) No 726/2004. Available at https://www.ema.europa.eu/en/documents/scientific-guideline/guideline-scientific-application-practical-arrangements-necessary-implement-commission-regulation-ec/2006-conditional-marketing-authorisation-medicinal-products-human-use-falling_en.pdf

EMA (2017). European Medicines Agency. Guideline on multiplicity issues in clinical trials (Draft). Available at https://www.ema.europa.eu/en/documents/scientific-guideline/draft-guideline-multiplicity-issues-clinical-trials_en.pdf

Fedorov V, Leonov S. (2013). Optimal Design for Nonlinear Response Models: CRC Press.

Fitzmaurice GM, Laird NM, Rotnitzky AG (1993). Regression Models for Discrete Longitudinal Responses (with discussion). Statistical Science, 8: 248-309.

Fitzmaurice GM, Laird NM, Ware JH (2011). Applied Longitudinal Analysis, Second Edition. John Wiley and Sons, Inc.

Fitzmaurice G, Davidian M, Verbeke G and Molenberghs G (2009). Longitudinal Data Analysis. Boca Raton, FL: Chapman and Hall/CRC Press.

Friede T, Parsons N, Stallard N. (2012). A conditional error function approach for subgroup selection in adaptive clinical trials. Statistics in Medicine, 31(30):4309-20.

Friedman LM, Furberg CD, DeMets DL, Reboussin DM, Granger CB (2015). Fundamentals of Clinical Trials. 5th Edition. Springer, New York.

De Glas, NA, Kiderlen M, Vandenbroucke JP, de Craen AJM, Portielje JEA, van de Velde CJH, Liefers GJ, Bastiaannet E, Le Cessie S (2016). Performing Survival Analyses in the Presence of Competing Risks: A Clinical Example in Older Breast Cancer Patients. Journal of National Cancer Institue, May; 108(5): 10.

Gould AL, ed. (2015). "Statistical Methods for Evaluating Safety in Medical Product Development." Chichester, United Kingdom: John Wiley & Sons Ltd.

Hall DB (2001). Zero-Inflated Poisson and Binomial Regression with Random Effects: A Case Study. Biometrics, 56(4):1030-1039.

He W, Pinheiro J, Kuznetsova O (2014). Practical Considerations for Adaptive Trial Design and Implementation. Springer, New York.

Hilbe JM (2007). Negative Binomial Regression. Cambridge, UK: Cambridge University Press.

Hochberg Y, Tamhane AC (1987). Multiple Comparison Procedures. Wiley, New York.

Hsu JC (1996). Multiple Comparisons, Theory and Methods. Chapman & Hall/CRC

Hu F, Rosenberger WF (2006). The Theory of Response-Adaptive Randomization in Clinical Trials. Wiley Series in Probability and Statistics.

Huang X, Tamura RN (2010). Comparison of test statistics for the sequential parallel design. Statistics in Biopharmaceutical Research 2:42–50.

Huber PJ (1964). Robust Estimation of a Local Parameter. Annals of Mathematical Statistics, 35: 73-101.

Huber PJ (1967). The Behavior of Maximum Likelihood Estimates Under Nonstandard Conditions. Proceedings of 5th Berkeley Symposium, 1: 221-233.

Hughes S (2014). The prevention of missing data. In: O'Kelly M. and Ratitch B., eds. "Clinical Trials with Missing Data, A Guide for Practitioners". Wiley, Statistics in Practice. John Wiley & Sons, Ltd, United Kingdom.

ICH E5 (1998). International Council for Harmonisation of Technical Requirements for Pharmaceuticals for Human Use. E5(R1) Guideline: Ethnic Factors in the Acceptability of foreign Clinical Data. Available at https://www.ich.org/fileadmin/Public_Web_Site/ICH_Products/Guidelines/Efficacy/E5_R1/Step4/E5_R1__Guideline.pdf

ICH E8 (1997). International Council for Harmonisation of Technical Requirements for Pharmaceuticals for Human Use. E8 Guideline: General Considerations for Clinical Trials. Available at https://www.ich.org/fileadmin/Public_Web_Site/ICH_Products/Guidelines/Efficacy/E8/Step4/E8_Guideline.pdf

ICH E9 (1998). International Council for Harmonisation of Technical Requirements for Pharmaceuticals for Human Use. E9 Guideline: Statistical Principles in Clinical Trials. Available at https://www.ich.org/fileadmin/Public_Web_Site/ICH_Products/Guidelines/Efficacy/E9/Step4/E9_Guideline.pdf

ICH E9 R1 (2017). International Council for Harmonisation of Technical Requirements for Pharmaceuticals for Human Use. E9(R1) Draft Guideline: Estimands and Sensitivity Analysis in Clinical Trials. Available at https://www.ich.org/fileadmin/Public_Web_Site/ICH_Products/Guidelines/Efficacy/E9/E9-R1EWG_Step2_Guideline_2017_0616.pdf.

ICH E10 (2001). International Council for Harmonisation of Technical Requirements for Pharmaceuticals for Human Use. E10 Guideline: Choice of Control Group and Related Issues in Clinical Trials. Available at https://www.ich.org/fileadmin/Public_Web_Site/ICH_Products/Guidelines/Efficacy/E10/Step4/E10_Guideline.pdf

ICH E17 (2017). International Council for Harmonisation of Technical Requirements for Pharmaceuticals for Human Use. E17 Guideline: General Principles for Planning and Design of Multi-Regional Clinical Trials. Available at https://www.ich.org/fileadmin/Public_Web_Site/ICH_Products/Guidelines/Efficacy/E17/E17EWG_Step4_2017_1116.pdf

Ivanova A, Qaqish BF, Schoenfeld D (2011). Optimality, sample size and power calculations for the sequential parallel comparison design. Statistics in Medicine, 30: 2793–2803.

Ivanova A, Tamura RN (2015). A two-way enriched clinical trial design: Combining advantages of placebo lead-in and randomized withdrawal. Statistical Methods in Medical Research, 24: 871–890.

Ivanova A, Marchenko O, Jiang Q & Zink RC. (2019). Safety Monitoring and Analysis in Oncology Trials. In: Roychoudhury S & Lahiri S, eds. "Statistical Challenges in Oncology Clinical Development". Boca Raton, Florida: CRC Press.

Izem R, Sanchez-Kam M, Ma H, Zink RC, and Zhao Y (2018). Sources of safety data and statistical strategies for design and analysis: Postmarket Surveillance. Therapeutic Innovation & Regulatory Science52 (2): 159-169.

Jenkins M, Stone A, Jennison C (2011). An adaptive seamless phase II/III design for oncology trials with subpopulation selection using correlated survival endpoints. Pharmaceutical Statistics 10: 347–356.

Jennison C, Turnbull BW (2000). Group Sequential Methods with Applications to Clinical Trials. Boca Raton, Florida: CRC Press.

Jiang Q, Xia HA, eds. (2014). Quantitative Evaluation of Safety in Drug Development: Design, Analysis and Reporting. Boca Raton, Florida: CRC Press.

Kauermann G and Carroll RJ (2001). The Sandwich Variance Estimator: Efficiency Properties and Coverage Probability of Confidence Intervals. Journal of the American Statistical Association, 96: 1387-1396.

Kleinbaum DG and Klein M (2012a). Survival Analysis: a Self-learning Text, 3rd Edition, New York, NY: Springer, New York.

Kleinbaum DG and Klein M. (2012b). Recurrent Event Survival Analysis. In: Survival Analysis. Statistics for Biology and Health. Springer, New York, NY

Krause A, O'Connell M (2012). A Picture Is Worth a Thousand Tables: Graphics in Life Sciences. New York, NY: Springer.

Lachin JM (1981). Introduction to sample size determination and power analysis for clinical trials. Control Clin. Trials, 2: 93–113.

Lachin JM (1988). Statistical Properties of Randomization in Clinical Trials. *Control Clin Trials*, 9: 289-311.

Lai TL, Robbins H (1978). Adaptive design in regression and control. Proceedings of the National Academy of Sciences of the United States of America, 75: 586–587.

Lambert D (1992). Zero-Inflated Poisson Regression, with an Application to Defects in Manufacturing. Technometrics. 34 (1): 1–14.

Lan KG, DeMets DL (1983). Discrete Sequential Boundaries for Clinical Trials, *Biometrika*, 70 (3):659–663.

LaVange LM (2013). The Role of Statistics in Regulatory Decision Making. Therapeutic Innovation & Regulatory Science, 48: 12–19.

LaVange LM, Permutt T (2016). A Regulatory Perspective on Missing Data in the Aftermath of the NRC Report. Statistics in Medicine, 35(17), 2853-64.

LaVange LM (2019). Statistics at FDA: Reflections on the Past Six Years, Statistics in Biopharmaceutical Research, 11:1, 1-12.

Li Z, Durham SD, Flournoy N (1995). An adaptive design for maximization of a contingent binary response: Adaptive Designs, Flournoy N, Rosenberger WF (eds.). Institute of Mathematical Statistics, pp.179–196.

Liang KY and Zeger SL (1986). Longitudinal Data Analysis Using Generalized Linear Models, Biometrica, 73: 13-22.

Liang KY and Zeger SL (1995). Inference based on estimating functions in the presence of nuisance parameters. Statistical Science, 10(2):196–199.

Lipkovich I, Dmitrienko A, Denne J & Enas G (2011). Subgroup identification based on differential effect search—A recursive partitioning method for establishing response to treatment in patient subpopulations. Statistics in Medicine 30: 2601–2621.

Lipkovich I, Dmitrienko A, D'Agostino BR (2017). Tutorial in Biostatistics: Data-driven subgroup identification and analysis in clinical trials. Statistics in Medicine, 36:136-196.

Little R and Rubin D (2002). Statistical Analysis with Missing Data. 2nd Edition. John Wiley & Sons, Inc., Hoboken, New Jersey.

Machin D, Campbell MJ, Tan SB, Tan SH (2008). Sample Size Tables for Clinical Studies, 3rd edition. Wiley-Blackwell.

Mallinckrodt C, Lipkovich I (2017). Analyzing Longitudinal Clinical Trial Data, A Practical Guide. CRC Press, Taylor and Francis Group, Boca Raton, FL.

Marchenko O, Jiang Q, Chakravarty A, Ke C, Ma H, Maca J, Russek-Cohen E, Sanchez-Kam M, Zink R, Chuang-Stein C (2015) Evaluation and Review of Strategies to Assess Cardiovascular Risk in Clinical Trials in Patients with Type 2 Diabetes Mellitus. *Statistics in Biopharmaceutical Research,* 7 (4): 253-266

Marchenko O, Jiang Q, Ke C, Ma H, Maca J, Levenson M, Liu L, Mehta C, Park S, Russek-Cohen E, Sanchez-Kam M, Zink R, Chuang-Stein C (2017). Statistical Considerations for Cardiovascular Outcome Trials in Patients with Type 2 Diabetes Mellitus. Statistics in Biopharmaceutical Research, 9, 4: 347-360.

Marchenko O, Russek-Cohen E, Levenson M, Zink RC, Krukas M & Jiang Q (2018). Sources of safety data and statistical strategies for design and analysis: Real World Insights. Therapeutic Innovation and Regulatory Science, 52 (2): 170-186.

Matange S (2016). Clinical Graphs Using SAS. Cary, North Carolina: SAS Institute Inc.

McGlothlin AE, Lewis RJ (2014). Minimal clinically important difference: defining what really matters to patients. JAMA, 312(13):1342-3.

O'Kelly M, Ratitch B (2014). Clinical Trials with Missing Data, A Guide for Practitioners. Wiley, Statistics in Practice. John Wiley & Sons, Ltd, United Kingdom.

O'Quigley J., Pepe, M., Fisher, L. (1990). Continual reassessment method: a practical design for phase I clinical trials in cancer. Biometrics, 46 (1): 33-48.

Panel on Handling Missing Data in Clinical Trials, National Research Council (2010). The Prevention and Treatment of Missing Data in Clinical Trials, National Academies Press.

Permutt, T., LaVange, L.M., Wilson, S., Lin, D.T.Y., Sridhara, R., Chakravarty, A. (2016a) "A Taxonomy of Estimands for Regulatory Clinical Trials with Discontinuations, Statistics in Medicine, 35(17), 2865-75.

Permutt, T., LaVange, L.M., Hung, H.M.J., Wilson, S., Lin, D.T.Y., Sridhara, R., Chakravarty, A. (2016b). "Sensitivity Analysis for Missing Data in Regulatory Submissions," Statistics in Medicine, 35(17), 2876-79.

Permutt, T. and Li, F. (2016) "Trimmed Means for Symptom Trials with Drop-Outs," Pharmaceutical Statistics, 16(1), 20–28.

Pierce DA and Peters D (1992). Practical use of higher order asymptotics for multiparameter exponential families. Journal of the Royal Statistical Society. Series B (Methodological), 54 (3):701-737.

Piantadosi S. (2017). Clinical Trials. A Methodologic Perspective. Third Edition. Wiley Series in Probability and Statistics.

Proschan MA, Lan KKG & Wittes JT (2006). Statistical Monitoring of Clinical Trials. New York, New York: Springer.

Quan, H, Li, M, Chen, J (2010). Assessment of consistency of treatment effects in multiregional clinical trials. Drug Inf J., 44:617–632.

Rao, C R (1973) Linear Statistical Inference and its Applications: 2nd Edition. New York: Wiley.

Rosenberger, W.F., Lachin, J.M. (2002). Randomization in Clinical Trials, Theory and Practice. John Wiley & Sons, Ltd.

Rutherford A (2011). ANOVA and ANCOVA: A GLM Approach, 2nd Edition. John Wiley & Sons, Inc., Hoboken, New Jersey.

Schuck RN, Woodcock J, Zineh I, Stein P, Jarow J, Temple R, Permutt T, LaVange L, Beaver JA, Charlab R, Blumenthal GM, Dorff SE, Leptak C, Lemery S, Rogers H, Chowdhury B, Litwack D, Pacanowski M. (2018). Considerations for developing targeted therapies in low-frequency molecular subsets of a disease. Clinical Pharmacology and Therapeutics, DOI: https://doi.org/10.1002/cpt.1041.

Snedecor GW and Cochran WG (1980). Statistical Methods. Seventh Edition. The Iowa State University Press.

Spiegelhalter DJ, Abrams KR, and Myles JP (2004). Bayesian Approaches to Clinical Trials and Health-Care Evaluation. Wiley, Statistics in Practice. John Wiley & Sons, Ltd, United Kingdom.

Stallard N. (2010). A confirmatory seamless phase II/III clinical trial design incorporating short-term endpoint information. Statistics in Medicine. 29:959–971.

Sweeney, Haslett, and Parnell (2018). A General Framework for Modeling Zero Inflation. Preprint.

Tamhane A and Gou J (2017). Hochberg Procedure under Negative Dependence. Statistica Sinica 28(1).

Thall, P.F., Cook, J.D. (2004). "Dose-finding based on efficacy-toxicity trade-offs", Biometrics, 60: 684-693.

US Food and Drug Administration (2006). Guidance for Clinical Trial Sponsors. Establishment and Operation of Clinical Trial Data Monitoring Committees. Available at https://www.fda.gov/media/75398/download

US Food and Drug Administration (2011). Brilinta (Ticagrelor) Tablets for Oral Use Label. Available at https://www.accessdata.fda.gov/drugsatfda_docs/label/2015/022433s017lbl.pdf. Revised Sep., 2015.

US Food and Drug Administration (2014a). Guidance for Industry. Expedited Programs for Serious Conditions – Drugs and Biologics. Available at https://www.fda.gov/files/drugs/published/Expedited-Programs-for-Serious-Conditions-Drugs-and-Biologics.pdf

US Food and Drug Administration (2014b). Pulmonary-Allergy Advisory Committee Meeting Materials. Available at http://www.fda.gov/AdvisoryCommittees/CommitteesMeetingMaterials/Drugs/Pulmonary-AllergyDrugsAdvisoryCommittee/ucm420669.htm

US Food and Drug Administration (2015a). Briefing Information for the May 12, 2015Meeting of the Pulmonary-Allergy Drugs Advisory Committee. Available at https://wayback.archive-it.org/7993/20170404155605/https://www.fda.gov/AdvisoryCommittees/CommitteesMeetingMaterials/Drugs/Pulmonary-AllergyDrugsAdvisoryCommittee/ucm446192.htm.

US Food and Drug Administration (2015b). Guidance for industry: safety Assessment for IND safety reporting (draft). Available at https://www.fda.gov/downloads/drugs/guidances/ucm477584.pdf.

US Food and Drug Administration (2017a). Briefing Information for the June 20, 2017 Meeting of the Endocrine-Metabolic Drugs Advisory Committee. Available at https://www.fda.gov/AdvisoryCommittees/CommitteesMeetingMaterials/Drugs/EndocrinologicandMetabolicDrugsAdvisoryCommittee/ucm563333.htm

US Food and Drug Administration (2017b). Guidance for Industry on Multiple Endpoints. Available at https://www.fda.gov/downloads/drugs/guidancecomplianceregulatoryinformation/guidances/ucm536750.pdf

US Food and Drug Administration (2017c). FDA Expands Approved Use of Kalydeco to treat Additional Mutations of Cystic Fibrosis. Press Release, available at https://www.fda.gov/NewsEvents/Newsroom/PressAnnouncements/ucm559212.htm

US Food and Drug Administration (2017d). Guidance for Industry Developing Targeted Therapies for Low-Frequency Molecular Subsets of a Disease. Available at https://www.fda.gov/ucm/groups/fdagov-public/@fdagov-drugsgen/documents/document/ucm588884.pdf

US Food and Drug Administration (2019a). Guidance for Industry. Enrichment Strategies for Clinical Trials to Support Determination of Effectiveness of Human Drugs and Biological Products. Available at https://www.fda.gov/media/121320/download

US Food and Drug Administration (2019b). Guidance for Industry on Adaptive Designs for Clinical Trials of Drugs and Biologics. Available at https://www.fda.gov/media/78495/download

Wainwright, C.E., Elborn, J.S., Ramsey, B.W., Marigowda, G., Huang, X., Cipolli, M., Colombo, C., Davies, JC, De Boeck K, Flume PA, Konstan MW, McColley SA, McCoy K, McKone EF, Munck A, Ratjen F, Rowe S.M., Waltz, D., and Boyle, M.P. (2015). "Lumacaftor-Ivacaftor in Patients with Cystic Fibrosis Homozygous for Phe508del CFTR," New England Journal of Medicine, 373, 220-231.

Wald A (1943). Tests of statistical hypothesis concerning several parameters when the number of observations is large. Transaction of the American Mathematical Society, 54(3): 426–482.

Wassmer, G and Brannath, W (2016). *Group Sequential and Confirmatory Adaptive Designs in Clinical Trials*. Springer series in pharmaceutical statistics, New York: Springer.

Willks, S S (1938). The Large-Sample Distribution of the Likelihood Ratio for Testing Composite Hypotheses. The Annals of Mathematical Statistics, 9, 1, 60-62.

Wellentin, L., Becker, R. C., Budaj, A., Cannon, C. P., Emanuelsson, H., Held, C., Horrow, J., Husted, S., James, S., Katus, H., Mahaffey, K. W., Sirica, B. M., for the PLATO Investigators (2009), "Ticagrelor versus Clopidogrel in Patients with Acute Coronary Syndromes," New England Journal of Medicine, 361, 1045-1057.

Woodcock, J. & LaVange, L. M. (2017) "Master Protocols to Study Multiple Therapies, Multiple Diseases, or Both," New England Journal of Medicine, 377,62-70. https://doi.org/10.1056/NEJMra1510062.

Yang S, Puggioni G, Harlow L, Redding C (2016). A Comparison of Different Methods of Zero-Inflated Data Analysis and an Application in Health Surveys. Journal of Modern Applied Statistical Methods, 16 (1), Article 29.

Yuan Y, Nguyen HQ, and Thall PF (2016). Bayesian Designs for Phase I-II Clinical Trials. CRC Press, Taylor and Francis Group, Boca Raton, FL.

Zink RC, Wolfinger RD and Mann G (2013). Summarizing the incidence of adverse events using volcano plots and time windows. Clinical Trials 10: 398-406.

Zhou Y, Ke Chunlei, Jiang Q, Shahin S & Snapinn S (2015). Choosing appropriate metrics to evaluate adverse events in safety evaluation. Therapeutic Innovation and Regulatory Science 49: 398-404.

Zink RC, Marchenko O, Sanchez-Kam M, Izem R, Ma H & Jiang Q (2018). Sources of safety data and statistical strategies for design and analysis: Clinical Trials. Therapeutic Innovation & Regulatory Science, 52 (2): 141-158.

Chapter 2
Pharmacometrics: A Quantitative Decision-Making Tool in Drug Development

Yan Xu and Holly Kimko

2.1 Background

2.1.1 What Is Pharmacometrics

Pharmacometrics is a bridging science that applies quantitative models representing physiology, pharmacology, and disease to describe and quantify interactions between drugs and patients (and pathogens) (Ette and Williams 2007). This involves the modeling of pharmacokinetics (PK) and pharmacodynamics (PD) with a focus on population and variability in order to characterize, explain, and predict PK and PD behaviors of therapeutic drugs. Variability may be predictable (e.g., due to differences in body weight) or apparently unpredictable (reflection of a knowledge gap).

2.1.2 Evolution of Pharmacometrics

To better understand the role of pharmacometrics in drug development, the major milestones in the growth of pharmacometrics are presented in Fig. 2.1, which reflects its evolution in utility. The journey of pharmacometrics started in the 1920s. The use of a one-compartment model to describe pharmacokinetics was introduced as early as 1924 (Widmark and Tandberg 1924); the use of a multi-compartment model

Y. Xu (✉)
Janssen Research and Development LLC., Spring House, PA, USA
e-mail: yxu115@its.jnj.com

H. Kimko
Janssen Research and Development LLC., Spring House, PA, USA
Present Address: AstraZeneca, Gaithersburg, MA, USA

© Springer Nature Switzerland AG 2020
O. V. Marchenko, N. V. Katenka (eds.), *Quantitative Methods in Pharmaceutical Research and Development*, https://doi.org/10.1007/978-3-030-48555-9_2

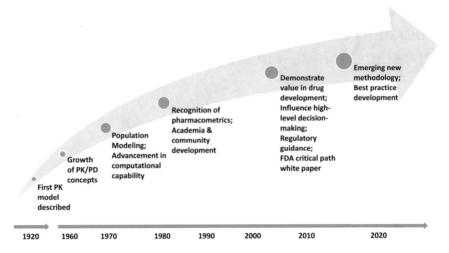

Fig. 2.1 Evolution of pharmacometrics (Modified from Gobburu 2013). *PK* Pharmacokinetics, *PK/PD* pharmacokinetics/pharmacodynamics

incorporating biological and physiological components for the simulation of PK data was introduced by Teorell in 1937. The latter is regarded as the first *physiologically based PK model* (PBPK).

The great growth of PK and PD, two core concepts of pharmacometrics, happened during the 1960s and 1970s (Forschungsinstitut et al. 1962; Levy 1966). For PK, the first symposium with the term *pharmacokinetics* (entitled as "*Pharmakokinetik und Arzneimitteldosierung* (Pharmacokinetics and Drug Dosage)") was held in Borstel, Germany, in 1962 (Forschungsinstitut et al. 1962), and *clinical pharmacokinetics* began to be recognized in the mid-1970s (Gibaldi and Levy 1976; Wagner 1981). For PD, the concept of *biophase compartment* was first introduced by Segre in 1968, which was reintroduced to drug development as *hypothetical effect compartment modeling* by Sheiner et al. in 1979. In 1964, Ariens provided the earliest description of drugs acting through *indirect mechanism*, and a model describing this was provided by Nagashima et al. (1969) 5 years later. Further systematic development and applications of the models for characterizing indirect pharmacodynamic responses came from Jusko's group later (Dayneka et al. 1993; Jusko and Ko 1994; Sharma and Jusko 1998).

An important focus in drug therapy is to understand the variability of a response among individuals in a population, which may be caused by both PK and PD. To address this, a *population modeling* approach was introduced by Sheiner et al. in 1972 (Sheiner et al. 1972). They proposed the use of *non-linear mixed effects* (NLME) regression models to analyze patient data pooled over all sampled individuals, allowing for the quantification of between-subject and within-subject variability. This analytical approach led to the development of a computer program, *NONMEM*. NONMEM was first released by Beal and Sheiner in 1980 (for the

IBM mainframe) and became exportable for all computers in 1984 (NONMEM 77). Since then, there has been a great deal of work in population PK/PD modeling using the NLME approach, both in method and in application.

In the early 1980s, the term *pharmacometrics* first appeared in the *Journal of Pharmacokinetics and Biopharmaceutics* (Rowland and Benet 1982). Pharmacometrics was then recognized as a unique branch of quantitative science; distinct sections for pharmacometrics were created in peer-reviewed journals, and advanced PK/PD modeling trainings were offered in academia. A few professional conference series have been established in the field of pharmacometrics, such as the Population Approach Group Europe Meeting (*PAGE*; since 1997), American Conference of Pharmacometrics (*ACoP*; since 2008), World Conference of Pharmacometrics (*WCoP*; since 2012), and so forth.

The importance of pharmacometrics in drug development has been increasingly recognized since the conference "The Integration of Pharmacokinetic, Pharmacodynamic, and Toxicokinetic Principles in Rational Drug Development" held in 1991 (Peck et al. 1992). As such, pharmaceutical companies and regulatory agencies began to pay attention to such integration-based modeling approaches in regulatory submissions for drug approvals. From the late 1990s to early 2000s, several excellent review papers from pharmaceutical companies highlighted the value of pharmacometrics in enabling scientific and strategic decision-making in drug development (Reigner et al. 1997; Olson et al. 2000; Chien et al. 2005). Model-based findings were recognized to be able to influence high-level decisions such as trial design, drug approval, and drug labeling. Such concepts were also well accepted by academia and regulatory agencies. For example, in a white paper published in 2004, the US Food and Drug Administration (FDA) underscored the importance of a *model-based drug development*, where pharmacometrics is believed to play a critical role (FDA 2004). Indeed, there has been a huge increase in the application of pharmacometrics in drug development over the last two decades. A survey from 2000 to 2008 shows that the drug approval and labeling decisions of more than 60% of the submissions for new drug applications (NDA) to US FDA were influenced by pharmacometric analysis (Lee et al. 2011). Systematic compilation of pharmacometrics has also been made in a few books (Kimko and Duffull 2003; Ette and Williams 2007; Kimko and Peck 2010; Bonate 2011).

Pharmacometrics is an evolving science with continuous advancement in novel modeling approaches and applications. Recently, physiologically based PK (and PK/PD) modeling has gained much widespread applications (Jones and Rowland-Yeo 2013), predominantly driven by major technological advances and increasing confidence in this approach. *Quantitative systems pharmacology* (QSP) is another fast-growing area (Sorger et al. 2011; Mager and Kimko 2016). It allows for predictions of the efficacy and safety of drugs based on known or possible mechanisms of action in pharmacology, pathology, or physiology. In addition, *model-based meta-analysis* (MBMA) (Mandema et al. 2011) has been advocated to leverage existing *big data* in making rational comparative risk/benefit assessment.

With the increasing application and acceptance of pharmacometrics in drug development, several regulatory guidelines and documents concerning *industry best practices* have been issued. This started in the late 1990s (FDA 1999; Holford et al. 1999) and continues thereafter (FDA 2003; EMA 2008, 2016) with the most recent position paper published in March 2016 (EFPIA MID3 Workgroup 2016).

2.1.3   Role of Pharmacometrics in Drug Development

In the past two decades, pharmacometrics—PK/PD modeling and simulation (M&S)—has developed into one of the most essential tools for the integration and interpretation of large and diverse pools of preclinical and clinical data, translating them into informative knowledge. It is beneficial not only for industry professionals in informing internal decision-making at critical drug development stages (e.g., first-in-human, proof-of-concept, pivotal trial, etc.) but also for regulatory authorities in compiling and analyzing data for approval and labeling.

There is no doubt pharmacometrics is playing an increasingly important role in improving R&D investment by facilitating applications of the *learn-and-confirm* paradigm proposed by Sheiner (1997). As a molecule moves through the drug development process, rational models are developed and refined using accumulated data and knowledge available at each stage to predict what is likely to happen in the next stage, thereby guiding research investment. Of note the impact of pharmacometrics on decision-making and risk management is dependent on the availability and quality of data accessible at a certain stage of drug development. Framing the right questions and capturing the key assumptions are critical components of the learn-and-confirm paradigm and are essential for the delivery of high-value pharmacometric results. This is particularly important at the early stage of drug development when data are limited.

This chapter aims to provide an overview on pharmacometrics with a focus on *drug model* (i.e., PK and PK/PD models). *Disease progression model* (i.e., quantification of the relevant biological [physiological] system in the absence of drug) and *trial model* (e.g., characteristics of enrolled study subjects, dropout and/or compliance) will not be discussed in detail; the reader can refer to the excellent review by Gobburu and Lesko (2009) and references therein for more information.

In the following sections, commonly employed PK and PK/PD analytical approaches will be introduced, followed by the software used for analyses, analysis work flow, and major model components with a focus on the population modeling. Four case studies will be illustrated to highlight the broader applications of pharmacometrics in drug development, from the translational stage to the early and late stage in clinical development.

2.2 Pharmacometric Analysis Approaches

2.2.1 PK Models

PK, in popular terms, is often described as *what the body does to the drug*. PK models characterize how a drug passes through the body by using concentrations in various areas of the body as a function of time. In order to build mathematical models to describe how the concentration changes with time, the body is conveniently divided into parts, called *compartments*, and in each compartment, the drug is assumed to behave in the same manner. Thus, each compartment is homogeneous and is described with a single representative concentration at any point in time, i.e., *well-stirred model* (Pang and Rowland 1977). Each compartment can be a real physiological space in the body. For example, the compartment where the concentration is usually measured is the bloodstream, which is called *central compartment*. However, compartments are typically abstract concepts that do not necessarily represent particular regions of the body. Additionally, a certain PK compartment might represent different tissue types depending on the characteristics of a given molecule. For example, lipophilic compounds are more likely to distribute into adipose tissue, while hydrophilic compounds are more likely to stay in the bloodstream. Therefore, *peripheral compartment* (into which the compounds may distribute) may represent different tissues for these two types of compounds.

Compartments have proven to be fundamental building blocks of PK models (and PK/PD models) with the difference between models being defined by the number of compartments and the way the compartments are connected. The drug amount in a compartment can be described with parameters of rate constant parameters that are estimated preferentially as ratios of clearance (CL) and volume (V) in data fitting. The parameterization using CL and V has the advantage of interpreting an estimated parameter with physiological meaning, and it is used throughout this chapter unless otherwise indicated. Figure 2.2 presents exemplary compartment PK systems and their associated, typical concentration-time curves.

The one-compartment system is the most basic PK model, which only includes a central compartment and an absorption compartment that are necessary for oral administration. This model is appropriate if the drug is distributed to accessible areas of the body instantly as in the case of direct intravenous bolus injection or infusion into the bloodstream (Fig. 2.2a), whereas extravascular administration requires an absorption compartment in addition to the central compartment (Fig. 2.2b).

Mathematically, for a drug administered as a bolus dose, the rate of drug elimination that governs the drug concentration in the one compartment model can be written as

$$dA2/dt = -CL/V2 \cdot A2, \tag{2.1}$$

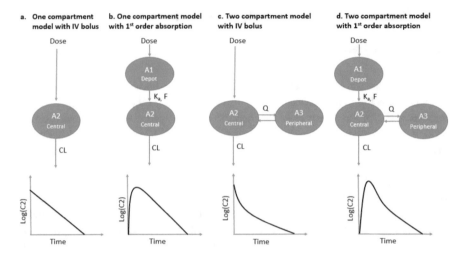

Fig. 2.2 Compartment pharmacokinetic model examples. (**a**) One-compartment model with IV bolus. (**b**) One-compartment model with first-order absorption. (**c**) Two-compartment model with IV bolus. (**d**) Two-compartment model with first-order absorption. *A1* Amount of drug at the extravascular absorption site, *A2* amount of drug in central compartment, *A3* amount of drug in peripheral compartment, *C2* concentration of drug in central compartment, *CL* clearance from central compartment, *F* bioavailability, *IV* intravenous, K_a first-order absorption rate, *Q* inter-compartment clearance

$$C2 = A2/V2, \tag{2.2}$$

where A2 and C2 are the amount and concentration, respectively, of the drug in the central compartment, CL is the clearance, and V2 is the volume of distribution in the central compartment.

In the case of extravascular dosing, the rate of change in the absorption compartment can usually be described with first-order kinetics, resulting in the following differential equations:

$$dA1/dt = -ka \cdot A1, \tag{2.3}$$

$$dA2/dt = ka \cdot A1 \cdot F - CL/V2 \cdot A2, \tag{2.4}$$

where A1 is the amount of the drug in the absorption compartment, k_a is the first-order absorption rate constant, and F denotes the bioavailability that is the fraction of the dose reaching the central compartment. Definitions of A2, CL, and V2 are the same as described above. The drug concentration in the central compartment, C2, can be estimated using the same equation as described in Eq. 2.2.

For multi-compartment models, the system typically consists of (1) a central compartment, representing the bloodstream and the rapidly equilibrated organs; (2) one or more peripheral compartments, representing more slowly equilibrating tissues; and (3) in the case of extravascular administration, an absorption compartment. The processes can also be described mathematically using differential equations. For example, the system shown in Fig. 2.2c can be described as

$$dA2/dt = -\ CL/V2 \cdot A2 + Q/V3 \cdot A3, \tag{2.5}$$

$$dA3/dt =\ CL/V2 \cdot A2 - Q/V3 \cdot A3. \tag{2.6}$$

And the system shown in Fig. 2.2d can be described as

$$dA1/dt = -ka \cdot A1, \tag{2.7}$$

$$dA2/dt = ka \cdot A1 \cdot F - CL/V2 \cdot A2 + Q/V3 \cdot A3, \tag{2.8}$$

$$dA3/dt =\ CL/V2 \cdot A2 - Q/V3 \cdot A3, \tag{2.9}$$

where A2 and A3 represent the amounts in the central compartment and the peripheral compartment, respectively, Q is the inter-compartment clearance, and V3 is the volume of distribution in the peripheral compartment. Definitions of A1, k_a, and F are the same as described above. And the drug concentrations in central compartment (C2) and peripherical compartment (C3), respectively, can be described as

$$C2 = A2/V2, \tag{2.10}$$

$$C3 = A3/V3. \tag{2.11}$$

The following three aspects should be carefully evaluated during the development of a PK compartment model:

- *Number of compartments*: During the decision-making on the number of compartments, it should be noted that too few compartments would not fit the data well, whereas too many compartments may show trivial improvement in curve fitting with poor precision parameter estimates. Typically, a multi-compartment system looks like a piecewise linear function in a plot of the concentration on a logarithmic scale versus time (Fig. 2.2c, d), while a one-compartment shows one linearly decreasing line (Fig. 2.2a, b).
- *Absorption kinetics*: A first-order process is a valid starting assumption in most extravascular administration cases. However, zero-order process has also been used to describe the absorption profile (e.g., controlled release), and inclusion of a delayed absorption time and non-linearity in absorption kinetics is not uncommon. If supported by the observed data, more sophisticated model should be considered to better capture the absorption profile (e.g., parallel or sequential zero-order plus first-order absorption processes) (Zhou 2003).
- *Elimination kinetics*: Many drugs are eliminated following a first-order elimination process. However, it is not unusual that some drug elimination pathways may be saturated at a high dose, which may be revealed from data collected across a wide dose range. This non-linear elimination is often described by Michaelis-

a. One compartment model with IV bolus and linear elimination kinetics

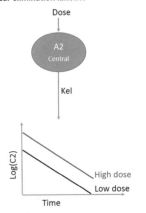

b. One compartment model with IV bolus and Michaelis–Menten type non-linear elimination kinetics

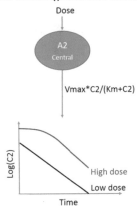

Fig. 2.3 Linear versus non-linear elimination kinetics. Elimination kinetic of drug from central compartment can be captured using a first-order elimination rate constant of K_{el} in the case of linear kinetic (Panel **a**) or a Michaelis-Menten kinetics type equation, $V_{max} \times C2/(K_m + C2)$, in the case of non-linear kinetics (Panel **b**). (**a**) One-compartment model with IV bolus and linear elimination kinetics. (**b**) One-compartment model with IV bolus and Michaelis-Menten-type non-linear elimination kinetics. *A2* Amount of drug in central compartment, *C2* concentration of drug in central compartment, K_m rate to achieve 50% maximum elimination rate, K_{el} linear elimination rate constant, *IV* intravenous, V_{max} maximum elimination rate

Menten kinetics type of equations as described in Fig. 2.3 (Gabrielsson and Weiner 2007). For the linear elimination kinetics, there is proportionality in the drug concentration kinetic following low-dose and high-dose administrations (black and red curves in Fig. 2.3a). In the case of the non-linear capacity-limited elimination kinetics, such proportionality disappears (Fig. 2.3b).

2.2.2 PK/PD Models

Contrary to PK, PD is described as *what the drug does to the body*. PK/PD models aim at linking dose and PK information to certain measures of biomarkers or response endpoints. The wide variety of possible efficacy and safety outcomes of a clinical trial or a preclinical experiment makes it difficult to generalize all cases of PK/PD modeling approaches with a few models. This section will focus on the most commonly used PK/PD models for continuous response variables. For discrete response variables, models often use logistic equation to convert the response to a probability that changes with a PK exposure metric.

Table 2.1 Basic concentration-effect relationship models

Model	Description	Equations	Comments
Linear	Linear and direct proportionality between drug concentration and effect	$E = Slope \cdot C$	The simplest model Sometimes useful when the range of concentration is relatively narrow and the drug effect is well below E_{max}
Log-linear	Linear and direct proportionality between log-transformed drug concentration and effect	$E = Slope \cdot \log(C)$	Extension of linear model Typically applies for concentrations over a wide range Cannot represent the case where concentration is zero
E_{max}	Define drug concentration and effect relationship using potency (EC_{50}) and maximum response (E_{max})	$E = \frac{E_{max} \cdot C}{EC_{50} + C}$	Most commonly used concentration-effect model Derived from the receptor theory (binding of a single drug to a single receptor)
Sigmoidal E_{max}	An extension of the E_{max} model, where the parameter N (Hill's coefficient) controls the steepness of the curve	$E = \frac{E_{max} \cdot C^N}{EC_{50}{}^N + C^N}$	A more general form of the E_{max} model Derived from the receptor theory where there is allosteric inhibition or stimulation of binding The larger the value of N, the steeper the line around EC_{50} (middle part of the curve)

C Concentration, *E* effect, E_{max} maximum achievable effect, EC_{50} concentration at which E is 50% of E_{max}, *N* Hill's coefficient

2.2.2.1   Basic Concentration-Effect Relationships

The center of a PK/PD modeling exercise is to figure out the appropriate concentration-effect relationship. The model should describe the observed data well while reasonably reflect the mechanism of action to exert the pharmacological effect at a given concentration. Table 2.1 summarizes the four commonly employed concentration-effect models, including linear, log-linear, maximum effect (E_{max}), and sigmoidal E_{max} models (Gabrielsson and Weiner 2007). A comparison of these fundamental concentration-effect relationships is shown in Fig. 2.4. A concentration-effect model is chosen depending on the type of the pharmacological response, and the most physiologically relevant model should be used to characterize such a response, data permitting. It should be noted that "concentration" could be any metric describing drug exposure, such as area under the curve (AUC), peak concentration, trough concentration, etc. When the drug acts by the inhibition of an effect, E_{max} and the concentration at which E is 50% of E_{max} (EC_{50}) may be referred

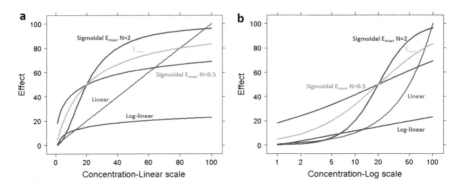

Fig. 2.4 Representative basic concentration-effect relationships. Panel (**a**), concentration in linear scale; Panel (**b**), concentration in log scale. Equations associated with the representative curves are as follows: (1) linear, $E = C \times 1$ [slope $= 1$]; (2) log-linear, $E = \log10(C) \times 5$ [slope $= 5$]; (3) simple E_{max}, $E = 100 \times C/(C + 20)$; (4) sigmoidal E_{max}, $N = 2$, $E = 100 \times C^2/(C^2 + 20^2)$; and (5) sigmoidal E_{max}, $N = 0.5$, $E = 100 \times C^{0.5}/(C^{0.5} + 20^{0.5})$ [$E_{max} = 100$ and $EC_{50} = 20$ for scenarios 3–5]. E Effect, C concentration, N Hill's coefficient

to as I_{max} and IC_{50}, where the effect ("E"—often by stimulation of a mechanism) terminology is transposed to inhibitory ("I"—the inhibition of a mechanism). The discussion below is applicable to both stimulatory and inhibitory cases.

The concentration-effect models shown in Table 2.1 and Fig. 2.4 assume the drug effect is zero when the drug concentration is zero. However, a more common scenario is that the effect has a baseline (e.g., pre-dose endogenous biomarker value). In this case, the observed effect during drug treatment would be a combination of drug effect (E_{drug}) and the baseline (E_{base}). To mathematically describe this, two relationships are commonly employed—additive or proportional:

$$E = E_{base} + E_{drug}, \tag{2.12}$$

$$E = E_{base} \cdot (1 + E_{drug}). \tag{2.13}$$

Both relationships should be considered during model building unless there is an established mechanistic understanding or certain prior information is known. The additive relationship (Eq. 2.12) yields the same magnitude of effect change given the same concentration regardless of the baseline measurement, whereas the proportional relationship (Eq. 2.13) indicates that a subject with a higher baseline results in a higher effect change.

2.2.2.2 Direct Effect

The concentration in the central blood compartment may be *directly* linked with the pharmacological effect in PK/PD modeling when the apparent biophase equilibrium

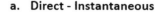

a. Direct - Instantaneous   **b. Indirect - Delayed**

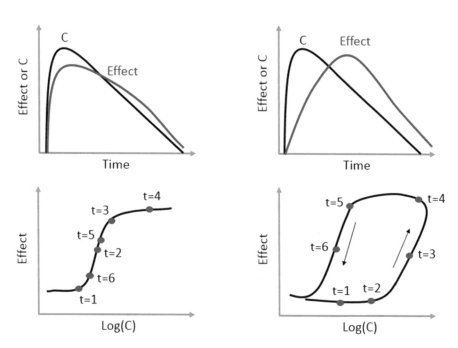

Fig. 2.5 Direct versus indirect concentration-effect schemes. (**a**) Direct—instantaneous. (**b**) Indirect—delayed. Upper panel, blood concentration (C) and effect versus time of a direct effect system (upper left) and a system with delayed effect (upper right); lower panel, effect versus concentration (C) for the direct effect system (lower left) and delayed effect system (lower right). Time labels t1– t6 and the arrows in the lower right plot indicate the time sequence of the response

is sufficiently rapid relative to the drug distribution (Fig. 2.5a) and can be described using the representative modeling scheme in Fig. 2.6a.

2.2.2.3 Link/Effect Compartment Model

In many situations there is a time delay between the drug concentration in blood and the drug effect. As such, the observed response is not apparently related to the blood concentration, and a hysteresis loop would present in the plot of response versus drug concentration in the blood (Fig. 2.5b).

This temporal displacement may be due to time to reach target site (i.e., drug tissue distribution), time for pharmacology to become available (e.g., active metabolite formation), or time to develop pharmacology (e.g., a slow ligand-receptor on/off time course or a cascade). In the case of distributional delay, it can be numerically handled by introducing a hypothetical *effect compartment* with a target site concentration representing the concentration at the site of action (C_e), which is

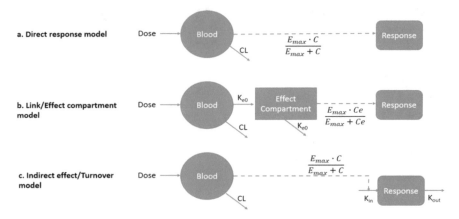

Fig. 2.6 Representative pharmacokinetic/pharmacodynamic model scheme. Drug effect is described using a simple E_{max} model. Other basic concentration-effect models may be used when appropriate. (**a**) Direct response model. (**b**) Link/effect compartment model. (**c**) Indirect effect/ turnover model. C Systemic concentration, Ce concentration in effect compartment, CL drug clearance, E_{max} maximum achievable response, EC_{50} concentration at which response is 50% of E_{max}, K_{e0} first-order effect compartment rate constant, K_{in} zero-order rate constant for the production of the response, K_{out} first-order rate constant for the loss of the response

assumed to drive the drug effect (Fig. 2.6b) (Sheiner 1997). The effect compartment (biophase) model was the first model structure that had been used to account for time delays in drug effects. Historically, it has often been applied inappropriately without recognizing that various other processes may contribute to such delays.

A first-order rate constant (k_{e0}) is typically used to describe the time delay from the systemic concentration (C_p) to the target site concentration (C_e). In order to avoid an identifiability problem due to unknown hypothetical effect compartment volume, the same k_{e0} value is used as an elimination rate constant for the effect compartment. A smaller k_{e0} value means the effect compartment equilibrates slower and that there is more of a time lag in drug distribution to effect compartment (hence "delayed effect"). The effect compartment model can be described as

$$\frac{dC_e}{dt} = k_{e0} \cdot C_p - k_{e0} \cdot C_e. \tag{2.14}$$

2.2.2.4 Indirect Response/Turnover Model

When the time delay between drug concentration and effect is due to the time required to trigger pharmacological response(s) rather than distributional delay, the *indirect response* model is frequently used (Fig. 2.6c). The term, *turnover* model, is sometimes used interchangeably, but it is often used to describe the homeostasis-maintaining, biochemical responses in body without drug intervention. Indirect

Table 2.2 Overview of indirect response/turnover models

Model	Scheme	Equation[a]
I: Inhibition of production		$\frac{dR}{dt} = K_{in} \cdot \left(1 - \frac{I_{max} \cdot C}{IC_{50} + C}\right) - K_{out} \cdot R$
II: Inhibition of removal		$\frac{dR}{dt} = K_{in} - K_{out} \cdot \left(1 - \frac{I_{max} \cdot C}{IC_{50} + C}\right) \cdot R$
III: Stimulation of production		$\frac{dR}{dt} = K_{in} \cdot \left(1 + \frac{E_{max} \cdot C}{EC_{50} + C}\right) - K_{out} \cdot R$
IV: Stimulation of removal		$\frac{dR}{dt} = K_{in} - K_{out} \cdot \left(1 + \frac{E_{max} \cdot C}{EC_{50} + C}\right) \cdot R$

Drug inhibition or stimulation effect is described using a simple E_{max} model. Other basic concentration-effect models may be used when appropriate, e.g., sigmoidal E_{max} model. C Concentration, R response, E_{max}/I_{max} maximum achievable drug effect ($0 < I_{max} \leq 1$ and $E_{max} > 0$), $EC_{50}/IC50$ concentration at which drug effect is 50% of E_{max}/I_{max}, I inhibition, S stimulation, K_{in} production rate, K_{out} dissipation rate

responses occur by perturbing the homeostasis (i.e., the inhibition or stimulation of the production or removal of endogenous mediators controlling the measured responses). In these cases, mechanistic delay happens even after the drug reaches the site of action.

The basic premise of the indirect models is that the observed PD effect is governed by a net balance between the rate of production and the rate of removal of an endogenous mediator that is perturbed by the drug:

$$\frac{dR}{dt} = k_{in} - k_{out} \cdot R, \qquad (2.15)$$

where k_{in} represents the apparent zero-order rate constant for the production of the response, k_{out} defines the first-order rate constant for the loss of the response, and R is the response variable, which is assumed to be stationary with an initial value of R_0 (k_{in}/k_{out}). In data fitting with the indirect response model, R is often assumed to be directly proportional to the unmeasured endogenous mediator quantity. A smaller k_{out} value results in a longer turnover time ($1/k_{out}$), i.e., longer time for a new steady state to be established following a change of the turnover system.

A drug can affect the net turnover system by the four mechanisms shown in Table 2.2 (Dayneka et al. 1993; Sharma and Jusko 1998). If production rate (k_{in}) increases or removal rate (k_{out}) decreases, then the value of the response variable increases, and vice versa.

Both the effect compartment model and the indirect response model may fit a given dataset well, but it is highly recommended that the model selection should rely on mechanistic understanding of whether the time delay is more due to a biophase equilibration (effect compartment model) or the need to develop a response (indirect response model). These processes might be concurrent, but rarely is there enough information in the observed data to support a combination of the two. Several other PK/PD models for continuous responses have been developed to better describe the data observed in certain scenarios such as the transit model, the tolerance and rebound model, and so forth. Readers can refer to the review by Csajka and Verotta (2006) for more information.

2.2.3   Emerging Approaches

Over the last several years, great progress has been made in pharmacometric analysis. New methodologies have been applied in drug development such as the physiologically based pharmacokinetic (PBPK) model, quantitative systems pharmacology (QSP), and model-based meta-analysis (MBMA).

2.2.3.1   Physiologically Based PK Modeling

The concept of physiologically based pharmacokinetic (PBPK) modeling is not new, as reviewed in Sect. 2.1.2. However, until recently, the application of PBPK models in drug development had been limited, mainly due to the computational complexity of the models and the necessity to collect various physiological or pharmacological data as inputs for the models. Currently, PBPK modeling is being used throughout drug discovery and development as a tool in assessing drug-drug interaction, designing appropriate formulations, and predicting PK in special populations such as pediatrics. The increased application in PBPK has been mainly facilitated by (1) the increased understanding of systems biology, pharmacology, genetics, and genomics, (2) the advancement of computation technology, and (3) the availability of commercial platforms for PBPK modeling, such as Simcyp simulator (Certara, Sheffield, UK), GastroPlus (Simulations Plus, California, USA) and PK-Sim (Bayer Technology Services, Leverkusen, Germany), and so forth.

Compared to data-driven empirical *top-down* modeling, PBPK model strives to be mechanistic by mathematically transcribing anatomical, physiological, physical, and chemical descriptions of the complex processes governing the fate of the drug in the body (i.e., *bottom-up*). It consists of multi-compartments corresponding to different tissues in the body and connected by the circulating blood system, where each compartment is defined by a volume (or weight) and blood flow specific to a given tissue. The parameters that describe the body system are refereed as *system-related input parameters*. Typically, compartments in PBPK models comprise of major tissues of the body such as adipose, muscle, skin, brain, gut, heart, liver, kidney, lung, spleen, etc. However, sometimes a reduced model is developed, by grouping organs or tissues with similar blood perfusion rate and lipid content, in order to reduce the overall complexity of the model.

To simulate the fate of a drug substance in the body, additional *drug-specific input parameters* are required, e.g., physicochemical characteristics determining drug permeability through membranes, partitioning to tissues, binding to plasma proteins and affinities to certain metabolizing enzymes or transporters, etc. Combined with *study design input parameters* (e.g., dose and dosage regimen, food intake, etc.), a PBPK model is expected to provide a more mechanistic insight of the various factors influencing PK (e.g., non-linearity) and thus a better understanding of the behaviors of a drug molecule in situations or populations that have not yet been investigated clinically. Its utility becomes more significant in the cases where it is difficult or not ethical to conduct clinical trials, such as trials with neonates or subjects with renal failure.

2.2.3.2 Quantitative Systems Pharmacology

Quantitative systems pharmacology, covering both efficacy and safety of a drug, has been introduced recently as a novel approach to link drug responses to physiological processes operating at molecular, cellular, tissue and organ levels. Compared to traditional PK/PD models, which focus on *confidence in pharmacologic agent*, QSP emphasizes *confidence in target* (Vicini and van der Graaf 2013). QSP models represent hybrid, multi-scale structures reflecting an understanding of fundamental mechanistic relationships of endogenous biomarkers affected by a pharmacologic agent and focusing on the dynamic interplay among the constituents of a system that manifests as emergent responses. As a result, QSP models allow for the exploration of questions in the absence of direct information because models (1) are based on best known understanding of physiology/pharmacology, (2) incorporate assumptions about drug and disease mechanisms, and (3) address drug action in the context of disease. For example, QSP models can be used to predict exposure-response or dose-response relationships for hypothesis generation. It can also be used to predict clinical outcomes with a new regimen and/or in a new population/indication. Moreover, it can test hypotheses when unexpected biological/pharmacological results are observed (Crawford 2016).

Although conceptually appealing due to its realistic representation of the body, the actual development and implementation of QSP models is often viewed as a practically difficult task. In particular, due to its complexity, QSP model development may not easily match timelines to address questions for fast-paced drug development. QSP models used to be developed in academia over decades, typically with a single lab focusing on a specific pathway of interest. To be of value in drug development, models must be developed rapidly and efficiently, because the time scale is being measured in weeks/months not years. It is, therefore, suggested to start with a fit-for-purpose, smaller model and then to build on it over time. This would avoid a long developmental period requiring a lot of effort with limited immediate impact, and long-term investment of QSP models is being increasingly appreciated in pharmaceutical industry. It is considered that QSP models, once developed, can be rapidly extended within their physiological and pharmacological fields in order to provide inferences on questions that empirical models have limited capability to answer, such as population selection, biomarker response explanation, off-target effect prediction, combinational therapy optimization, and so forth.

2.2.3.3 Model-Based Meta-analysis

Model-based meta-analysis (MBMA) has been recognized as an innovative data enrichment strategy to make efficient use of internal and external data sources, resulting in increased knowledge and more precise decision-making in drug development (Mandema et al. 2011). This strategy involves a systematic search and tabulation of summarized results from public and confidential clinical studies, followed by a regression analysis that may attribute variability in the study results to the differences in the study population or trial conduct. It provides a quantitative framework that leverages valuable existing data into the decision-making process for a drug candidate—e.g., a quantitative understanding of how a new compound will perform relative to existing standard of care and/or compounds in development.

To better understand the utility of MBMA, it is worth mentioning the key assumptions of MBMA. First, it assumes all drugs with a similar mechanism of action share the similar onset of action and a common maximum effect. Secondly, true (relative) treatment effects are considered to be "exchangeable" across studies, i.e., given the same treatments, each study would estimate the same, exchangeable treatment effects. Thirdly, heterogeneity, due to, for example, random unexplained study-to-study difference, can be accounted for by study-specific random effect models. An inadequate fulfillment of these assumptions would lead to bias during result interpretation.

Like any meta-analysis, MBMA requires a careful review of literature and an assessment of potential publication bias. Readers can refer to the standard procedures described in the *Preferred Reporting Items for Systematic Reviews and Meta-Analyses* (PRISMA) statement (http://www.prismastatement.org).

2.3 Pharmacometric Analysis Methodology

This section describes modeling aspects related to non-linear mixed effect population modeling, one of the most widely applied analysis tools in drug development. The book by Bonate (2011) details the methodology.

2.3.1 Software

From a historical perspective, it is noticeable that the development of personal computers together with software combining differential equation solvers with non-linear minimization routines accelerated the progress made in pharmacometrics. NONMEM (Beal and Sheiner 1984) was the first software available for population modeling. After its first release in the early 1980s, continuous improvements were implemented with the advancement of statistical and estimation techniques. There has been a series of updates (http://www.iconplc.com/innovation/nonmem/). At the same time, several other pharmacostatistical programs have been developed to handle NLME PK/PD modeling such as WinBUGS (http://winbugs-development. mrc-bsu.cam.ac.uk/), Monolix (http://lixoft.com/products/monolix/), Phoenix NLME (https://www.certara.com/software/pkpd-modeling-and-simulation/phoe nix-nlme/), nlme and nlmixr packages in R (https://www.r-project.org/), proc nlmixed in SAS (https://www.sas.com/), and many more. It is important that the software used for population analysis should be adequately validated and maintained. User-written model codes, subroutines, and scripts are usually provided for review as part of the regulatory submission.

2.3.2 Pharmacometric Analysis Work Flow

A schematic work flow for the development of a population PK or PK/PD model is provided in Fig. 2.7. The key associated activities are briefly described below.

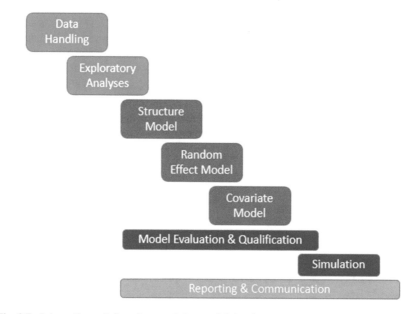

Fig. 2.7 Schematic work flow for population model development

- *Data handling*: Before any modeling analysis can take place, some form of data handling will be required to assemble the data into the appropriate format. It is advised to obtain access to data as early as possible so that data quality can be assured before analysis. This is extremely helpful for time-sensitive analyses.
- *Exploratory analyses*: Analysis is initiated with various exploratory analyses to better understand the data and potential difficulties associated with the modeling. Also, some aspects of data handling (e.g., imputation of missing data) may depend on the results of exploratory analyses. Both graphical and numerical methods (such as tabulation) may be applied.
- *Structural model*: The first modeling step pertains to structural model development (see Sect. 2.3.3.1), which looks for the optimal structure form for the fixed effects. The choice of a structure model will be largely driven by prior knowledge and results from exploratory analyses. Random effects need to be included in order to allow the refinement of the structure model.
- *Stochastic random effect model*: The next step is random effect model development (see Sect. 2.3.3.2). Both between-subject and within-subject random effect models are optimized in this step. In order to precisely estimate the fixed effects in a model, the random effects have to be properly accounted for.
- *Covariate model*: The base model developed from the above procedures is then used for covariate model development, if applicable. After selection of the final covariate model, the appropriateness of the random effect model should be reassessed. For example, a parameter describing between-subject variability should be reduced upon inclusion of a covariate effect. The resulting model is then considered as the final model.
- *Model evaluation and qualification*: The final model should be subjected to purpose-driven, model qualification. Model qualification should provide a sufficiently complete characterization of the model's behavior to better understand its potential limitations in future use.
- *Simulation*: In many instances the last component of a pharmacometric analysis is simulation, for example, to predict the responses to treatment regimens that have not yet been tested. Variability and parameter uncertainty should be carefully considered depending on the purpose of the simulation (see Sect. 2.3.5).
- *Reporting and communication*: Appropriate reporting and communication of the modeling results is essential for any pharmacometric analysis in support of drug development. This is of particular importance for analyses intended for regulatory review.

2.3.3   Model Development

Population models are comprised of several components: the structural model, statistical model, and covariate model (Mould and Upton 2012; Mould and Upton 2013; Upton and Mould 2014). Development of each component will be discussed below.

2.3.3.1 Structural Model

The structural model describes the relationships between the PK and PD variables for a typical individual. It can be represented as algebraic functions or differential equations.

For example, the simple one-compartment PK model for a drug being administrated as a IV bolus dose can be described using the algebraic function below:

$$C(t) = \frac{Dose}{V} \cdot e^{-\frac{CL}{V} \cdot t} \tag{2.16}$$

where C(t) is the systemic concentration at time t. Dose, CL (clearance), and V (volume of distribution in the central compartment) are parameters to define the relationship between C(t) and time. Alternatively, this one-compartment PK model can be written as a differential equation, as already discussed in Sect. 2.2.1 (Eqs. 2.1 and 2.2).

Compared to an algebraic function, which states the relationship between a dependent variable (i.e., systemic concentration) and an independent variable (i.e., time) explicitly, a differential equation describes the rate of change of a variable, e.g., the rate of change in concentration with respect to time. Many complex pharmacometric systems cannot be stated as algebraic functions, and instead they are comprised of differential equations using a set of typical parameter estimates (i.e., fixed effects) to quantify the mass transfer between compartments.

Identification of an appropriate structural model is the first step in population model development. It is usually guided by the exploratory analyses to determine the key characteristics of the structure model, for example:

Pharmacokinetics

- Is there an absorption lag time?
- Does the absorption follow a first-order or zero-order process, or some combination thereof?
- How many apparent distribution/elimination phases are there?
- Are there linear or non-linear PK processes (in the absorption or elimination phases) with respect to dose and/or over time?

Pharmacodynamics

- Is there a time delay between drug exposure and response?
- Are the data following a linear or non-linear PK/PD relationship?
- Is there an endogenous baseline component?
- Is there a placebo response over time?
- Is there a diurnal variation (circadian rhythm)?

Only plausible models should be tested. For instance, if the concentration versus time plot shows two distinct distribution/elimination phases, then a one-compartment model that describes a monophasic decreasing profile is not appropriate. For the mechanistic or semi-mechanistic PK/PD models, all tested models should be in agreement with the mechanisms of action of the drug.

Once a structural model provides an adequate goodness-of-fit, it is recommended to evaluate additional models with reduced complexity to avoid over-parameterization. If the omission of complexity does not result in a significant deterioration of model performance, then the reduced model should be chosen as the final model according to the principle of *parsimony*.

2.3.3.2   Statistical Model

The statistical models describe random effects, i.e., variability around the structural model parameters. There are two primary sources of variability in population modeling: between-subject variability (BSV), which is the variance of a parameter across individuals, and the residual unexplained variability (RUV), which is the unexplained variability, after controlling for other sources of variability, including within-subject variability (WSV), measurement error, etc. In some situations, between-occasion variability (BOV) is also employed to describe variability among multiple different measurement periods within a single subject. Population models usually have fixed effects as well as random effect parameters and are therefore called *mixed effect* models.

Figure 2.8 depicts the concepts associated with different levels of variability. Considering a drug being administrated as a single bolus dose, its typical or population mean concentration-time profile can be described using Eq. 2.16 (blue solid line in Fig. 2.8). However, the PK parameters for this model such as CL and V are not constant across all individuals, i.e., each individual subject has his/her unique CL and V values, as described by Eq. 2.17:

$$P_i = \theta_{pop} \cdot e^{\eta_i}, \tag{2.17}$$

Fig. 2.8 Source of random effects. *BSV* Between-subject variability, *RUV* residual unexplained variability, η_i deviation from the population mean for the ith subject, ε_{ij} residual errors in the jth observed concentration for the ith subject

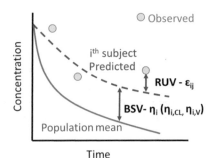

where P is the parameters of interests such as CL and V, i is the ith subject, θ_{pop} is the estimate of the population mean parameter value, and η_i is the deviation from the population mean for the ith subject under the assumption of $\eta \sim N (0, \omega_i^2)$. A log-normal function is used in Eq. 2.17 to describe the distribution of η values because CL and V, like most PK parameters, must be positive and are often right-skewed. An individual concentration-time profile (red dashed line in Fig. 2.8) is described with subject-specific values of CL_i and V_i using the same one-compartment structural model (Eq. 2.16).

Concentration measurements are affected by errors such as assay error, dosing history error, sampling time error, etc. As such, population models include RUV, which reflects the difference between the observed data and the model predictions, to capture these errors as well as WSV, model misspecification-related errors, and other unexplained variability. Such residual variability for drug concentrations can be assumed to follow a normal distribution and described by

$$Y_{ij} = C_{ij} * (1 + \varepsilon_{ij}), \tag{2.18}$$

where Y_{ij} is the jth observed concentration for the ith subject, C_{ij} is the corresponding model predicted concentration, and ε_{ij} are the residual errors under the assumption of $\varepsilon \sim N (0, \sigma^2)$.

In addition to the proportional residual variability model shown in Eq. 2.18, additive or combinational proportional and additive residual variability models are also often used to describe RUV.

Parameterization of the statistical model is usually based on data range being evaluated and the properties of the variables being analyzed. For example, an exponential BSV model is often used for estimation of the concentration to achieve the half maximum effect (EC_{50}) in order to avoid a negative value, which is not plausible for concentration measures. In contrast, BSV of some baseline clinical outcomes may be captured using an additive BSV model to ensure a normal distribution. Developing an appropriate statistical model is important for covariate evaluations (see Sect. 2.3.3.3) because covariates identification may be confounded by the BSV and RUV parameterizations used in the model to evaluate covariates. Moreover, results from simulation (see Sect. 2.3.5) depend highly on the choice of the statistical model. It is recommended that statistical models should be evaluated early during structural model development and monitored for adequacy throughout model development via multiple diagnostic tools as presented in Sect. 2.3.4.

2.3.3.3   Covariate Model

Covariates are defined as individual subject-specific factors including demographics (such as weight, age, and gender), baseline disease characteristics, laboratory measures (such as hepatic functional enzyme), co-medications, comorbidities, and life styles (such as smoking) that might affect the PK and/or PD characteristics of a drug.

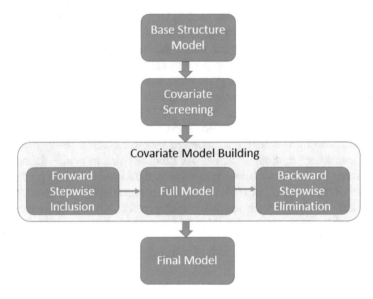

Fig. 2.9 Covariate model development

The identification of covariates which explain variability is an important objective in population modeling analysis. During drug development, questions such as "How much does drug exposure vary with covariates such as body weight?" can be answered through a dedicated clinical trial via enrolling subjects who have low and high body weights. However, such information can also be opportunistically assessed though the population modeling analysis of studies that are not specifically planned to answer such a question. Population modeling allows for the investigation of relationships between covariates (e.g., weight) and parameters of interests (e.g., clearance) as fixed effects. BSV estimates in models involving covariates would reduce when compared to estimates from the base model.

Figure 2.9 outlines the common approach used for covariate model development. In general, good structural and statistical error models are prerequisites for covariate analysis; when a covariate is known to have a large influence on the model parameters, as seen with body weight for pediatric subjects, this covariate can be included in the structural model (a structure covariate). Scientific and clinical relevance should guide the selection of potential covariates to be tested. Because run times can sometimes be extensive with multiple covariates and multiple base model parameters of interests, it is often necessary to limit the number of covariates evaluated in the model. Screening of covariate correlations is typically conducted to reduce the number of covariates to be tested so that covariate effects can be reliably estimated from the analysis dataset.

Several well-recognized covariate search methods (automated or manual) are available (Hutmacher and Kowalski 2015). All covariates can be tested stepwise (one at a time; forward selection and/or backward elimination) on all model parameters. Alternatively, covariates can be tested on select parameters, based on physiological plausibility, e.g., creatinine clearance on clearance (one of the most important parameters for exposure determination) for renally excreted drug, body weight on clearance and volume for pediatric subjects based on principles of allomeric scaling. The inclusion or exclusion of a covariate is usually determined via the likelihood ratio test with a pre-specified significance level (e.g., forward addition at the 5% significance level and backward elimination at the 1% level). Moreover, the addition or deletion of a covariate should be based on clinical and pharmacological experience and overall model goodness-of-fit. The models built via stepwise procedures can suffer from selection bias due to the order of covariates evaluated, and thus other covariate search approaches may be considered, e.g., a full model with all potential covariates incorporated followed by backward elimination.

A covariate can be included in the model in several ways, e.g., multiplicatively as a power model (continuous covariates; Eq. 2.19) or as a conditional effect relative to groups (categorical covariates; Eq. 2.20). Other covariate parameterizations can also be applied such as exponential and linear functions when appropriate.

$$\text{Continuous: } P_j = \theta_0 \cdot \left(\frac{X_{ij}}{M(X_j)} \right)^{\theta_j}, \tag{2.19}$$

$$\text{Categorical: } P_j = \theta_0 \cdot \theta_i^{X_{ij}}. \tag{2.20}$$

where P_j is the jth population estimate of parameters, X_{ij} is the covariate of subject i for the parameter P_j, $M(X_j)$ is the median (or standard reference) of covariate X for the population, θ_0 is the typical value of the parameter P_j, and θ_i is a constant that reflects the covariate's effect on the parameter.

2.3.4   Model Evaluation and Qualification

The objective of model evaluation and qualification is to examine whether the model is a good description of the dataset in terms of its behavior and the application proposed (*fit-for-purpose*). Model selection in general should be based on a combination of model performance, mechanistic plausibility, and clinical relevance (FDA 1999). And for model performance, three basic sets of criteria are used, model stability (e.g., bootstrap, condition number, etc.), predictive performance (e.g., visual prediction check [VPC]), and model sensitivity (e.g., influence of outlier, key assumption, etc.).

There are many diagnostics tools developed for model selection, and further details can be found in a review by Karlsson and Savic (2007). Some commonly used tools include statistical significance criteria (e.g., change in objective function value, Akaike information criterion, etc.), precisions in parameter estimates, diagnostic plots, and so forth. A VPC, stratified by significant covariates included in the final model, is usually recommended to be conducted to ensure that the models perform adequately well across various subgroups including different dose groups, disease populations, age and weight groups, etc. Alternatively, prediction corrected VPC (pcVPC) can be generated to check model performance. Ideally, the final model should satisfy the following criteria:

- Provides a good description of the observed data
- Has no apparent trend in the relevant goodness-of-fit diagnostics
- Is consistent with existing clinical/pharmacological/physiological knowledge
- Has a successful termination of the covariance step and/or is adequately stable

The parsimony principle should be applied to guide model selection whenever applicable. There may be reasons to select a more complex model instead of a parsimonious one despite lack of statistical significance. For instance, although mechanistic models require a high level of complexity, they take into account physiological processes and/or a mechanism of action to yield more plausible simulation results from the models.

2.3.5 Simulation

The quality of the simulation depends on the quality of the model in addition to prior information on drug attributes and the system. Simulations are most often used to explore the implications of a population model under differing assumptions and/or circumstances compared to those used for model building—i.e., beyond the scope of existing data. In these instances, it is important to define and disclose all assumptions for model building and simulation and to perform a sensitivity check to investigate the impact of the assumptions. Simulation results should be interpreted with a clear understanding of the limitations and assumptions inherent in the model.

2.3.5.1 Stochastic Simulation

Stochastic simulations using a mixed effect (fixed effects and random effects) population model are more complex than non-stochastic simulations using a model with fixed effects only. Random effect parameters describe variability in the population of interest and must be accounted for in simulations when understanding population variability is important for decision-making, e.g., designing future studies. This is implemented using a random number generator (available in most modeling software) to sample parameter values from a distribution. Simulations are repeatedly executed so that the distributions of the simulated output can be summarized (e.g., median and 5th and 95th percentiles). A common "rule of thumb" is that at least 200 simulation replicates are needed when summarizing data as mean values and at least 1000 to include their associated confidence intervals (Mould and Upton 2012).

2.3.5.2 Parameter Uncertainty

The precision of parameter estimates is limited by current knowledge and the input dataset. Parameter uncertainty is crucial to consider when running simulations. Large uncertainty in general indicates low model robustness and thus low confidence in model projection. By excluding parameter uncertainty, while including only between-subject-variability estimates, the simulation results underestimate the overall range in model prediction.

2.3.5.3 Simulation Approach Selection

Questions to consider in the determination of a simulation approach include:

- For model evaluation or inference?
- For interpolation (within the boundary of the original dataset) or extrapolation (outside of the boundary of the original dataset)?
- Interested in population mean or individual responses with associated variability?
- Time constraint for simulation analysis?

Depending on the objective of a simulation study, variability and uncertainty of parameter estimates may or may not be included, and Table 2.3 summarizes common simulation scenarios with their respective application conditions.

Table 2.3 Simulation scenarios

Scenario	Between-subject variability	Parameter uncertainty	Examples of applications
I	No	No	Simple, quick simulation for a typical subject Can be used for early-phase exploration or sensitivity analysis
II	No	Yes	To understand population mean response in early phase exploration Between-subject variability usually could not be well characterized in early phase studies
III	Yes	No	Model quantification (e.g., visual prediction check) Simulation for the same population with no extrapolation May be used for extrapolation when there is a time constraint for the scenario IV simulation below
IV	Yes	Yes	Design of future trials or support of label claim of the condition that has not been studied

2.4   Case Studies

Modeling and simulation tools have been widely applied to address critical questions in drug development in an efficient way. This section highlights such applications via four case studies where modeling and simulations have been used:

1. To identify a translational PK target to guide early clinical development (via MBMA)
2. To optimize dosing regimens for an efficacious and safe dose-finding trial design (via population PK/PD modeling)
3. To support regulatory approval and to alleviate the need for additional clinical trial (via population PK/PD modeling)
4. To guide early pediatric formulation development by determination of doses to be investigated in pediatrics (via PBPK)

In each example, the critical question to be answered will be introduced, followed by a pharmacometric analysis work flow, key outcomes, and the impacts on decision-making.

2.4.1   Translational Development

To guide the development of a novel anti-HIV-1 (human immunodeficiency virus type 1) agent, particularly the early clinical development, it is critical to have a good understanding of the target drug exposure that must be achieved clinically to ensure a robust long-term viral suppression (i.e., PK target). Using an MBMA approach, class-specific exposure-response models were developed for anti-HIV drugs of non-nucleoside reverse transcriptase inhibitors (NNRTIs) and integrase strand transfer inhibitors (INSTIs). These models linked viral load kinetics to potency-normalized steady-state trough plasma concentrations by retrospectively analyzing pooled internal/external data from the early-phase short-term monotherapy trials (phase 1b) and the in vitro potency measurements (Xu et al. 2016). Given the apparent existence of a class-specific common exposure-response relationship within a given drug class, this modeling approach was considered reasonable. Simulations were then conducted using these models to simulate viral load inhibition following doses that have a long-term efficacy based on literature reports. This led to the determination of steady-state trough concentrations of 6.2 and 2.2-fold above the in vitro potency for NNRTIs and INSTIs, respectively, as the PK targets (Fig. 2.10).

The models developed and the PK targets selected were used to guide compound selection during preclinical development, and to informe proof-of-concept trial design in subjects with HIV-1 for new antiretroviral agents. The models provided a reasonable prediction of the dose-response relationship for an investigational anti-HIV agent and enabled the comparisons against existing and emerging treatment

Critical Question: What is the target drug exposure which must be clinically achieved to ensure robust long term viral suppression (i.e., PK target)?

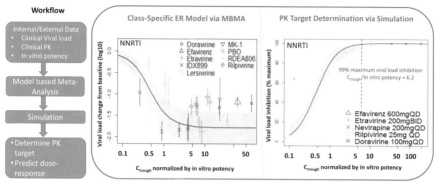

Fig. 2.10 Identification of pharmacokinetic targets for HIV-1 antiretrovirals by characterizing class-specific exposure-response via model-based meta-analysis (Modified from Xu et al. 2016). *ER* exposure-response, *PK* pharmacokinetics, *MBMA* model-based meta-analysis, *NNRTI* non-nucleoside reverse transcriptase inhibitor, C_{trough} trough concentration, *QD* once daily, *BID* twice daily

options. This MBMA modeling approach serves as an effective path forward to increase the probability of success in achieving conclusive trial outcomes.

2.4.2 Early Clinical Development

Guselkumab is a human IgG1 monoclonal antibody (mAb) in clinical development, which specifically blocks human interleukin (IL)-23. Understanding the exposure-response relationship of guselkumab is important to guide dose selection for phase 2 study in patients with moderate-to-severe psoriasis. However, at the time of designing a phase 2 study, limited information was available from patients; population PK/PD modeling and simulation were used to bridge the data gap in order to select the optimal phase 2 doses (Hu et al. 2014).

A population semi-mechanistic exposure-response modeling of guselkumab was conducted to evaluate the association of guselkumab exposure with Psoriasis Area and Severity Index (PASI) scores using a Type I indirect response model with an empirically modeled placebo effect (Fig. 2.11). A model was initially developed based on a small dataset from a phase 1 study of 47 healthy subjects and a phase 2 study of 24 patients with psoriasis who received various doses of guselkumab. A natural consequence of limited patient efficacy data was substantially high uncertainty in the resulting model. The simulated PASI75 (a 75% improvement in PASI score from the baseline) response rates were considered higher than expected, based

Critical Question: What is the optimal dosage regimen(s) for the gulselkumab phase2b dose-ranging study in patients with psoriasis?

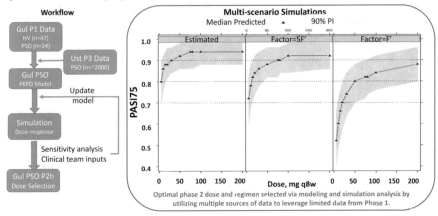

Fig. 2.11 Phase 2 dose selection of guselkumab in patients with psoriasis by utilizing multiple data sources via population PK/PD modeling and simulation (Modified from Hu et al. 2014). *Gul* Guselkumab, *HV* healthy volunteers, *P1* phase 1, *P2b* phase 2b, *P3* phase 3, *PASI75* 75% improvement in PASI score from the baseline, *PSO* psoriasis, *q8w* every 8 weeks, *Ust* ustekinumab

on prior experience with ustekinumab, another human mAb with a similar mechanism of action (IL-12 and IL-23 blockage).

Upon feedback from the clinical team, the model was subsequently updated, first by incorporating data from psoriasis patients who received a placebo (n = 765) and from patients actively treated with ustekinumab (n = 1230) in two ustekinumab phase 3 trials. The similarity in mechanisms of actions between guselkumab and ustekinumab suggests that they may share similar exposure-response model parameters, except for IC_{50} (concentration to reach 50% maximum inhibition), where an additional parameter RC_{50}, defined as the ratio of IC_{50} of ustekinumab over that of guselkumab, was included. Inclusion of additional ustekinumab data and the consequent adjustment to the specific model parameter substantially reduced uncertainties in all model parameters. Simulations of various scenarios were then conducted using the final model to select optimal doses and regimens. Sensitivity analyses were also performed with a few tentative RC_{50} values to evaluate the impact on the regimen decision.

Upon discussion with the clinical team, the final dose regimens were recommended for the phase 2b study. After the completion of the phase 2b study, the data observed were consistent with the model prediction, and an optimal phase 3 dose was then selected for further development.

2.4.3 Late Clinical Development

Canagliflozin is a sodium-glucose transporter-2 (SGLT2) inhibitor approved for the treatment of type 2 diabetes with the recommended dose being 100 or 300 mg once daily (QD). For patients requiring a combined treatment with metformin and canagliflozin, the use of a fixed-dose combination (FDC) tablet may improve patient convenience and compliance. Because metformin immediate release is typically administered twice daily (BID) for patients with type 2 diabetes, the FDC was developed to be BID where the canagliflozin was divided into 50 and 150 mg to provide the same currently approved total daily dose (100 and 300 mg).

Glycated hemoglobin (HbA1c) lowering (the efficacy measures for diabetes therapy) with 100 and 300 mg QD doses (not FDC) in two clinical studies was seen to be somewhat greater than those with 50 and 150 mg BID doses in a third study; however, there were differences in some factors between the studies that would limit the utility of such cross-study comparisons (most notably, baseline HbA1c was lower in the BID than in the QD studies). To address this, a population PK/PD analysis (de Winter et al. 2016) was conducted to provide a robust model-based solution that could account for differences in study populations. In the absence of directly comparable long-term study results, the analysis was used to assess whether there were clinically significant differences in the efficacy between QD and BID regimens of canagliflozin at the same total daily dose.

An established population PK model was used to predict full, 24 h PK profiles from measured trough concentrations. The PK/PD model was then developed using pooled data from all three aforementioned studies, incorporating an E_{max}-type model relationship between 24 h canagliflozin exposure and HbA1c-lowering efficacy (Fig. 2.12). Internal and external model validation demonstrated that the model adequately predicted HbA1c lowering for canagliflozin QD and BID regimens. Simulations using the final PK/PD model demonstrated the absence of clinically meaningful between-regimen differences in efficacy. This result supported the regulatory approval of a canagliflozin-metformin FDC tablet and eliminated the need for an additional clinical study.

2.4.4 Pediatric Development

CPD-1, a non-nucleoside reverse transcriptase inhibitor for the treatment of HIV-1 infection, was in phase 2 development. To support pediatric formulation development, it is important to understand the dose levels likely to be investigated in children. A PBPK modeling approach was undertaken (Xu et al. 2014) to provide a computational framework for predicting PK exposure in children to guide dose

Critical Question: Are there differences in the efficacy between once-daily (QD) and twice-daily (BID) regimens of canagliflozin at a same total daily dose (TDD)?

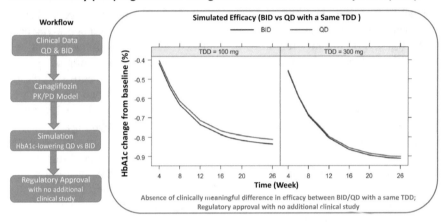

Fig. 2.12 Support of regulatory approval of canagliflozin-metformin fixed-dose combination via population PK/PD modeling and simulation (Modified from de Winter et al. 2016). *QD* Once daily, *BID* twice daily, *TDD* total daily dose

selection. Such PBPK model incorporated the physicochemical properties of the drug, the system, and the known enzyme maturation trajectories.

An adult PBPK model was initially constructed in Simcyp® and translated to pediatrics by applying complex built-in maturation functions including drug-related (e.g., enzyme ontogeny etc.) and system-related physiological parameters (e.g., organ size, blood flow, etc.). CPD-1 is primarily eliminated by hepatic metabolism mediated by CYP3A4 and a 100% CYP3A4 metabolism was assumed to facilitate PK scaling from adults to children. The pediatric PBPK model was used to simulate exposures in virtual pediatric populations to guide dose selection in children: the proposed dose levels must provide steady-state exposures that are sufficient for efficacy (i.e., steady-state trough concentration $\geq 0.88\ \mu M$) but within the safety exposure limit (i.e., steady-state AUC [area under the curve] during 24 h dosing interval $< 66.5\ \mu M{\cdot}h$). Based on model based dose projections in children, a suspension formulation was selected for younger children <6 years old, while scored tablets that allow flexibility in dosing (i.e., split dose) based on the adult formulation were selected for children ≥ 6 years old (Fig. 2.13).

It is anticipated these formulation/dose combinations should provide dosing flexibility in children while streamlining the supply chain of CPD-1, shortening its development timeline, and reducing the costs associated with potential dosing waste.

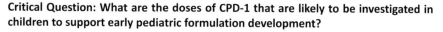

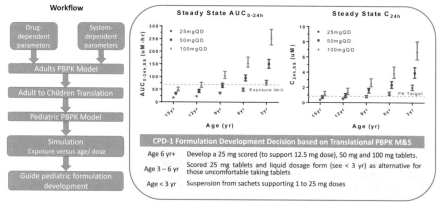

Fig. 2.13 Decision-making in pediatric formulation development via physiologically based PK modeling (Modified from Xu et al. 2014). AUC_{0-24h} Area under the curve during 24 h dosing interval, $C_{24h,SS}$ steady-state trough concentration at 24 h, QD once daily, yr year

2.5 Concluding Remark

Pharmacometrics is an evolving, multifaceted science pertaining to pharmacokinetic and pharmacodynamic modeling and simulation. Its value in quantitative integration of available information in drug development has been increasingly appreciated. This is beneficial to inform decision-making at critical drug development stages such as first-in-human, proof-of-concept, and pivotal trials, along with drug approval and labeling. Indeed, pharmacometrics is considered a valuable tool for the improvement of R&D return on investment.

The use of pharmacometrics in drug development requires adequate resources and experts with sufficient training. Continuous education is critical with the emergence of new modeling approaches. A good pharmacometrician must see his/her role extending beyond developing models: a model, complex or simple, should translate data into knowledge about a drug candidate and support quantitative decision-making. A pharmacometrician's job is to influence drug development decisions, not to simply develop models.

References

Ariens EJ (ed.) (1964) Molecular Pharmacology: The mode of action of biologically active compounds. Academic Press, New York.

Beal S, Sheiner LB (1984) NONMEM I Users Guide. Technical Report, Division of Clinical Pharmacology, University of California at San Francisco.

Bonate PL (ed.) (2011) Pharmacokinetic-pharmacodynamic modeling and simulation, Springer, New York.

Chien JY, Friedrich S, Heathman MA, et al. (2005) Pharmacokinetics/pharmacodynamics and the stages of drug development: role of modeling and simulation. AAPS J 7:e544-59.

Crawford M (2016) The when and why of quantitative systems pharmacology. AAPS News Magazine. December.

Csajka C, Verotta D (2006) Pharmacokinetic-pharmacodynamic modelling: history and perspectives. J Pharmacokinet Pharmacodyn 33:227-79.

Dayneka NL, Garg V, Jusko WJ (1993) Comparison of four basic models of indirect pharmacodynamic responses. J Pharmacokinet Biopharm 21:457-78.

De Winter W, Dunne A, Woot deTrixhe X, et al. (2016) Dynamic population PK/PD modeling and simulation supports similar efficacy in HbA1c response with once or twice-daily dosing of canagliflozin. Br J Clin Pharmacol doi: https://doi.org/10.1111/bcp.13180.

Ette EI, Williams PJ (2007) Pharmacometrics: impacting drug development and pharmacotherapy. In: Ette EI, Williams PJ (eds.) Pharmacometrics: The science of quantitative pharmacology, John Wiley & Sons, Inc., New Jersey, p 1-21.

EFPIA MID3 Workgroup (2016) Good practices in model-informed drug discovery and development: practice, application, and documentation. CPT Pharmacometrics Syst Pharmacol 5:93-122.

EMA (2008) Reporting the results of population pharmacokinetic analyses. http://www.ema.europa.eu/ema/index.jsp?curl=pages/regulation/general/general_content_001284.jsp&mid=WC0b01ac0580032ec5. Assessed 28 Jan 2017.

EMA (2016) Guideline on the qualification and reporting of physiologically based pharmacokinetic (PBPK) modelling and simulation. http://www.ema.europa.eu/docs/en_GB/document_library/Scientific_guideline/2016/07/WC500211315.pdf. Assessed 28 Jan 2017.

FDA (1999) Guidance for Industry: Population Pharmacokinetics. Food and Drug Administration. http://www.fda.gov/downloads/drugs/guidances/UCM072137.pdf. Assessed 28 Jan 2017.

FDA (2003) Guidance for Industry: Exposure-Response Relationships—Study Design, Data Analysis, and Regulatory Applications. Food and Drug Administration. http://www.fda.gov/downloads/drugs/guidancecomplianceregulatoryinformation/guidances/ucm072109.pdf. Assessed 28 Jan 2017

FDA (2004) Challenge and Opportunity on the Critical Path to New Products. Food and Drug Administration. http://www.fda.gov/downloads/ScienceResearch/SpecialTopics/CriticalPathInitiative/CriticalPathOpportunitiesReports/UCM113411.pdf. Assessed 28 Jan 2017

Forschungsinstitut B, Dettlti L, Freerksen E, et al. (1962) Pharmakokinetik und Arzneimitteldosierung (Pharmacokinetics and Drug Dosage). Kolloquium im Forschungsinstitut Borstel vom 25. bis 27. Oktober 1962. In: Antibiot Chemother. vol. 12, Karger Publishers, Basel, Switzerland (1964)

Gabrielsson J, Weiner D (2007) Pharmacokinetic concepts. In: Gabrielsson J, Weiner D (eds.). Pharmacokinetic and pharmacodynamic data analysis: concepts and applications, 4th Edition. Swedish Pharmaceutical Press, Stockholm, Sweden, p 11-224.

Gibaldi M, Levy G (1976) Pharmacokinetics in clinical practice: 1. Concepts. JAMA 235:1864–1867.

Gobburu JV, Lesko LL (2009) Quantitative disease, drug, and trial models. Annu Rev Pharmacol Toxicol 49: 291-301.

Gobburu JV (2013) Intermediate PKPD Modeling. Course: PHAR747, University of Maryland School of Pharmacy.

Holford NHG, Hale M, Ko H, et al. (1999) Simulation in drug development: good practices. Originally published by the Centre for Drug Development Science http://holford.fmhs.auckland.ac.nz/docs/simulation-in-drug-development-good-practices.pdf. Assessed 28 Jan 2017

Hu C, Wasfi Y, Zhuang Y, et al. (2014) Information contributed by meta-analysis in exposure-response modeling: application to phase 2 dose selection of guselkumab in patients with moderate-to-severe psoriasis. J Pharmacokinet Pharmacodyn 4:239-50.

Hutmacher MM, Kowalski KG (2015) Covariate selection in pharmacometric analyses: a review of methods Br J Clin Pharmacol 79:132-47

Jones H, Rowland-Yeo K (2013) Basic concepts in physiologically based pharmacokinetic modeling in drug discovery and development. CPT Pharmacometrics Syst Pharmacol 14:e63

Jusko WJ, Ko HC (1994) Physiologic indirect response models characterize diverse types of pharmacodynamic effects. Clin Pharmacol Ther 56:406-19

Karlsson MO, Savic RM (2007) Diagnosing model diagnostics. Clin Pharmacol Ther 82:17-20.

Kimko H, Duffull S (eds.) (2003) Simulation of clinical trials in drug development. Marcel-Dekker, New York.

Kimko H, Peck C (eds.). (2010) Clinical trial simulations: applications & trends. AAPS Advances in the Pharmaceutical Sciences Series, Springers, New York.

Lee JY, Garnett CE, Gobburu JV, et al. (2011) Impact of pharmacometric analyses on new drug approval and labelling decisions: a review of 198 submissions between 2000 and 2008. Clin Pharmacokinet 50:627–635.

Levy G (1966) Kinetics of pharmacologic effects. Clin Pharm Ther 7:362–372.

Mager DE, Kimko H (eds.) (2016) Systems pharmacology and pharmacodynamics. AAPS Advances in the Pharmaceutical Sciences Series, Springers, New York.

Mandema JW, Gibbs M, Boyd RA, et al. (2011) Model-based meta-analysis for comparative efficacy and safety: application in drug development and beyond. Clin Pharmacol Ther 90:766-9.

Mould DR, Upton RN (2012) Basic concepts in population modeling, simulation, and model-based drug development. CPT Pharmacometrics Syst Pharmacol 26:e6.

Mould DR, Upton RN (2013) Basic concepts in population modeling, simulation, and model-based drug development-part 2: introduction to pharmacokinetic modeling methods. CPT Pharmacometrics Syst Pharmacol 17:e38.

Nagashima R, O'Reilly R, Levy G (1969) Kinetics of pharmacologic effects in man: the anticoagulant action of warfarin. Clin Pharmacol Ther 10:22–35.

Olson SC, Bockbrader H, Boyd RA, et al. (2000) Impact of population pharmacokinetic-pharmacodynamic analyses on the drug development process: experience at Parke-Davis. Clin Pharmacokinet 38:449-59.

Pang S, Rowland M (1977) Hepatic clearance of drugs. I. Theoretical considerations of a "well-stirred" model and a "parallel tube" model. Influence of hepatic blood flow, plasma and blood cell binding, and the hepatocellular enzymatic activity on hepatic drug clearance. J Pharmacokinet Biopharm 5:625-53.

Peck C, Barr WH, Benet LZ, et al. (1992) Opportunities for integration of pharmacokinetics, pharmacodynamics and toxicokinetics in rational drug development. Clin Pharm Ther 51: 465-473.

Reigner BG, Williams PE, Patel IH, et al. (1997) An evaluation of the integration of pharmacokinetic and pharmacodynamic principles in clinical drug development. Experience within Hoffmann La Roche. Clin Pharmacokinet 33:142-52.

Rowland M, Benet L (1982) Pharmacometrics: a new journal section. J Pharmacokinet Biopharm 10:349–350.

Sharma A, Jusko WJ (1998) Characteristics of indirect pharmacodynamic models and applications to clinical drug responses. Br J Clin Pharmacol 45: 229–239.

Sheiner L, Rosenberg B, Melmon K (1972) Modeling of individual pharmacokinetics for computer-aided drug dosage. Comput Biomed Res 5:441–459.

Sheiner LB, Stanski DR, Vozeh S, et al. (1979) Simultaneous modeling of pharmacokinetics and pharmacodynamics: application to d-tubocurarine. Clin Pharmacol Ther. 25:358-71.

Sheiner L (1997) Learning versus confirming in clinical drug development. Clin Pharmacol Ther 61:275–291.

Segre G (1968) Kinetics of interaction between drugs and biological system. Farmaco Sci 23:907–918.

Sorger PK, Allerheiligen SRB, Abernethy DR, et al. (2011) Quantitative and systems pharmacology in the postgenomic era: new approaches to discovering and understanding therapeutic drugs and mechanisms. An NIH White Paper from the QSP Workshop Group, http://www.nigms.nih.gov/Training/Documents/SystemsPharmaWPSorger2011.pdf. Assessed 28 Jan 2017

Teorell T (1937) Kinetics of distribution of substances administered to the body. The extravascular modes of administration. Arch Int Pharmacodyn Ther 57:205–255.

Upton RN, Mould DR (2014) Basic concepts in population modeling, simulation, and model-based drug development: part 3-introduction to pharmacodynamic modeling methods. CPT Pharmacometrics Syst Pharmacol 2:e88.

Vicini P, van der Graaf PH (2013) Systems pharmacology for drug discovery and development: paradigm shift or flash in the pan? Clin Pharmacol Ther 93:379-81.

Wagner JG (1981) History of pharmacokinetics. Pharmacol Ther 12:537-62.

Widmark E, Tandberg J (1924) Uber die bedingungen fur die akkumulation indifferenter narkoliken theoretische bereckerunger. Biochem Z 147:358–369.

Xu Y, Hartmann G, Gibson C, et al. (2014) Utility of physiologically based pharmacokinetics in pediatric drug development. In: Abstracts of the 5th American Conference of Pharmacometrics. Las Vegas, NV, 12-15 October 2014.

Xu Y, Li YF, Zhang D, et al. (2016) Characterizing class-specific exposure-viral load suppression response of HIV antiretrovirals using a model-based meta-analysis. Clin Transl Sci 9:192-200.

Zhou H (2003) Pharmacokinetic strategies in deciphering atypical drug absorption profiles. J Clin Pharmacol. 43:211-27.

Chapter 3
Genomics and Bioinformatics in Biological Discovery and Pharmaceutical Development

Wendell Jones

3.1 Introduction: Bioinformatics—A Confluence of Molecular Biology, Genetics, Statistics, and Computing

3.1.1 What Is Bioinformatics

Bioinformatics is a cross-disciplinary area that requires skills and knowledge in molecular biology, computer science, and statistics. Specialists in this area generally have academic training in one or two of these areas and professionally develop the remaining area(s) related to their particular needs. Bioinformatics is heavily used in translational medicine, the study of nucleic acids (DNA/RNA/smRNA), pharmacogenomics, proteomics, and other areas of cellular biology. Common features of bioinformatics application areas include highly parallelized data processing, quantitative and comparative analysis, data management, dimension reduction and classification, merging and coordinating initially disparate datasets, assembly (of genomes), and distilling information in useful visualizations, graphs, and tables. Bioinformatics data contexts are often large and span whole genomes or transcriptomes for potentially hundreds to tens of thousands of subjects. Biostatistics has many areas of overlap with bioinformatics, especially conducting statistical tests, developing biomarkers, or creating predictive/classification models for outcomes. Biostatistics is also a more mature discipline covering many areas of macro-, micro-, and molecular biology. Bioinformaticians may be more familiar with particular esoteric statistical methods in their application domain (e.g., multiple testing correction, empirical Bayes methods for high dimensional problems, specific specialized graphs), while biostatisticians may be more familiar with a breadth of analysis

W. Jones (✉)
EA Genomics, A Business Unit of Q² Solutions, Morrisville, NC, USA
e-mail: wendell.jones@q2labsolutions.com

© Springer Nature Switzerland AG 2020
O. V. Marchenko, N. V. Katenka (eds.), *Quantitative Methods in Pharmaceutical Research and Development*, https://doi.org/10.1007/978-3-030-48555-9_3

methods, statistical power estimation, adaptive trials, and foundational methods. Computational biology is a closely related field that overlaps certain areas of bioinformatics and which may be more focused on computer and mathematical models of biological systems as well as simulations of these systems.

3.1.2 Two Sides of the Same Coin: Genomics and Proteomics

Genomics (the study of nucleic acids such as DNA/RNA/smRNA) and proteomics (the study of proteins and enzymes important for cellular function) are two sides of the same coin. There is a strong "symbiotic" relationship between nucleic acids and proteins as:

- Cellular proteins require the DNA code and the RNA template to produce new copies and versions of proteins.
- DNA is propagated (copied) and managed/regulated primarily through proteins. RNA combined with proteins are sometimes a vehicle for inserting new material into DNA.
- RNA is created (with the help of proteins) from DNA and then spliced/modified by other proteins into its final form before being translated into a protein.

3.1.3 Important Concepts

Genomics differentiates from genetics in a few ways. Genetics is mostly concerned with individual genes and heredity. In genomics, we wish to examine all of the genes at once within an organism to understand how the genes and other DNA structures relate to each other, what are its products, how did it evolve, what are its functions, how it can malfunction, and possibly how it can be repaired. The transcriptome is a closely related concept to the genome, as all transcribed products are based on DNA templates but which manifest as a related nucleic acid (RNA). In this chapter, we will consider transcriptomics as an important component of genomics due to the similar characteristics of RNA and DNA (they are both nucleic acids; thus, biotechnologies that measure one generally can measure the other) and due to RNA being an immediate product of DNA. Therefore, we will use the term "genomics" to cover both areas, but "proteomics" will refer to cellular proteins and enzymes.

The basic complexities of DNA are generally known gene content, junk DNA, double helix, and chromatin structures. However, RNA also has a rich complexity in that many RNA code for proteins (messenger RNA, or mRNA) but others serve other functions, primarily regulatory. There are many classes of non-coding RNA (ncRNA) including small RNA (smRNA) [which can be divided further into micro RNA (miRNA), piwi RNA (piRNA), small nuclear RNA (snRNA), and transfer

RNA (tRNA)], long non-coding RNA (lncRNA), and certain ribosomal RNA (rRNA).

The association of genetics with certain inherited diseases has long been recognized. The association of genomics with other non-Mendelian diseases has been more recent. We now recognize that autoimmune disorders often have very obvious genomic characteristics that can be readily identified via RNA (Li et al. 2010). Cancer is now recognized as a genomic disease. There may be multiple paths that lead to cancer: viruses, radiation, toxins, inherited variants, random events during cell division, and others. However, it is generally understood that all of these paths had a beginning with one or more key genomic alterations in one or more cells.

Traditionally, cancers have been analyzed and treated based on their tissue of origin, their cell morphology, and the transitions from early-stage malignant neoplasia to later-stage large-scale growth and metastasis. The traditional tumor staging and classification manual (UICC-TMN) has been a widespread historical reference for decades related to the recognition, classification, and treatment of cancer, but that perspective is changing (Mason 2006). Today it is understood that there is widespread variation in event-free and overall survival as well as response to therapies for cancers with the same stage classification; in particular, stage rarely predicts response to therapy. In addition, clearly there are other factors, such as the presence of TIL (tumor-infiltrating leukocytes) that also play a significant role in cancer outcomes (Galon et al. 2012). Finally, with the onslaught of genomic and molecular information that has arisen since the beginning of the human genome project, a valid question arises as to whether we need to think about cancer in a radically different way. In particular, bioinformatics has enabled medical science and pharmacology to classify distinct cancers in terms of genomic variants and gene expression profiles in addition to previous established categorizations. These new methods are demonstrating more appropriate and personalized approaches to treatment and more accurate assessments of response to therapy.

For this chapter, an analyte is defined as a particular instance of a genomic-related substance being measured. An analyte in gene expression would usually be an exon, transcript, gene, or gene fusion. An analyte in DNA measurement could be a genome position, genomic locus or region, a gene, or even larger regions of importance which reflect germline variants, somatic mutations, insertions or deletions (indels) of various sizes, structural variants (including translocations, or other rearrangements), and copy number status. In methylation, an analyte may be a specific locus (i.e., a genomic base position) or methylation site. In proteomics, an analyte may be a protein, protein product, or phosphorylation status of a protein. In current practice, genomic datasets may yield thousands to millions or even billions of analytes per specimen.

This chapter is focused on bioinformatic practices primarily in genomic studies. On occasion, closely related methods in proteomics and other areas may be identified. However, this chapter should not necessarily be viewed as a comprehensive review of current or previous bioinformatic and computational biology methods and techniques in proteomics due to its genomics focus.

3.2 Pharmaceutical Analytics

3.2.1 Bioinformatics in Clinical Practice

Clinical practice often requires examining both proteomics and genomics. The reasons for this are straightforward. In particular, the etiology of diseases and treatments show that many begin with single or multiple variants or mutations in DNA or its organization which may result in the following (that are not mutually exclusive):

1. Malformed and aberrant functional proteins within cells
2. Dysregulation of gene networks
3. Loss of important cellular functions due to, e.g., loss of DNA material or silencing
4. Out-of-control cell proliferation, especially in cancer
5. Cell dysregulation, especially autoimmune disorders
6. Combinations of issues due to cumulative errors including the inability of the cell to repair DNA damage or initiate apoptosis when damaged

Bioinformatics plays various roles in clinical research. For pre-clinical testing, the same techniques used for genomic measurement in humans can be applied to model organisms either usually involving rats (for toxicity) or mice for functional genomic and pharmacodynamic testing. Therefore bioinformatics is often an important part of pre-clinical testing. As the genomes of many of these model organisms are often highly controlled (e.g., most experiments utilize nearly genomically identical rodents), often the RNA is of primary interest. Gene expression profiles are measured to examine pathways affected by treatment. Are the drug targets having their intended effect? Are there off-target consequences? Usually, these measurements are from tissue most relevant to the therapy, for example, heart or arterial tissue related to cardiovascular disease (CVD) or liver tissue related to toxicity. These measurements and results then feed into the greater analysis within pre-clinical assessment of therapies.

In phases I–III of clinical trials, genomics may play key roles in different phases for different reasons. For example, in oncology and some inherited diseases, it may be beneficial to pre-screen patients for enrollment regarding one or more genomic features. In addition, in some complex trials such as basket trials, genomic testing may be indispensable in assigning patients to different treatment arms. The testing may ideally utilize whole blood tissue or serum (for inherited, hematopoietic, and autoimmune diseases—possibly oncology from using circulating tumor DNA) or other tissue including tumor mass (biopsy or surgery). In phase I, there may be more focused (i.e., several analytes) genomic testing to verify that, for example, as dose escalates, the therapy is having the intended biologic effects. In phase II and especially phase III, there is often retrospective genome-wide analysis (tens of thousands of analytes) to determine genomic biomarkers for treatment response, drug resistance, serious adverse events, etc. These tests may involve whole genome, exome, or transcriptome analysis of each subject. As the genomic tests and the data that result from these tests grow larger or are more complex, bioinformatics is required to assimilate, evaluate, and analyze the data. Genomic biomarkers derived from previous trials may sometimes be used to enroll patients especially for new phase II/III trials or to assign patients to cohorts. We will discuss particular examples of studies, genomic tests, and analysis methods in later sections.

3.2.2 General Motivation and Need for Bioinformatics

Downstream cell functions occur from DNA, primarily through protein-protein, protein-DNA, and sometimes protein-RNA interactions. Thus, the amount, content, and ultimate structure (which can sometimes be determined from its content) of the transcribed RNA intermediaries and the translated protein products that result provide clues as to the nature, prognosis, and potential treatment (as well as potential drug resistance) for the disease even if the DNA were somehow inaccessible. Often the DNA is amenable to isolation and measurement but does not provide enough insight for certain diseases as the root causes may be diffuse within the DNA, yet result in similar gene expression dysregulation (sometimes termed an expression profile). For most molecular studies associated with pharmaceuticals, it is frequently a matter of determining which individual or collections of molecules (nucleic acids or proteins) provide the quickest, safest, most economic, most accessible, and most accurate means for determining biological states or transitions, evaluating the pharmacodynamics of the therapy, understanding the biologic pathways impacted, identifying therapy targets, or evaluating treatment response.

The challenge even today is that although the first draft normal human genome reference was completed in 2001 (IHGSC 2001, 2004; Venter et al. 2001), more than a decade later, we are still learning many fundamental aspects of our genome and cellular and nuclear processes including the complex networks of DNA, RNA, and protein interactions. Bioinformatics plays an important role in helping understand the interplay of these complex processes. As such, it is an important interdisciplinary complement to biostatistics, computational biology, computer science, molecular biology, biochemistry, genetics, and clinical research. One additional aspect that makes bioinformatics complex is the scale at which observational data and processing needs to occur. Due to the size of the potential information in our genome, transcriptome, proteome, etc. and the fact that this information can change from cell to cell, bioinformatic methods are best leveraged with large collections of molecular and endpoint data. We have transitioned from megabyte and gigabyte levels of data in the 1990s to terabyte and petabyte levels by 2010. Some organizations currently or soon will generate data at near exabyte levels (10^{18} bytes). As a result, certain aspects of computer science such as programming and management of large datasets and large computing systems (high-performance computing) are a natural skill required in bioinformatic organizations. Similarly, characterizing and inferring knowledge from this complex collection of data is best performed with sufficient knowledge of statistics. As a result, some feel that for pharmaceutical practice, bioinformatics must be multidisciplinary involving the fields mentioned earlier (molecular biology, genetics, computer science, and statistics).

Most functional genomics studies must still be initiated or at least validated through laboratory bench work, even if relatively accurate complex computational biology models are available. Our models for gene and protein interactions cannot yet simulate complete processes occurring within even one cell, much less multiple distinct cells, including intercellular signaling, cell products (including exosomes), and cellular heterogeneity. Bioinformatics has emerged as an important discipline to complement the "wet bench" both by providing potential insight for a functional genomic experiment or by confirming that the experiment had the intended effect. For example, an observational study may lead to a hypothesis that one of a handful of genes is directing a biological process. The analysis of this initial discovery-oriented study may have been genome-wide and may have used bioinformatic methods to narrow the list of important gene candidates. However, to determine which of the genes are truly critical to the biological process of interest, investigators often return to (e.g.) an animal model where they will attempt to control these genes, often one at a time, through a variety of breeding, transfection, and gene knockout techniques and then examine the effects controlling each factor one by one. Since the effects are also potentially genome-wide, bioinformatics methods are then used to confirm or describe the effect. So, whether in genomic discovery or confirmatory modes after functional testing, bioinformatics plays an important role.

3.3   Bioinformatic Methods

3.3.1   Introduction

Bioinformatics is notorious for its many algorithms, methods, and pipelines which manifest themselves in computer programs. To understand what drives their formation and use, it is important to consider the full cycle of genomic studies as shown in Fig. 3.1.

Bioinformaticists play a role in helping answer genomic questions at all levels as they must utilize their knowledge of genomic characteristics to direct the question to the most appropriate assay and technology. This step is often conducted with both clinical and molecular biologists to ensure the proper cells and nucleic acids are collected and preserved in the proper amount and handled with the appropriate protocol to address the question (an experimental design aspect that can be easily underappreciated). After the assay is completed, it is the primary responsibility of the bioinformaticist to carry out appropriate computationally driven analysis of that data in support of the greater statistical analysis that also must be conducted as part of the clinical study.

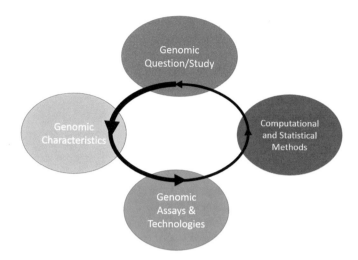

Fig. 3.1 Bioinformatics cycle—genomic questions and studies have to be combined with current knowledge of general genomic characteristics so that the appropriate genomic assay can be designed and the appropriate technology can be utilized for specimen testing and data collection. Once the genomic assay is processed, then appropriate computational and statistical methods must be executed to address the question and complete the study, which often yields a new question and study

The genomic questions in a study are often many and varied. Does the patient have relevant polymorphisms that would lead to fast metabolism of the drug? Is this autoimmune disorder driven by T cells or exogenous antigens? Is this cancer driven by a particular mutation in a particular gene (e.g., BRAF V600E)? Does the gene expression profile of this breast tumor suggest it is aggressive? Is there a reason why multiple myeloma patients have highly variable response to a new therapy? Do the responses of human cell lines to certain drugs mimic the behavior of actual tissues in vivo? All of these questions may have discernible answers once we design appropriate assays and conduct appropriate tests.

3.3.2 Important Genomic Characteristics and Concepts Related to Bioinformatics

The following items are important general genomically related characteristics having relevance to cellular biology, disease, assay design, specimen processing in the lab, and bioinformatics:

1. Cell Structure—Mammalian cells have important structures.

- Nucleus vs. the cytoplasm. The RNA contents of each can be very different (Barthelson et al. 2007). DNA is primarily in the nucleus (mitochondrial DNA being the exception).
- There is a fixed amount of DNA per cell in normal cells; however, the amount of RNA varies greatly. Messenger RNA (mRNA) is a small amount of the total RNA (2–5%).

2. Genomic Structure—The genome itself has important structures. Here are two:

- Centromeres and telomeres (middles and ends of chromosomes, respectively).
- Genes are a small portion of the sequence of mammalian genomes.

3. Genomic Repetition—Many regions of the genome are repetitive in different ways at different scales for different reasons.
4. Genomic Content Similarity—Many regions of mammalian genomes have content similarity of different types and scales for different reasons that go beyond simple repetition.

- Human genes have various levels of similarity with genes from primates, other mammals including rodents, and even yeast, due to common ancestry.
- Individual human chromosomes have high similarity between chromosomal pairs due to meiosis and reproduction.
- A subset of genes within our genome have high similarity with each other (paralogous genes) due to duplication events within species.
- Large regions of the genome have similarity to each other due various reasons including a putatively common infectious event long ago. Structures having similarity across the genome include long terminal repeat retrotransposons (LTRs), long interspersed nuclear elements [LINEs], and short interspersed nuclear elements [SINEs]). Together, LTRs, SINEs, and LINEs may comprise nearly ½ of the human genome (Burns 2017).

5. Hybridization (Complementary Base Pairing)—Within the basic genomic alphabet (A, C, G, T, U), individual A and T bases (or A and U in the case of RNA) will favorably bind or hybridize to each other, and likewise G and C bases will favorably bind to each other (thus each base pair is termed complementary bases). Many genomic methods and measurement technologies are based on hybridization and base pairing.
6. Genomic Plasticity—Although we tend to think of the genome as quite rigid, the functional genome is flexible in multiple ways. Here are a few:

- Genes, when expressed into RNA, may be alternatively spliced, may have alternative start and stop regions, and sometimes undergo post-transcriptional editing when creating mRNA.
- DNA sections can break, reshuffle, and reintegrate with other DNA sections for a variety of reasons both normally (transposons and adaptive immunity genes) and related to damage and disease (chromothripsis and translocations). Some of these translocations are drivers of cancer.

– Secondary and tertiary structures of DNA change and guide regulation and expression.

7. Genomic Nucleotide Content—The human genome is a mosaic of GC-rich to GC-poor regions which has an impact on the ability to efficiently and effectively measure them. In particular, higher eukaryotes have protein-coding regions (or exons) that are enriched for GC content.
8. Regulation and Networks—The cell and the cellular system regulates itself using nucleic acids and proteins (which are chains of amino acids). These systems are in essence cellular networks that are chemically connected and are often correlated (statistically) in their amount and activity.
9. Polymerases—Polymerases are a class of general enzymatic tools used both within our cells and by our molecular labs to synthesize DNA/RNA strands from a DNA/RNA template based on base pairing. It a core tool for both our cells and most laboratory genomic assays.

3.3.3 Genomic Assays and Technologies

Genomic assays generally fall into a few categories. The primary category is whether the assay is targeting DNA vs. RNA as this determines much of the required molecular chemistry. However, there is complexity beyond the target molecule. Of primary importance is the number of different analytes to be measured as testing a few analytes often implies different methods than interrogating analytes genome-wide. Other requirements dictate the next steps. Is the required output qualitative in nature (such as a genotype, SNV, or detection of an RNA molecule) or quantitative (DNA copy number or RNA expression level)? Still other issues relate to detecting rare or isolated genomic events, such as structural rearrangements in DNA and fusions or certain splice variants in RNA. Finally, the preservation of the tissue from which the nucleic acids are isolated also has an impact on the assay. For example, many RNA measurement platforms have protocols that require intact (non-degraded) RNA. Therefore, isolated RNA from tissue that is preserved and fixated using formalin (aka FFPE, which degrades nucleic acids considerably), a common preservation method for tumors in clinical practice, are incompatible with these methods. Another important component is the amount of required input material for the assay. For some biological specimens, it is relatively easy to isolate hundreds of nanograms of nucleic acids; for others it may not be. It is important in clinical practice to consult with a genomic laboratory before determining the suitable assays given the genomic study, especially given the rapid evolution of the technology.

Also of primary importance is the fact that most molecular measurement is not in vivo but in vitro (i.e., in a laboratory). The long and sometimes chemically tortuous paths that flow from the in vivo collection of tissue, cells, and/or biofluids to their in vitro measurement are often filled with peril unless performed by trained clinicians and laboratories. A poor understanding of these protocols and chemical interactions inevitably leads to poor control over the steps within protocols, yielding biased, non-reproducible, or erroneous results. There have been several publications that highlight this difficulty (e.g., Prinz et al. 2011; Casadevall and Fang 2010). Moreover, there is plenty of blame to go around; lack of suitable laboratory control material and improperly manufactured reagents, poor analysis methods, confirmation bias, publication bias, administrative data handling errors, and fraud all contribute to this issue (Ioannidis 2005; Cyranoski 2017; RetractionWatch.com 2015).

The following are a condensed version of current genomic technologies. Some, such as PCR and next-generation sequencing, can be extremely flexible and can be modified to accommodate a large number of disparate assays. Others such as pre-fabricated microarrays are less flexible but can be relatively inexpensive (due to economies of scale in manufacturing) and are often designed to measure analytes genome-wide.

3.3.3.1   PCR (Polymerase Chain Reaction)

PCR is a flexible assay with the following variations: allele-specific (DNA), reverse transcriptase (RT), quantitative or real-time, digital, and digital droplet. Different PCR methods are used for DNA/RNA and for scale (assays and samples). Generally, PCR assays are very sensitive and specific and are most cost-efficient when relatively few analytes are being interrogated. PCR platforms are many and varied. Common platforms and reagents are provided by Thermo Fisher (formerly Life Technologies/Applied Biosystems), Fluidigm, Qiagen, and others.

PCR assays are straightforward to validate. In fact, PCR is an accepted in vitro diagnostic (IVD) platform approved in various forms by the FDA. As mentioned previously, polymerases are a core laboratory tool and thus have a wide variety of applications to DNA and RNA measurement. They are sometimes a trusted assay unto themselves, or they may create intermediates for a more complex assay such as genomic sequencing. Bioinformatic methods with PCR-based tests are utilized for multi-analyte RNA measurement and DNA genotyping. For example, for RNA, the bioinformaticist may assist with both the design of primers for PCR and determining appropriate reference genes. Historically, reference genes are called "housekeeping" genes as some of the first genes utilized for this purpose performed core cellular functions. However, their actual purpose is to provide an invariant quantitative reference control for the general level of RNA in the cell as the molecular reactions associated with the specific test can vary in efficiency from specimen to specimen. Reactions for all target genes are compared to this reference. Having suitable numbers of reference genes in addition to the target genes provides a superior level of quality in the resulting quantitative gene expression level output. Although PCR-based tests for both DNA and RNA can be easily designed to be of high quality, custom assays may be difficult to efficiently scale to a large number of analytes and may be costly to initiate even with small studies (e.g., a phase 1 study) as one often must purchase PCR reagents for each analyte in large quantities.

3.3.3.2   Microarrays and Other Hybridization-Based Platforms

Microarrays and other hyb-based methods can generally measure both DNA and RNA genome-wide or in a more focused manner. DNA platforms interrogate common single nucleotide polymorphisms (SNPs) with Illumina and Affymetrix (now part of Thermo Fisher) as two of the main platform providers. Illumina's BeadChips have various designs interrogating ~240,000 exome SNPs to ~5,000,000 genomic SNPs. Affymetrix's SNP arrays also have semi-customized designs that vary from >100,000 to >1,000,000 loci. Agilent provides array platforms based on comparative genomic hybridization (CGH) that interrogate both SNPs and copy number (CN) variants.

Microarrays are organized grids or arrays of oligonucleotides (typically DNA, thus the name DNA microarrays, although many actually measure RNA as the RNA target is frequently converted into DNA and termed cDNA) that have known content. Each microarray cell or position within the grid contains probes of a specific oligonucleotide. If lab processes are followed consistently, then microarrays can provide reasonable *relative* quantification of individual RNA species in a collection of biological cells when properly processed, normalized, and analyzed. Absolute quantification is extremely difficult as microarray probe or probe set design and protocols have numerous opportunities for bias in the reverse transcription, amplification, selection, attachment of reporter molecules, and hybridization steps. These biases are generally consistent for experienced and qualified laboratories and various microarray platforms so long as protocols and equipment/array types remain consistent (MAQC Consortium 2006, 2010). However, over time, even highly qualified laboratories have processing "drift" (differential biases due to gradual changes in reagents, equipment, ambient temperature, protocols, and personnel practices), and "batch" biases continue to plague microarray analysis even after 20 years of advancements in probe design, protocol design, and array miniaturization (probe density). RNA-Seq (discussed later) is also subject to batch biases but not nearly to the same degree, which is one reason why RNA-Seq methods are preferred for clinical studies. These batch biases, when not accounted for, can lead to false positive results: apparent differential changes in biology that are actually due to technical factors alone. This propensity for batch biases with RNA measurement implies that microarrays for clinical trials are best suited for retrospective studies where all specimens can be assayed together simultaneously.

NanoString is an FDA 510(k)-approved device for IVD applications. It utilizes capture probes (via hybridization) to measure strands of RNA. This device can measure up to several hundred distinct RNA analytes with one assay. It is also robust to sample preservation method (FFPE samples are assayable) and requires 100 ng input of total RNA. As it is hybridization-based, it is subject to batch biases as any other hyb-based system. However, the system does not require amplified target material, which eliminates one source of potential assay bias.

FISH (fluorescent in situ hybridization) is another genomic measurement method based on hybridization. Its primarily applications are threefold: detecting specific genes within chromosomes (both location and count), determining whether individual cells are missing or have extra chromosomes, and creating a color map of a cell's chromosomes (karyotyping). While FISH tests have been somewhat replaced by other tests, they are still used for specific applications. Again, as with most hyb-based methods, it is important to strictly follow protocols and have experienced or well-trained technicians for accurate results.

3.3.3.3 Sequencing

Sanger Sequencing—This method provides accurate DNA sequencing with intermediate-sized reads (500–800b) which were used to construct the first high-quality human genome. Sanger sequencing is inexpensive for a gene or exon but expensive at scale, and next-gen methods offer more flexibility (e.g., RNA-Seq) and much cheaper options. Nevertheless, Sanger is often viewed as the gold standard in sequencing although that view is evolving (Beck et al. 2016). Sanger sequencing is primarily available through Thermo Fisher (formerly Applied Biosystems/Life Technologies) and Promega platforms.

Next-Generation Sequencing—In the mid to late 2000s, several sequencing platforms became generally available that extended the applications of sequencing in several ways. First, throughput greatly increased, enabling the affordable sequencing of much larger collections of genomic targets or to sequence some targets more deeply (e.g., to detect lower-frequency alleles including somatic variants). The increase in the level of throughput cannot be understated: five orders of magnitude ($100,000\times$) per machine since 2004. Genomic assays that once were unthinkable for a clinical trial are now common. Second, protocols were developed to assay a wide variety of genomic-related content including WGS (whole genome sequencing), Exome-Seq (sequencing of the coding regions, i.e., the exome, only), RNA-Seq (mRNA-, total RNA-, miRNA-specific protocols), ChIP-Seq (protein-binding DNA sites), Rep-Seq (human immune repertoire sequencing), focused DNA panels where a relative few genes or exons are sequenced, Methyl-Seq (methylation sites), and still others. Other next-gen or third-generation technologies have enabled long reads ($>10,000$ bases in length) which sequence through repetitive regions allowing relatively easy assembly of complete genomes, especially bacteria and other small genomes.

Illumina, Thermo Fisher (formerly Life Technologies), and PacBio are the current major next-gen platform providers with still others, such as Oxford Nanopore, continuing to emerge. Sequencing kits that create the genomic target material for sequencing, which are known as libraries, are made by a larger assortment of manufacturers (e.g., Agilent, Roche, Illumina, Thermo Fisher, NuGEN, Qiagen, NEB, Rubicon Genomics). By 2015, most new development efforts in bioinformatics were in support of genomic assays performed on next-gen sequencing platforms and methods.

Many of the wet-lab protocols for molecular testing have common components. Typically DNA and RNA are isolated using common methods across testing platforms. Often RNA needs to be converted into cDNA (complementary DNA) before processing. However, there are differences, advantages, and disadvantages offered by various platforms. In general, when using targeted PCR and microarray assays, one has already pre-identified genomic targets to measure. With this pre-identification follows certain assumptions, often very exact, regarding what could be seen. Sequencing is more hypothesis-free, or better stated, sequencing has fewer assumptions regarding what will be seen. Thus, sequencing is the primary technology available to perform genomic or transcriptome assembly. If there are unexpected or unknown insertions, deletions, or fusions in DNA, one must generally sequence them to detect them. These unexpected genomic constructs are also challenging bioinformatically as much effort is invested in detecting and separating actual genomic events from technical artifacts. Nevertheless, the capability of detecting novel genomic constructs combined with laboratory technology and bioinformatic advances (and due to frequent deficiencies that microarrays have had historically with respect to batch effect sensitivity) has caused a dramatic shift in DNA and RNA molecular technologies toward sequencing for intermediate to larger-scale genome/transcriptome measurement over the last 10 years.

3.3.3.4 Platform Combinations

Sequencing, especially whole genome sequencing, can be hypothesis-free (i.e., no predefined manufactured probes or baits) and use unamplified material. However, the constraints and limitations that exist with most clinical tests with respect to the amount of cells or nucleic acids available require that the starting DNA or RNA material be amplified through PCR methods. Also, to provide more economical and focused assays, frequently hybridization methods are combined with amplification to enrich the target material for specific important genomic regions such as exons. Therefore, hybridization methods for sample target enrichment of important regions and sequencing to determine its content are a frequent platform combination assay. This combination has enabled high-throughput whole exome sequencing (WES), focused cancer gene panels, focused inherited disease panels, and focused RNA and fusion testing. Similarly, amplicon-based sequencing (artificially created constructs created through PCR techniques) can also be used to enrich targets for important genomic regions. However, for somatic mutation detection, amplicon-based methods present challenges due to the inability to identify whether the resulting sequences come from the same or independent molecular fragments. To reduce bias in measurement, it is strongly preferred to measure independent fragments of DNA from the original sample to overcome PCR biases that may obscure the true variant profile of the sample.

3.3.4 Bioinformatic Algorithms, Pipelines, and Methods

3.3.4.1   Algorithms

Bioinformatics is replete with algorithms, often due to the magnitude of genomic data and the need to make the processing of that data efficient. However, much is also driven by the biological mechanisms at work and the technical aspects of their measurement. For example, in next-generation sequencing, large stacks of sequence reads (tens to hundreds of millions) frequently need to be aligned to a large (gigabase) reference per sample. Bioinformaticists and computer scientists have put much effort into developing efficient algorithms for performing this alignment where a well-defined activity (find where a sequence exists in a reference genome) is repeated over and over again, independent of previous and future alignments. This is termed an "embarrassingly parallel" problem because, as problems go, these problems are relatively easy to solve by parallelization of tasks. Nevertheless, a single specimen with >10 gigabases of data may still take a few hours of total time to align even with multiple processors available. However, other problems, such as determining copy number status of DNA, are very positionally dependent. Data at one DNA locus provides important information regarding the copy number state of an adjacent locus. Therefore, algorithms that determine copy number from array or sequencing data should take this into account.

Algorithms are often used to help reduce overall noise, compensate for measurement bias, leverage prior or reference information, or leverage homology in various ways. Algorithms can also be specific to the biotechnology platform due to unique characteristics of their design. For example, Affymetrix microarrays have an inherent design attribute of using a large number of probes to measure one analyte such as a particular RNA molecule. Various researchers developed what eventually became a large selection of algorithms summarizing those probes for a given gene somewhat surprisingly without consensus as to which methods were optimal, as each method made different trade-offs.

Bioinformatic algorithms are often placed into larger programs that perform a specific function with well-defined inputs and outputs. These programs are written in a variety of languages: Perl, Python, C/C++, Java, R, SQL, and Linux shell script, depending on various factors. For larger efforts, individual programs are kept intact or converted to an executable for efficiency and then linked together (e.g., in a wrapper program using Perl or Python) to create a pipeline. Pipelines offer end-to-end or near end-to-end solutions for many genomic assays.

A list of only the primary bioinformatic algorithms and their contexts that are used in molecular biology and genomics would fill several pages, much less than what would be required to list and describe all published algorithms. Even reference books on bioinformatics algorithms soon become out-of-date due to the rapid change in technology and the fact that many algorithms are tied to specific technologies. Common journals where new algorithms/methods are published include

Bioinformatics, BMC Bioinformatics, Nature Biotechnology, Nature Genetics, Genome Research, and *Nature Methods.*

3.3.4.2   Bioinformatic Pipelines

As mentioned previously, bioinformatic pipelines are frequently constructed by stringing programs together mostly in series. The inputs and outputs of each program need to be well-defined so that the output of an earlier program can be fed into the input of the next program, similar in concept to the pipe function in UNIX/Linux ("l" as in "ls *.txt l grep –v hg19"). In fact, the need to facilitate creation of new pipelines is one reason why the Linux environment has been adopted by the majority of bioinformaticists and institutions that create and utilize massive data processing programs, often from next-generation sequencing. As pipelines have grown in both size, complexity, and utilization, frameworks for pipeline creation are emerging (Leipzig 2016). Pipelines often use common functional objects as programs even if the algorithms within these programs are specialized to the genomic assay or study. For example, alignment is a common functional concept in genomics. However, DNA alignment is often handled differently than RNA alignment due to the plasticity of RNA. An RNA aligner must be aware of gaps that can occur in RNA sequence relative to the template DNA sequence due to splicing activity.

The following are illustrations of simple pipelines which are color coded by common functional objects. The implemented algorithms within each object may be specialized or tuned to the specific context. The colors of each object are intentional. Objects with the same color have the same or similar function across methods or assays. Only the algorithms inside may be different.

1. Pipeline for single-nucleotide variant (SNV) and small indel calling from focused or exome-based sequencing

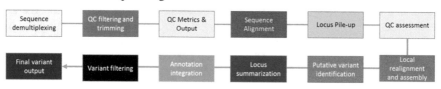

2. Pipeline for RNA quantitation from RNA-Seq

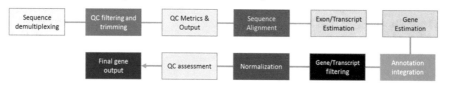

3. Pipeline for fusion/translocation detection from RNA or DNA sequencing

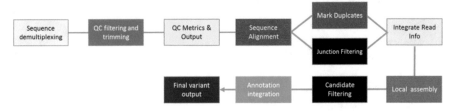

Common themes are obvious within just these three pipeline examples. Some will be discussed in later sections. Frequently appearing objects within pipelines include methods for QC filtering and trimming of reads, sequence alignment, sequence or candidate filtering, annotation integration, and QC metrics of basic data. Other complex pipelines include pipelines for genomic assembly either using a reference genome or without reference, transcriptome assembly, meta-genomics classification, and determining the state of DNA methylation sites from sequencing.

Biomarker development is another bioinformatics and statistics area that may utilize pipelines. However, the complete path of development is usually composed of several phases each of which has one or more pipelines. Within or at the end of each phase, intermediate results are reviewed before transitioning to the next phase. Based on the results, one may choose to possibly reiterate the current phase by transforming the data or adding new data items. Biomarker development may occur from genomics data alone. Other biomarkers may benefit from utilizing concomitant information, such as subject age or medical state. Even when using genomic-related information, a question remains as to whether a biomarker should use different types of genomic data (such as DNA variants and expression) as this may require complex and comprehensive testing. There is no single right answer to this question for every study. Simplicity and predictive accuracy should be the guiding principles to any biomarker. If an equivalent biomarker can be made using fewer genes or one molecular type, then that is generally preferred. Some clinical/general characteristics of subjects, such as age and gender, should also be considered if they are useful. For example, age is often strongly associated with many types of survival (event-free survival (EFS), overall survival (OS)) and with methylation status of many loci.

3.3.4.3 Bioinformatic Methods

The following are methods that are common in bioinformatics. Some have a statistical testing component. We will also describe statistical methods common with genomic and bioinformatic data in Sect. 3.4.

Filtering

Filters are a primary class of methods heavily used in bioinformatics. Bioinformatic filters are commonly used to remove irrelevant information (e.g., unimportant or false variants), simplify data (e.g., identify analytes invariant in a study), reduce noise (e.g., remove analytes with high measurement error), or adjust context (e.g., identifying samples associated with a particular disease within a compendium).

For example, each person may have roughly three million or more variants compared to the reference human genome (Drmanac et al. 2010; Fujimoto et al. 2010). The vast majority of these variants are less important and contribute to benign variety. Only a few may lead directly or indirectly to disease. Cancer cells generally introduce new variants (mutations) both benign and otherwise, and common preservation methods for cancer cells (fixation via formalin) introduce additional damage to the DNA that was not present before preservation that can be mistaken for a variant. Sequencing of the DNA often creates technical errors. Putting all of these factors together, that is, the large number of inherited variants and somatic variants, biased and error-contributing assays, and small numbers of actual and useful genomic targets, the adage of finding the needle in the haystack becomes an appropriate analogy for many genomic sequencing assays. In particular, in clinical reporting, when creating a summary report of relevant genomic variants from a focused cancer panel identifying putative mutations within 10–300 genes, care must be taken to adjust filters based on the needs of the report or clinical study. Current standards employ summarizing potential variant information in *vcf* (variant call format) files. These files, when combined with proper annotation, can be filtered based on whether the putative variant:

- Is intergenic or intragenic:

    If intergenic, if it is near important genes or possibly in a regulatory region of genes such as the promoter region
    if intragenic, if it is in a untranslated region (UTR), exon, or intron, and whether the variant leads to:

        A potential amino acid change (nonsynonymous variant)
        A change in gene splicing (alternatively spliced transcript isoform)

- Has an association with important genes or other variants
- Is pathogenic, benign, or of unknown significance (ACGM standards; Richards et al. 2015)
- Has an existing or potential drug target associated with it (ClinVar: Landrum et al. 2015)
- Is a common variant (based on current knowledge) in one or more population groups implying it may be germline
- Is a SNV or indel (and its size)
- Indicates the person is from a particular family or population group
- Has high measurement quality. That is, the putative variant:

Has sufficient depth (multiple measurements) of the non-reference allele
Is not biased relative to the measured strand
Is mapped to the genome appropriately
Is derived from analytes of sufficient quality

This filtering may either be an important step in creating a clinical report (e.g., filtered for pathogenic or drug targets) or creating a list of exploratory variants (e.g., variants with unknown significance) that may be associated with clinical response to new therapies in a larger study.

Statistical filters are another common tool in bioinformatics. These filters frequently remove irrelevant or invariant information or prioritize information that potentially has the most importance. For example, to alleviate multiple testing penalties (a common hurdle in genomics which is expressed in more detail in another section), analytes are often filtered before statistical testing begins. This is proper so long as the filtering is done without knowledge of any outcomes or experimental groups. Pertinent examples include filtering undetected or invariant genes in gene expression studies (which can often be 1/3 to 2/3 of all genes), filtering genomic loci with low or very high alternative allele frequency in SNP studies (10–50% of all SNPs depending on the study and platform), and poorly called SNP genotypes (e.g., loci from control samples that fail to meet Hardy-Weinberg Equilibrium assumptions (Anderson et al. 2010)).

Quality-based filtering, often related to probe characteristics, is common with some assays. For example, genome-wide assessments of copy number variants and alterations can have poor reproducibility of copy number calls and have been a historical challenge (Hester et al. 2009), especially in the case of small alterations or in the presence of low tumor purity. Quality filtering is also common with next-generation sequence reads as ends of reads with poor base quality are often trimmed to reduce false positive variant calls (Del Fabbro et al. 2013). Consolidating duplicate sequence reads in DNA sequencing is also a common practice as most are thought to come from one fragment source. Bioinformaticists also commonly filter gene expression results based on either significance, effect sizes, or both to then utilize the filtered gene list for various types of enrichment testing relative to biological pathways to discern relevant biological activity.

Clustering and Correlated Genes

Clustering is a general mathematical and statistical method that is based on two ideas: a measure of similarity or equivalently of dissimilarity between two objects and a mechanism or rule for two or more objects to join together to be one cluster. Although there are more advanced methods that allow clustered objects to be split apart and join with other clusters, we will only examine the more straightforward methods that are in common practice. Consult *Cluster Analysis* (Everitt et al. 2011) for a more comprehensive examination of clustering techniques and applications.

In genomics, the analysis of gene expression is a natural fit with clustering methods. Due to the large number of genes ($>$10,000 in mammal) and that these genes are typically co-regulated in some manner, clustering of gene expression is useful both in understanding and simplifying the relevant biological mechanisms manifesting within the study. Within these studies, a small to large number of genes and specimens (tens to thousands) are typically hierarchically clustered to discern primary, secondary, and tertiary effects, potential common regulation or function, "guilt-by-association" (if several genes in a cluster are involved in a cellular pathway or network, it is likely the other genes have some role in the pathway as well), and variability within the expression (are some genes and samples near opposites of other genes/samples?). Gene expression clustering in practice is typically hierarchical and agglomerative due to an early publication and free software provided by Eisen et al. (1998). However, other methods, such as k-means and self-organizing maps are also used. When combined with corresponding graphics, such as dendrogram-enhanced heat maps, clustering can be very effective in demonstrating the level of co-expression of collections of genes and how they relate to the patients or subjects studied. For example, Fig. 3.2 shows a clustered heat map of genes and ovarian cancer patients illustrating the coordinated expression (or lack thereof) of various genes that commonly express in immune cells.

Clustering of sequences is also used to compare organisms. Phylogenetic trees indicate the potential evolutionary history of related organisms based on clustering sequences. In addition, sequence clusters can also simply show relatedness and similarity of genes, regions, or chromosomes. Figure 3.3 is an example of a phylogenetic tree. From this illustration, one can see why rats (*Rattus norvegicus*), mice (*Mus musculus*), and primates are candidates for human pre-clinical studies based on their relatedness genetically.

Linking Multiple Sources of Information

A pervasive approach in bioinformatics is linking, integrating, and then leveraging multiple sources of data and information to solve problems. The "magic" is often in finding the appropriate linking mechanism coupled with the computing knowledge needed to execute the link and the contextual knowledge to understand the appropriateness of the link and the resulting resolution.

For example, a common practice is to use sequence similarity of genes across species (i.e., identifying orthologs) to find functional links between organisms based on detailed functional knowledge of one or more organisms and emerging knowledge of another organism's genome to determine the function of specific genes in the poorly characterized genome. In addition, common sequence motifs within and between organisms are often discovered to have common regulatory purposes between genomes. Still other challenges are addressed by integrating multiple sources of genomic and clinical information. For a different example, in understanding the onset, progression, treatment, and survival of ovarian cancer patients, one should be aware of deleterious inherited genomic variants (such as in BRCA1 and

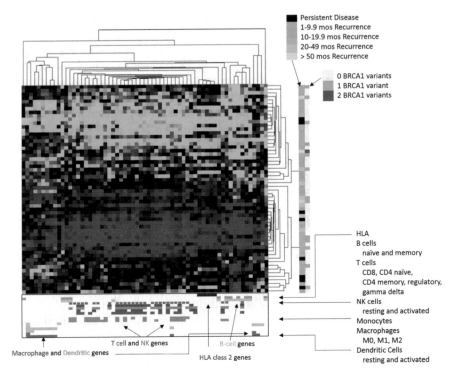

Fig. 3.2 A clustered heat map of ovarian tumor gene expression with annotations for event-free survival, BRCA1 pathogenic mutations, and different classes of genes associated with different immune cell types. Red indicates a very high level of expression, whereas green indicates relatively low expression. Black would indicate typical levels of expression. Just over 1/3 of these patients show relatively high levels of T-cell expression of the tumor sample indicating likely immune infiltration of the tumor

BRCA2); somatic mutations in these genes and also in NF1, RB1, and CDK12; certain copy number alterations; miRNA subtypes, expression profiles; and DNA methylation patterns (Cancer Genome Atlas Research Network 2011). This requires linking multiple distinct sources of genomic information. In short, complex disease and their treatments may involve multiple systems and therefore represent multiple opportunities for drug targets. Comprehensive analysis and understanding of complex diseases generally cannot be achieved by a single simple genomics or proteomics result.

In a more straightforward example of data and knowledge integration common in bioinformatics, suppose one would like to design an inexpensive genomic assay to track a patient's genomic testing results so that one could ensure that important clinical genomic tests detecting deleterious variants using a whole genome microarray, exome, whole genome sequencing, or RNA-Seq match the intended patient. It so happens only 24–48 higher allele frequency SNPs can assure uniqueness (aside from identical twins) in identifying an individual and thus enable complete

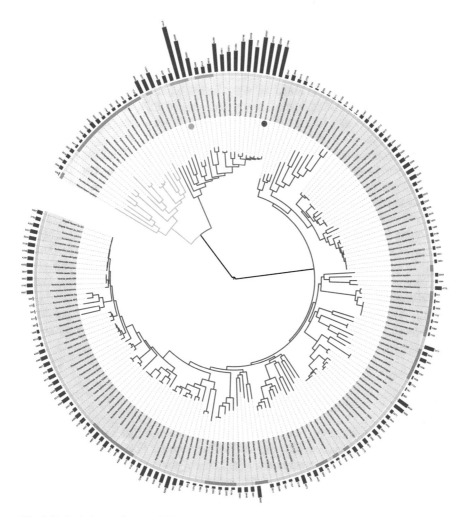

Fig. 3.3 A phylogenetic tree of life constructed entirely from genomic sequence data. The color gray represents bacteria, green represents archaea, and pink represents eukaryota which holds *Homo sapiens* and other mammals as well as plants. From a sequence similarity perspective, *Homo sapiens* are much closer to plants and insects than they are to bacteria. The graph is by Letunic and Bork (2007)

traceability of the patient's test result. However, which several dozen SNPs should be assayed from the greater than ten million population-based SNP candidates? Or can it be done at all? This is a classic bioinformatics question and is resolved by cross-referencing and linking detailed probe information regarding leading SNP microarray platforms (each platform has a manifest), detailed descriptions of the genomic regions of exon enrichment in a whole exome sequencing (WES) kit, determining a medium-sized collection of genes that are commonly expressed in most human tissues including blood, and then merging and cross-referencing that information to determine if there are 50 or so genomic loci that have sufficient variation in the human population that are detectable in each possible assay. If they exist, then once this SNP panel is designed, then no matter whether the primary laboratory clinical assay is based on WGS, WES, whole genome and exome SNP microarrays, or RNA-Seq, the relatively inexpensive PCR-based SNP assay can ensure that chain of custody was preserved during the processing of the clinical genomic assay.

Bioinformatics also leverages lists and unstructured data. For example, several genes have been identified in scientific publications as being associated with dysregulated pathways with their expression altered by disease or stimulus. Many of these have been consolidated into a database (Subramanian et al. 2005) which can be cross-referenced with pre-clinical or early-phase genomic test results to help determine both the biological pathways involved as well as to gain insight into whether the observed expression profiles have commonality with other experimental results from different tissues or different indications/conditions. Bioinformaticists also use text-mining techniques to peruse medical and research publications to find novel relationships between genotypes, phenotypes, and therapies. PharmGKB is an excellent resource for much of this information describing drug-oriented pathways, summaries of genes important in pharmacology, pharmacogenomics relationships with genotypes, and annotation of variants (Thorn et al. 2010).

Importance of Annotation

Bioinformatic methods make extensive use of annotations that are associated with genomic objects of many types. Annotations are used for linking, clustering, filtering, and interpreting information and results from genomic assays. The sources of annotation are extensive and growing, and the content within each source also continues to grow. For example, in 2001, dbSNP, a database containing annotations of known single nucleotide polymorphism in the human genome, contained less than two million non-redundant SNPs. In mid-2017, it contained more than 135,000,000 validated SNPs. The complete sources of annotation are too extensive to list here, but Table 3.1 provides a list of primary sources. For example, the human GeneCards

Table 3.1 Primary sources of genomic and proteomic annotation

Genomic reference sequence, gene names, gene sequence	NCBI, Ensembl, UCSC
Genomic variation	HGMD, dbSNP, dbVAR, 1000 Genomes, COSMIC, Broad GDAC Firehose
Proteomics	InterPro, PhosphoSitePlus, UnitProKB/Swiss-Pro
RNA sequence	UniGene, RefSeq, UCSC, Ensembl
Gene annotation	GeneCards, HGNC, EntrezGene, GO
Genes and phenotypes	PharmGKB, OMIM, ClinVar

database (http://www.genecards.org/), a compendium of other genomic and proteomic databases, lists over 100 sources of genomic and proteomic information that are
compiled to present information on a gene-by-gene basis.

3.3.5 Statistics in Bioinformatics

3.3.5.1 Mathematical and Statistical Methods

Some methods are not described in detail here, especially complex methods. Rather,
this section associates statistical methods within the greater context of bioinformatics
in clinical and genomic applications.

Bioinformatics has direct ties to many statistical and mathematical methods and
techniques due to the intrinsic nature of the domain. Some are simple but not always
used. For example, a particular gene's expression can vary by many orders of
magnitude in a collection of cells. Whenever gene expression measurements are
graphed in scatterplots or used as input into certain methods (such as principal
component analysis, a method discussed later), it is always advisable to perform
log transformations especially for platforms that measure expression either by
hybridization and scanning (such as microarrays and NanoString) or by counting
molecules (sequencing or flow cytometry). One platform, qPCR, naturally provides
measurements that are already on $\log_2$ scale due to its intrinsic properties, and thus
its output data does not require log transformation. The statistical tie-ins are evident
as PCR errors are not additive but multiplicative, justifying the log transformation
from an error stabilization and modeling viewpoint. Analysis and graphs of gene
expression will be much more meaningful using the log scale. Even biologists
typically discuss expression differences as being n-fold rather than n absolute
units. Log transformations of ratios of measured quantities are also used to discern
differences in target and reference material (DNA copy number and competitive
hybridization methods).

Regarding statistical methods, population-based hypothesis testing is widespread
due to the many different biological states that can exist in model organisms and
humans. In clinical development, these hypotheses are often related to measurable
cellular impacts of drug therapy or the pathways of various biological functions and
disease. As hypothesis testing is often genome-wide or for a large number of
analytes, methods are available that adjust p-values for proper inferences in the
presence of multiple testing of analytes (Noble 2009). These challenges are most
seen in tests associating genotypes, SNVs, gene expression, methylation, and protein
levels with treatments or clinical outcomes. Additional complexity with these
challenges includes proper handling of highly correlated systems of analytes (e.g.,
gene expression, protein levels, and to a lesser extent methylation levels). False
discovery rate (FDR) estimation methods, often using straightforward methods such
as Benjamini-Hochberg correction in RNA-Seq, or permutation-based reference
methods with expression microarrays (Tusher et al. 2001) are common practice.

Bonferroni adjustments are most frequently employed with initial genome-wide association studies (GWAS), a method to associate common population variants with disease or health, as most SNP analytes by design have less correlation due to optimized coverage of genomic variation. In gene expression, there is a trade-off between sensitivity, specificity, and reproducibility of differential expression (Shi et al. 2008). The large variations in effect size across the transcriptome have typically led researchers to prioritize analytes exhibiting a potentially larger effect size over small effects with high statistical significance.

As studies or designs become more complex, the statistical methods associated with them can likewise become more complex, leading to the use of linear or mixed models to account for the various factors. Genome-wide studies can be expensive even when a relatively small number of samples are tested. For pre-clinical testing (often examining gene expression) where many factors may be examined at once, the expression variance structure may also be complex and difficult to properly estimate. Therefore, the use of variance stabilization techniques such as empirical Bayes methods (Smyth 2004) has been adapted to address the level of parameterization with these studies. Other methods such as LIMMA (Ritchie et al. 2015) have been adapted for both microarray and RNA-Seq expression data and can be flexible to account for model complexity. However, whether microarray or RNA-Seq, a myriad of statistical methods have emerged to assess differential expression utilizing different assumptions and information under a variety of experimental designs.

Statistics also provides many techniques for describing multi-dimensional data common in genomic studies. The most used genomic dimension reduction method is principal components analysis (PCA). It performs several useful functions:

– It provides an overview of the genomic study and facilitates cluster and outlier identification. The relative distance of the samples, sample groups, or objects provides rough views of similar and highly contrasting samples or genomic structures.
– It illustrates the main effects in studies, especially pre-clinical animal studies or studies involving human cell lines. Sometimes the effects are obvious. It also quantifies the amount of variance associated with each common effect. Sometimes the primary dimensions reflect a technical factor, such as the laboratory or the reagent lot associated with sample clusters.
– It can also illustrate commonality (or lack thereof) of change if there are paired samples.
– Analysis of the associated gene loadings can also indicate the genes that are driving the common variation associated with the component.
– Sample groupings in different top components often directly relate to clustered groups of more highly varying genes in heat maps.

PCA is a universal tool applicable to gene expression, genotyping and GWAS, somatic variation, and methylation. An illustration of several of these characteristics is provided in Fig. 3.4, where miRNA-Seq data from flow cytometry-separated immune cells demonstrates that the miRNA profile for these cells is distinct and identifiable using principal components. This implies that there is sufficient co-expression of

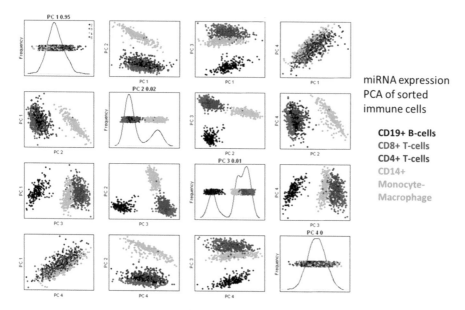

Fig. 3.4 Top four principal components of miRNA expression of four types of sorted immune cells. CD14+ cells clearly separate in the second component, while CD19+ B cells separate in the third component. CD4+ and CD8+ have less separation as they are both T cells

several miRNAs within specific immune cells that would allow relatively easy identification of the cells. If one examines the graph closely, one can spot outliers within each cluster. In fact, these were later found to be misclassified or mislabeled specimens. In this case, PCA detected outliers that were group outliers without necessarily being experimental outliers, a far more powerful and difficult task.

Expectation-maximization (EM) methods are another class of statistical methods that exist in more than one domain of genomic bioinformatics. It is a highly suitable method for maximum likelihood estimation in the presence of several different parameters that need to be estimated simultaneously. Perhaps it is best known for its use with gene quantification from RNA-Seq data. There have been several publications (Li et al. 2010; Li and Dewey 2011; Trapnell et al. 2010) regarding the use of EM in estimating isoform abundance from RNA-Seq short reads produced by Illumina and Life Technologies (now Thermo Fisher) next-generation sequencers. These methods resulted in two popular software implementations of EM for expression quantification, RSEM (RNA-Seq using expectation maximization) and Cufflinks. EM methods are also used in estimating haplotypes, which are genomic regions that are typically inherited together in a population. Identifying genomic motifs (disparately located regions having similar sequence characteristics) is another common application of EM methods which are typically combined with Markov models (Parida 2007). Methods for finding common motifs, putative genes, and haplotypes were heavily used before and during the Human Genome Project and the related sequencing and assembly of model human organisms.

Empirical Bayes (EB) methods are also commonly used in genomics information. An excellent example of this is its use in testing the large number of genes that may be differentially expressed in two or more biological conditions. In this case, EB methods may be used to borrow information from other genes to stabilize population variance estimates of individual genes especially when these genes have few counts. This method when combined with other statistical frameworks has been successfully used for differential expression testing for both expression microarray data (Smyth 2004) and RNA-Seq data (Leng et al. 2013).

In clinical trials and especially in terminal disease such as cancer, survival analysis is a common statistical method that evaluates the efficacy and response to therapy of different drugs or drug combinations. In one sense, survival analysis is not conducted any differently using genomic information than when a clinical trial or clinical study only utilizes traditional clinical parameters. However, genomic characteristics have been shown to be effective at explaining variation seen in patient responses. The genomic information may relate to inherited or somatic variants detected in tumors or to gene expression or methylation profiles of particular disease cells. A more recent development in understanding differential cancer survival rates in the presence of uniform adjuvant post-operative therapy is the utilization of knowledge of immune system activity in the tumor microenvironment. Various cancers have shown improved overall survival or event-free survival when tumor-infiltrating leukocytes (TILs) are present as shown in Fig. 3.5.

Survival analysis is greatly enhanced by biomarkers conjoined with clinical information. The biomarkers are sometimes simple proteomic markers, but increasingly more genomic markers are being used as the technology to measure them

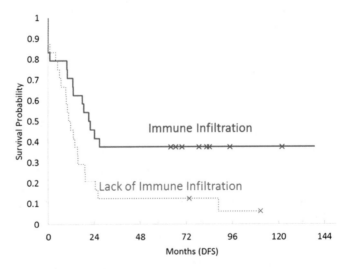

Fig. 3.5 Kaplan-Meier curves—an example of a statistically significant differences in response to therapy based on the immune infiltration status of the tumor. In this case, higher levels of immune infiltration within the tumor microenvironment (determined by bioinformatic methods) were associated with a higher likelihood of event-free survival (EFS)

becomes less costly and more widely available. Common genomic biomarkers are DNA variants and expression profiles. The variants can be of different types: germline and somatic SNVs, indels, copy number variants (CNVs) or alterations (CNAs), fusions, or other structural variants. Biomarkers for CNVs/CNAs are becoming more important as several indications show strong associations of copy number with treatment response (Bokemeyer et al. 2013; Wilson et al. 2016; An et al. 2014), especially in cancer where CNAs are common. However, there are challenges working with each variant type. For example, breakpoints for copy number variants and other structural variants are difficult to estimate precisely. Generally, once a particular variant's utility has been confirmed, then it may be used in clinical development as a supporting companion diagnostic (CDx). Designing tests for specific variants is relatively straightforward with many resources available to design PCR primers or various probes for enrichment or capture for other assays. Many platform providers have special tools available to design small custom panels to measure variants or may already have designed and tested methods to measure the variant of interest.

3.3.6 Informative Graphics

A number of informative graphics have been developed for displaying useful data from genomic studies. Some, such as heat maps, have been displayed earlier in this chapter. Other statistical graphics and methods such as principal components analysis have been adapted for use in bioinformatics analysis and were also illustrated earlier.

The following are some additional examples of interesting or novel graphics that are of general interest in bioinformatics. For example, Fig. 3.6 illustrates the overlay of variant allele frequency (VAF) information with the log ratio of sequence read depth, both of which are important measures at a genomic locus to determine copy number status of a sample at that locus. Historically captured somatic variants from cancer are illustrated in Fig. 3.7 for the gene PIK3CA. In this graph, certain positions in the gene are shown to be "hotspots" for variation. Major genomic structural changes, rearrangements, and translocations are often difficult to illustrate for various reasons. Figure 3.8 provides one way of illustrating and summarizing these changes via a circos plot as well as other positional information.

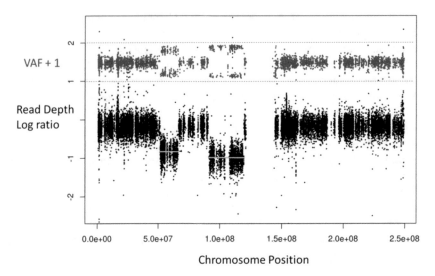

Fig. 3.6 Copy number diagnostic graph for a cancerous DNA sample for one of its chromosomes using exome sequencing. Black points are loci indicating the log ratio of the sequencing depth of the target specimen's cells relative a normal reference collection. Consistent deviations away from 0 indicate copy number changes. The points in red are measures of heterozygous VAF. Normal diploid values center around 0.5. Values deviating from 0.5 (or 1.5 for VAF + 1) indicate a copy number alteration for that region. In this case, there are at least two regions with obvious copy number loss (indicated by green lines)

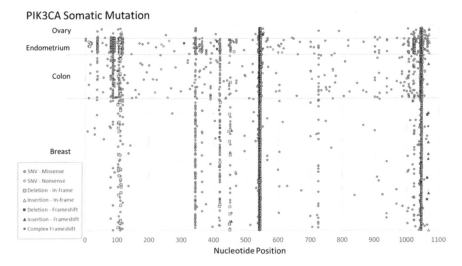

Fig. 3.7 Genomic variant plot showing loci within the PIK3CA gene that are hotspots for nonsynonymous variants in cancer cells. Note that some variants are more frequent in certain tissues while other variants go across many tissues. This graph uses data from the COSMIC (http://cancer.sanger.ac.uk/cosmic) database but is inspired by similar plots at http://www.tumorportal.org/ from the Broad Institute

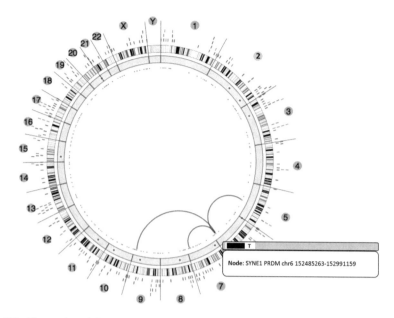

Node: SYNE1 PRDM chr6 152485263-152991159

Fig. 3.8 Circos plot of the genome indicating the nature and extent of structural chromosome abnormalities and translocations of an ovarian tumor as well information regarding mutations, expression, and methylation at a regional chromosomal level (from Boyle et al. 2012)

3.4 Case Studies in Genomic Bioinformatics with Associated Impacts to Treatment and Therapy

3.4.1 BRAF and NF1 Somatic Mutations Across Traditional Indications

As mentioned in the introduction, there are many research physicians, molecular biologists, and bioinformaticists who are thinking about cancer not as to where the disease arises or its stage, but what are the molecular mechanisms that are driving the cancer. Perhaps just as important, could these new classifications of cancer, such as BRAF V600E (a cancer having a nonsynonymous variant in the BRAF gene that causes an amino acid change from a valine (V) to a glutamic acid (E) in the 600th position), be more important than the tissue or stage from which the cells containing the variant arise?

For example, there have been a series of studies (Krauthammer et al. 2012; Hodis et al. 2012; Cancer Genome Atlas Network 2015) that demonstrate the role of particular somatic variants and other genomic features of BRAF, NRAS, NF1, and RAC1 (RAC1 variants being more recently found through exome sequencing) in melanoma oncogenesis. Different SNVs and genomic variations may interact with different pathways leading to melanoma. Bioinformatics methods combined with clinicians, molecular biologists, and other scientists have successfully identified the genes and mutations that drive most forms of melanoma. Many of these mutations lead to MEK or RAS pathway activation. Binimetinib, cobimetinib, and vemurafenib are all examples of targeted therapy MEK inhibitors that align with inhibiting specific activity due to mutations in these genes. However, the utility of bioinformatics does not end with one disease. Some of the same important BRAF mutations in melanoma have been observed in colorectal cancer and multiple myeloma by cross-linking of the sequencing data. In addition, the gene name, NF1, comes from neurofibromatosis type 1, a disease where certain inherited nonsynonymous variants result in 100% penetrance of a type of neurofibromatosis resulting in benign tumors of the nerves and skin. A bioinformatics-based discovery uncovered that some of the same germline mutations that play a role in inherited neurofibromatosis can, if a somatic variant, lead to NF1 functional loss, activate the RAS gene, and thus have implications for both prognosis and therapy in melanoma (Nissan et al. 2014). In this case, although the tissue plays a role in the expressivity of the variant, the variant is the driver of the disease. We now see connections between diseases that heretofore were unrelated. This connection has implications both in the diagnosis and the treatment of both constitutional and somatic variant-driven diseases.

3.4.2 Breast Cancer Subtypes

By the 1990s, it was known that certain inherited variants in the genes BRCA1/2 greatly increased a woman's risk for early-onset breast (and ovarian) cancer in adulthood although the great majority of these cancers are sporadic in nature. Hormone therapy using tamoxifen was demonstrated to be useful (sometimes alone) as a treatment for patients who had larger amounts of estrogen in cancer cells (so-called ER+ patients). Finally a subset of breast cancer patients overexpressed the HER2 gene, and Genentech in the 1990s developed one of the first targeted therapy drugs, Herceptin, explicitly for this condition. However, only a small percentage of women have these BRCA1/2 germline variants, and HER2+ breast cancer patients were a minority (<20%). While the morphology of breast cancer was known and that certain breast tumors responded to Herceptin and hormone-based therapy, there was not a detailed understanding of the molecular aspects of breast cancer. One of the first well-known biological insights enabled by expression microarray technology was the discovery of breast cancer subtypes at the molecular level (Perou et al. 2000; Sørlie et al. 2001). However, microarray technologies then did not have the quality that microarrays have now. Bioinformatic methods were still emerging regarding the proper way to analyze the expression patterns of thousands of genes simultaneously across a considerable number of subjects. As research progressed, biotechnology and bioinformatic methods improved, and the characteristics of these subtypes were reproduced at other genomic centers using different microarray technology. The intrinsic breast cancer molecular subtypes were then shown to have clinical relevance both related to their ability to predict aggressiveness and recurrence and to their ability to suggest appropriate therapies. One subtype, termed luminal A, was shown to be non-aggressive, and patients did not benefit from chemotherapy. Irrespective of treatment response, the risk of recurrence of breast cancer in patients was viewed as a useful clinical prognostic factor that could guide treatment decisions and therapy choice. Parker et al. (2009) developed a biomarker using statistical and bioinformatic tools that utilized the genes driving the intrinsic breast cancer subtypes, luminal A, luminal B, HER2, basal, and normal-like, to create a panel of 50 expression markers (called PAM50) that could classify the tumor's intrinsic subtype and provide a risk of recurrence score given the presence or absence of standard therapies such as neoadjuvant chemotherapy.

PAM50 had its roots in the early days of expression microarrays. However, microarrays have characteristics that do not provide robustness to variations in lab procedures, equipment, and personnel. They are also not as suited to measure RNA extracted from FFPE preserved tissue, a common preservation matrix for solid tumors. Finally, expression arrays are not FDA 510(k)-approved devices. To develop a clinical biomarker that would transition this research result into clinical practice, the biomarker development team decided to start with a subset of the relevant genes that had a demonstrated ability of providing concordant information when used with an orthogonal technology (such as qPCR or NanoString, which has devices that have achieved 510(k) clearance) and could reproduce the classifications when using degraded RNA from FFPE tissue. Out of the several hundred genes that were initially shown to have relevance with the various intrinsic subtypes, Parker used knowledge of co-expression of many of these genes combined with proper statistical methods for biomarker development: sufficiently powered study using hundreds of pertinent samples, independent training and test/validation datasets and phases, genes or features that passed performance testing for qPCR using FFPE material, n-fold cross-validation during training to optimize parameters and model selection, and selection of robust methods such as shrunken centroids for classification (Tibshirani et al. 2002). As development continued, the PAM50 classifier for breast cancer was ported to the NanoString device and marketed as the Prosigna® test. Since the initial publication, the PAM50 predictor has been found to provide superior prognostic value compared to standard immunohistochemistry (IHC) and other clinical endpoints (Nielsen et al. 2010; Wallden et al. 2015).

In summary, the successful development of both the breast cancer subtypes and the prognostic predictors of tumor aggressiveness and response to therapy all depended heavily upon biological insight, biotechnology platforms, and bioinformatics and statistical methods.

3.4.3 Characterizing Multiple Biological Systems Using Gene Expression Data

Important facets of characterizing tumor cells (breast cancer and other cancer sub-types) are related to (e.g.) cell motility; epithelial-mesenchymal transitions; migration, proliferation, and angiogenesis; and immune and therapy resistance. However, when tumors cells are collected by resection biopsy, nearby and internal stromal cells and possibly immune cells are also in the mix due to their proximity. These immune cells typically have genes that express nearly exclusively for the different types: T cells, B cells, dendritic cells, NK cells, and macrophages. Recent research has identified genes that are characteristic of these cells (Bindea et al. 2013; Newman et al. 2015). When the gene expression assay is transcriptome-wide, it is relatively easy to isolate the signals from these genes and produce a heat map. For example, the heat map in Fig. 3.2 is one such representation where ovarian cancer patients who had tumors removed prior to platinum-based chemotherapy show variations in the type and level of immune cell activity within and around the tumor cells. This figure is created through combining and filtering gene lists from different related experiments that may be from one platform (e.g., microarrays) and then utilizing them to filter data from these ovarian patients generated from a different platform (RNA-Seq). After selection, the gene signals are centered by gene and then clustered using correlation and hierarchical clustering methods. From this, a basic heat map is generated using standard bioinformatic tools and then overlaid with other important annotations. In this case, both clinical measurements (such as BRCA1 pathogenic mutational status and EFS data) and immune gene classes are added. Within this figure, one can see that roughly 1/3 of the patients seem to have consistent and larger immune cell activity. There is a small subset of patients in the lower right part of the graph that appear to have only B-cell activity, without accompanying activity of T or NK cells.

This pattern of a subset of patients having immune activity with tumor-infiltrating leukocytes (TILs) while other patients do not is common in ovarian cancer (Cancer Genome Atlas Research Network 2011; Konecny et al. 2014). This infiltration pattern also exists in other solid tumors (summarized by Iglesia et al. 2016). Samples with evidence of TIL activity are often inflamed and more amenable to certain classes of therapy. Tumors with TILs are also the best candidates for certain classes of immunotherapy drugs. In particular drugs that interfere with the PD1-PDL1 checkpoint or the B7/CTLA4 pathway theoretically will have the best opportunity to provide durable responses (Pardoll 2012). The importance of this information must be put in the context of the greater set of information available. The TIL expression is but one facet of the overall activity of the tumor microenvironment. As the previous case study has shown, expression patterns of the tumors cells themselves have relevance to diagnosis, prognosis, and therapy decisions. Now we discover that information regarding non-tumor cells in the same environment also has relevance to treatment decisions regarding the tumor. Regarding genomic assays, it is notable that we did not have to run a separate assay to uncover this important additional information of the immune component, which is somewhat independent measurement-wise from the tumor cells.

3.5 Current Challenges and Developments in Bioinformatics

3.5.1 RNA Versus DNA Biomarkers: Advantages and Disadvantages in the Clinical Space

An advantage of certain DNA biomarkers is that some can be relatively simple. In fact, many FDA-approved tests exist for specific mutations (germline or somatic). If a new therapy targets a particular gene with a particular mutation, development of a DNA biomarker may be relatively straightforward and economically implemented, but the speed at which the new test can be implemented may not be optimal, especially if one is implementing multiple individual tests at once. This has led some to create panels of genes so that a particular class of therapies could use a single panel. The panel would be designed, implemented, and validated once and thus could be used for several distinct therapies over time. In the long term, this may save both time and money as a panel that is used multiple times will gain efficiencies and reliability with continued use.

A disadvantage of DNA biomarkers is similar to the disadvantage of a software tester when restricted to only reviewing the computer source code (and not the actual running of the software) or to an airport controller when restricted to only the architect's drawings of the terminals and runway (and not a view of the airplanes in real time). In each case, the person may find a "fault" that may impact the system but will be unable to determine if it will lead to a "failure." The DNA test is examining a very static structure (i.e., the DNA itself) and not the dynamic aspect of the cell, much of which is embodied in the gene and protein expression.

RNA-based biomarkers have an advantage of capturing the dynamic nature of a possibly heterogeneous collection of cells. For example, in immuno-oncology applications, RNA biomarkers may be able to characterize the aggressiveness of the tumor and indicate the pathways responsible and whether there is immune activity in the tumor microenvironment, simply by examining the relative expression levels of different classes of genes. RNA can indicate certain structural variations (e.g., gene fusion events) better than targeted DNA tests and can discriminate important alternative splicing events, which DNA tests generally cannot do. RNA also indirectly reflects other characteristics such as methylation events, as well as general epigenetic changes to promoter regions or spatial proximity of enhancers. RNA is less effective than DNA at detecting specific variants, especially somatic mutations, due to less uniform coverage of the exome regions of genes when performing RNA-Seq and the inherent limitations of measuring individual bases using gene expression microarrays.

3.5.2   Emerging Methods in Immuno-oncology

New bioinformatics and laboratory developments are occurring in immuno-oncology. Bioinformatics has a role in developing new or reinterpreting existing genomic or proteomic tumor assays that characterize whether the tumor is inflamed, has evoked an immune response, or is nonimmunogenic. In immuno-oncology, having a well-characterized status of the tumor is important, as certain classes of drugs—such as immune checkpoint inhibitors and chimeric antigen receptor T-cells (CAR-T) therapies—are much more appropriate depending on this status. For example, immune checkpoint inhibitors work best if the immune system has already engaged the tumor microenvironment. Currently a common immunohistochemistry technique is used to assess tumor status by staining tumor slides for CD4+ and CD8+ cell activity. However, these techniques can have challenges with either sensitivity or specificity based on the specific mono- or polyclonal antibodies used. Separately, RNA-Seq has demonstrated proficiency at enumerating and deconvoluting cell populations for the potentially heterogeneous tumor microenvironment (Newman et al. 2015). This implies that bioinformatic methods combined with RNA-Seq data can be used to provide multiple information sets for a particular tumor specimen: general tumor expression profile; cell composition including immune-specific cells such as T cells, B cells, and dendritic cells; gene fusions; important mutations; and important splice variants. Utilizing current and emerging bioinformatic methods effectively will yield more information in these areas from a single assay.

If there is a noticeable immune response present and checkpoint inhibitors are a possibility, bioinformatic methods can be further leveraged to identify patients that are susceptible to autoimmunity-related adverse events (AEs) from particular therapies. The cause for the AE may be due to a combination of the nature of the therapy and genotypic characteristics of the patient, especially HLA type and variants associated with drug metabolism. For example, HIV-positive patients with the HLA-B*57:01 type have a hypersensitivity to certain antiretroviral medications (Hughes et al. 2004). Patients taking ipilimumab, a cytotoxic T-lymphocyte-associated protein 4 (CTLA-4) inhibitor immunotherapy, have encountered a high rate of adverse events (AEs) including colitis-related ailments. Whether the ipilimumab-related autoimmunity is due to HLA-DR-related alleles is currently unknown (Bertrand et al. 2016). Recent developments in bioinformatics have allowed investigators to determine HLA status with high precision from assays such as RNA-Seq that were not originally designed for that particular purpose (Buchkovich et al. 2016). Thus, if one is performing RNA-Seq for other reasons such as establishing expression profiles or detecting structural variants, the same raw results from this assay can now be used for safety and risk assessment of AEs by determining HLA types and performing correlative analysis.

3.6   Concluding Remarks

Bioinformatics is a relatively new field that requires a multidisciplined approach with computing and molecular biology as its foundations but which often requires statistical skills to be effective. It is evolving at a rapid pace due to ongoing rapid changes in biotechnology and molecular biological knowledge over the last 15 years. It has wide-ranging applications in pharmaceutical development, genomics, proteomics, molecular and cellular biology, and toxicology. As "-omic" analysis becomes more complex, we will be dependent on bioinformatic skills and methods to manage this complexity.

Bioinformatics has been effective during discovery phases for uncovering mechanisms, exposing subtypes and complexity, and linking seemingly disparate information sources to provide a more comprehensive view of biological systems and potential drug targets.

Genomics has the potential to revolutionize how we assess, diagnose, and treat patients for a wide variety of disease types by identifying and understanding disease in a more fundamental and individualized manner, leading to precision medicine. Biotechnology, genomics, and bioinformatic methods have revolutionized our understanding of many diseases but especially cancer and immune-related therapies. Bioinformatic methods are at the forefront in leveraging our emerging -omics knowledge to understand many diseases, choose appropriate therapies, monitor residual disease, and improve outcomes.

References

Li, Q-Z., et al. "Interferon signature gene expression is correlated with autoantibody profiles in patients with incomplete lupus syndromes." *Clinical & Experimental Immunology* 159.3 (2010): 281-291.

Mason, Emma. "Has TNM been overtaken by science?." *CANCER* (2006): 33.

Galon, Jérôme, et al. "Cancer classification using the Immunoscore: a worldwide task force" *Journal of translational medicine* 10.1 (2012): 205.

International Human Genome Sequencing Consortium. Initial sequencing and analysis of the human genome. *Nature* 409, 860–921 (2001)

International Human Genome Sequencing Consortium. Finishing the euchromatic sequence of the human genome. *Nature* 431, 931–945 (2004)

Venter, J. C., et al. The sequence of the human genome. Science 291, 1304–1351 (2001)

Burns, Kathleen H. "Transposable elements in cancer." Nature Reviews Cancer. 17.7 (2017): 415-424.

Barthelson, Roger A., et al. "Comparison of the contributions of the nuclear and cytoplasmic compartments to global gene expression in human cells." *BMC genomics* 8.1 (2007): 340.

Prinz, Florian, Thomas Schlange, and Khusru Asadullah. "Believe it or not: how much can we rely on published data on potential drug targets?." *Nature reviews Drug discovery* 10.9 (2011): 712-712.

Casadevall, Arturo, and Ferric C. Fang. "Reproducible science." *Infection and immunity*, (2010): 4972-4975.

Ioannidis, John PA. "Why most published research findings are false." *PLos med* 2.8 (2005): e124.

Cyranoski, David. "The secret war against counterfeit science." *Nature* 545.7653 (2017): 148-150. http://retractionwatch.com/2015/11/07/its-official-anil-potti-faked-data-say-feds/

MAQC Consortium. "The MicroArray Quality Control (MAQC) project shows inter-and intraplatform reproducibility of gene expression measurements." *Nature biotechnology* 24.9 (2006): 1151-1161.

MAQC Consortium. "The MicroArray Quality Control (MAQC)-II study of common practices for the development and validation of microarray-based predictive models." *Nature biotechnology* 28.8 (2010): 827-838.

Beck, Tyler F., et al. "Systematic evaluation of Sanger validation of next-generation sequencing variants." *Clinical chemistry* 62.4 (2016): 647-654.

Leipzig, Jeremy. "A review of bioinformatic pipeline frameworks." *Briefings in bioinformatics* (2016): bbw020.

Drmanac, Radoje, et al. "Human genome sequencing using unchained base reads on self-assembling DNA nanoarrays." *Science* 327.5961 (2010): 78-81.

Fujimoto, Akihiro, et al. "Whole-genome sequencing and comprehensive variant analysis of a Japanese individual using massively parallel sequencing." *Nature genetics* 42.11 (2010): 931-936.

Richards, Sue, et al. "Standards and guidelines for the interpretation of sequence variants: a joint consensus recommendation of the American College of Medical Genetics and Genomics and the Association for Molecular Pathology." *Genetics in Medicine* 17.5 (2015): 405-423.

Landrum, Melissa J., et al. "ClinVar: public archive of interpretations of clinically relevant variants." *Nucleic acids research* 44.D1 (2015): D862-D868.

Anderson, Carl A., et al. "Data quality control in genetic case-control association studies." *Nature protocols* 5.9 (2010): 1564-1573.

Hester, Susan D., et al. "Comparison of comparative genomic hybridization technologies across microarray platforms." *J Biomol Tech* 20.2 (2009): 135-151.

Del Fabbro, Cristian, et al. "An extensive evaluation of read trimming effects on Illumina NGS data analysis" *PloS one* 8.12 (2013): e85024.

Everitt, Brian S., et al. *Cluster Analysis, 5th Edition* (2011): 1-13.

Eisen, Michael B., et al. "Cluster analysis and display of genome-wide expression patterns." *Proceedings of the National Academy of Sciences* 95.25 (1998): 14863-14868.

Letunic I., Bork P. Interactive Tree Of Life (iTOL): an online tool for phylogenetic tree display and annotation, *Bioinformatics*, 2007, vol. 23 (pg. 127-128)

Cancer Genome Atlas Research Network. "Integrated genomic analyses of ovarian carcinoma." *Nature* 474.7353 (2011): 609-615.

Subramanian, Aravind, et al. "Gene set enrichment analysis: a knowledge-based approach for interpreting genome-wide expression profiles." *Proceedings of the National Academy of Sciences* 102.43 (2005): 15545-15550.

Thorn, Caroline F., Teri E. Klein, and Russ B. Altman. "Pharmacogenomics and bioinformatics: PharmGKB." *Pharmacogenomics* 11.4 (2010): 501-505.

Noble, William S. "How does multiple testing correction work?" *Nature biotechnology* 27.12 (2009): 1135-1137.

Shi, Leming, et al. "The balance of reproducibility, sensitivity, and specificity of lists of differentially expressed genes in microarray studies." *BMC bioinformatics* 9.9 (2008): S10.

Tusher, Virginia Goss, Robert Tibshirani, and Gilbert Chu. "Significance analysis of microarrays applied to the ionizing radiation response." *Proceedings of the National Academy of Sciences* 98.9 (2001): 5116-5121.

Smyth, Gordon K. "Linear models and empirical bayes methods for assessing differential expression in microarray experiments." *Stat Appl Genet Mol Biol* 3.1 (2004): 3.

Ritchie, Matthew E., et al. "Limma powers differential expression analyses for RNA-sequencing and microarray studies." *Nucleic acids research* (2015): gkv007.

Li, Bo, et al. "RNA-Seq gene expression estimation with read mapping uncertainty." *Bioinformatics* 26.4 (2010): 493-500.

Li, Bo, and Dewey, Colin N. "RSEM: accurate transcript quantification from RNA-Seq data with or without a reference genome." *BMC bioinformatics* 12.1 (2011): 323.

Trapnell, Cole, et al. "Transcript assembly and quantification by RNA-Seq reveals unannotated transcripts and isoform switching during cell differentiation." *Nature biotechnology* 28.5 (2010): 511-515.

Parida, Laxmi. *Pattern discovery in bioinformatics: theory & algorithms*. CRC Press, 2007.

Leng, Ning, et al. "EBSeq: an empirical Bayes hierarchical model for inference in RNA-seq experiments." *Bioinformatics* 29.8 (2013): 1035-1043.

Bokemeyer, Almut, et al. Copy number genome alterations are associated with treatment response and outcome in relapsed childhood ETV6/RUNX1-positive acute lymphoblastic leukemia. *haematologica* (2013): haematol-2012.

Wilson, Melissa A., et al. "Copy number changes are associated with response to treatment with carboplatin, paclitaxel, and sorafenib in melanoma." *Clinical Cancer Research* 22.2 (2016): 374-382.

An, Gang, et al. "Chromosome 1q21 gains confer inferior outcomes in multiple myeloma treated with bortezomib but copy number variation and percentage of plasma cells involved have no additional prognostic value." *Haematologica* 99.2 (2014): 353-359.2

Boyle, John, et al. "Methods for visual mining of genomic and proteomic data atlases." *BMC bioinformatics* 13.1 (2012): 58.

Krauthammer, Michael, et al. "Exome sequencing identifies recurrent somatic RAC1 mutations in melanoma." *Nature genetics* 44.9 (2012): 1006-1014.

Hodis, Eran, et al. "A landscape of driver mutations in melanoma." *Cell* 150.2 (2012): 251-263.

Nissan, Moriah H., et al. "Loss of NF1 in cutaneous melanoma is associated with RAS activation and MEK dependence." *Cancer research* 74.8 (2014): 2340-2350.

Cancer Genome Atlas Network. "Genomic classification of cutaneous melanoma." *Cell* 161.7 (2015): 1681-1696.

Perou, Charles M., et al. "Molecular portraits of human breast tumours." *Nature* 406.6797 (2000): 747-752.

Sørlie, Therese, et al. "Gene expression patterns of breast carcinomas distinguish tumor subclasses with clinical implications." *Proceedings of the National Academy of Sciences* 98.19 (2001): 10869-10874.

Parker, Joel S., et al. "Supervised risk predictor of breast cancer based on intrinsic subtypes", . *Journal of clinical oncology* 27.8 (2009): 1160-1167.

Tibshirani, Robert, et al. "Diagnosis of multiple cancer types by shrunken centroids of gene expression." *Proceedings of the National Academy of Sciences* 99.10 (2002): 6567-6572.

Nielsen, Torsten O., et al. "A comparison of PAM50 intrinsic subtyping with immuno-histochemistry and clinical prognostic factors in tamoxifen-treated estrogen receptor–positive breast cancer." *Clinical Cancer Research* 16.21 (2010): 5222-5232.

Wallden, Brett, et al. "Development and verification of the PAM50-based Prosigna breast cancer gene signature assay." *BMC medical genomics* 8.1 (2015): 54.

Bindea, Gabriela, et al. "Spatiotemporal dynamics of intratumoral immune cells reveal the immune landscape in human cancer." *Immunity* 39.4 (2013): 782-795.

Newman, Aaron M., et al. "Robust enumeration of cell subsets from tissue expression profiles." *Nature methods* 12.5 (2015): 453-457.

Konecny, Gottfried E., et al. "Prognostic and therapeutic relevance of molecular subtypes in high-grade serous ovarian cancer." *Journal of the National Cancer Institute* 106.10 (2014): dju249.

Iglesia, Michael D., et al. "Genomic analysis of immune cell infiltrates across 11 tumor types." *Journal of the National Cancer Institute* 108.11 (2016): djw144.

Pardoll, Drew M. "The blockade of immune checkpoints in cancer immunotherapy." *Nature Reviews Cancer* 12.4 (2012): 252-264.

Hughes, Arlene R., et al. "Association of genetic variations in HLA-B region with hypersensitivity to abacavir in some, but not all, populations." *Pharmacogenomics* 5.2 (2004): 203-211.

Bertrand, A. et al. Immune Related Adverse Events Associated with Anti-CTLA-4 Antibodies: Systematic Review and Meta-Analysis. *BMC Medicine* 13 (2015): 211. 6 Oct. 2016.

Buchkovich, M., Brown, C., and Robasky, K, HLAProfiler: a novel, allele sequence signature approach enabling HLA-typing for biomarker identification in gene expression data. Poster at ASHG 2016.

Chapter 4
Biostatistical Methods in Pharmacoepidemiology

Ana Filipa Macedo, Ana Maria Rodriguez, William Hawkes, and Alban Fabre

4.1 Introduction

4.1.1 Experiment vs. Observation

Pharmacoepidemiology is mostly categorized in two main types of studies. In general the objective is to test or observe a causal interpretation of the relationship between the exposure of a drug and an outcome of interest such as efficacy or safety.

These studies are differentiated between experimental (also called intervention studies) and observational. Intervention or experimentation involves attempting to change a variable in one or more groups of people. In experimental research, the investigator controls the management of the patient, and the allocation of the drug in most of the cases is randomized. Observation allows nature to take its course, so the investigator measures but does not intervene. In observational research, exposure to the drug is not dictated by the study protocol, and its use within the study has the advantage of mimicking the situation of real-life conditions.

Compared to observational research, the limitations of experimental research lay in the size of the study, for instance, it could be too small or too short in time to identify occurrences of rare outcome (e.g. long-term rare adverse reaction). The design of these studies does not address real-life condition effects due to their controlled nature, since under the experimental design the allocation of the exposure is defined by randomization.

On the other hand, the major challenge of observational research is to draw inferences about drug effects free from other factors observed in an uncontrolled environment. Observational research of drug effects is very challenging in Pharmacoepidemiology given the uncontrolled nature of its designs, which require

A. F. Macedo · A. M. Rodriguez · W. Hawkes · A. Fabre (✉)
IQVIA Real World Evidence Solutions, Biostatistics and Epidemiology,
Durham, NC, USA

© Springer Nature Switzerland AG 2020
O. V. Marchenko, N. V. Katenka (eds.), *Quantitative Methods in Pharmaceutical Research and Development*, https://doi.org/10.1007/978-3-030-48555-9_4

particular analytic methods to address methodological challenges in this area. For this reason, this is the main focus of this chapter.

4.1.2   Observational Studies

In observational research, we usually make a distinction between descriptive studies and etiologic studies.

4.1.2.1   Descriptive and Etiologic Studies

The objective of descriptive studies is to provide statistics to understand the health status of the population, without establishing a relationship with any risk factors. Most commonly, we use descriptive statistics to describe the frequency of disease occurrence in relation to variables such as person, place, and time (described in Sect. 4.2.1). Descriptive studies can suggest hypotheses about associations, which can be tested in etiologic studies.

The objective of etiologic studies is to compare groups of patients in order to identify an association between an exposure and an outcome and test a causal hypothesis. The demonstration of these associations should account for the real-life nature of the design, introducing different sources of variability (described in Sect. 4.2.2) involving particular statistical approaches (described in Sect. 4.4).

4.1.2.2   Designs in Etiologic Studies

In Pharmacoepidemiology, we observe three main study designs: cohort studies, cross-sectional studies, and case-control studies. Cohort and cross-sectional studies can be designed for both descriptive and etiologic objectives, whereas case-control studies will only address an etiologic objective.

In order to understand the concept of these designs, we need to introduce the notion of time, inclusion of patient, data collection, and start of the study.

In cohort studies, a group of people exposed to a risk factor and a group who are unexposed to the risk factor (or exposed to another risk factor) are followed over time to determine the occurrence of disease. In cohort studies, the start of the study will occur between the inclusion of patients and the data collection. When the start occurs at the time of patient inclusion, we talk about a prospective cohort (Fig. 4.1), whereas when the start of the study occurs at the time of data collection, we talk about retrospective cohort (Fig. 4.2).

In cross-sectional studies, the patients are included at the start of the study, the time at which the data is collected. Cross-sectional studies are also viewed as a snapshot of the situation at a certain defined time.

Fig. 4.1 Schematic design
of a prospective study

PROSPECTIVE

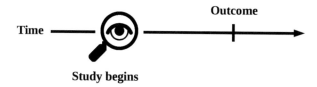

Fig. 4.2 Schematic design
of a retrospective study

RETROSPECTIVE

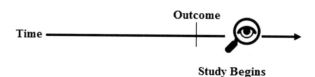

Table 4.1 Advantages and disadvantages of observational etiologic studies

	Advantages	Disadvantages
Cohort studies	Direct measurement of incidence Measurement of temporal relationships Multiple outcomes Rare exposures	High cost Can be time-consuming Open to bias due to losses to follow-up
Cross-sectional studies	Low cost Relatively quick to conduct No losses to follow-up Multiple outcomes Multiple exposures	No measurement of temporal relationships Prone to recall bias
Case-control studies	Multiple exposures Rare diseases Diseases with long latency Low cost Relatively quick to conduct	Can't estimate incidence Prone to selection bias and recall bias

The objective of case-control studies is to compare frequency of exposure among patients suffering from a disease (cases) versus healthy patients (controls). The exposure will occur prior to the disease being diagnosed (time of inclusion) for cases and before the time the control is included. By definition, a case-control study is always retrospective because it starts with an outcome and then traces back to investigate exposures (Fig. 4.2). Table 4.1 summarizes the main advantages and disadvantages of the major types of observational studies.

Cohort studies, also called incidence studies, provide the most direct measurement of the risk of developing a disease, although they may require long periods of follow-up, which makes them more prone to selection bias due to follow-up losses (when these are correlated with the exposure or outcome of interest). Cohort studies are particularly suited for assessing the effects of rare exposures or assessing multiple effects of a single exposure (Table 4.1).

As mentioned previously, cohort studies can be "prospective" or "retrospective" (also called *historical cohorts*) with regard to the timing of data collection. In a retrospective cohort study, both the exposure and outcome have already occurred at the study initiation. This type of cohort study is less time-consuming and costly than a prospective cohort study, but it depends on the availability of the relevant data, so it is more susceptible to reporting bias due to differential accuracy and completeness of data between the study groups.

An additional modification in the cohort design involves the selection of the cases and controls from a defined cohort (*nested case-control study*). This type of design can be particularly useful because it can lead to reduced exposure measurement costs and reduced selection bias (since cases and controls are sampled from the same population). For example, the UK Clinical Practice Research Datalink, a population-based cohort of primary care patients from the UK, can be used to perform a nested case-control analysis to determine whether high-intensity statin treatment is associated with reduced risk of rheumatoid arthritis (Tascilar et al. 2016).

Case-control studies are particularly efficient in terms of time and cost in relation to cohort studies. Cohort studies are particularly well suited for the evaluation of rare diseases or long latency diseases. The major potential problem of case-control studies is their susceptibility to selection bias (from the differential selection of the study cases or controls on the basis of their probability of exposure) and to recall bias (due to differential recall of exposure information between study groups, based on their disease status) (Table 4.1).

In cross-sectional studies, also known as *prevalence studies*, the measurements of exposure and effect are made at the same time. These studies may be purely descriptive and used to assess the prevalence of a particular disease in a defined population or may be used for generating hypotheses, by examining the relationship between a disease (or health outcome) and other variables of interest as they exist in a defined population at a single time point, for example, a cross-sectional study examining the prevalence, correlates, and sequencing of electronic cigarette and tobacco use among 11–16-year-olds in schools in Wales (de Lacy et al. 2017). Cross-sectional studies are relatively easy and inexpensive to conduct. The main disadvantage of cross-sectional studies is their inability to assess whether the exposure preceded or followed the outcome (temporal relationships cannot be demonstrated), because both exposure and outcome are assessed at the same time (Table 4.1).

4.2 Measures in Pharmacoepidemiology

4.2.1 Frequency Measures

The frequency is the number of times a particular value of a variable has been observed to occur. The frequency of a value can be expressed in different ways depending on the purpose. Common frequency measures are absolute frequencies, ratios, proportions, and rates:

Absolute Frequency describes the number of times n_i a particular value for a variable has been observed to occur. The simplest way to express a frequency is in absolute terms.

Ratio compares the frequency of one value n_i for a variable with the frequency of another value n_k for the variable. These frequencies may be related or totally independent. For example, in a study that included 20 men and 80 women, the ratio of men to women is 20:80 or 1:4, which indicates that for every man there are 4 women in the study.

Proportion describes the number of times n_i a particular value for a variable has been observed to occur (absolute frequency) in relation to the total number of values that might occur for that variable (N) in the same period (Eq. 4.1). It is a ratio in which the numerator (n_i) is included in the denominator (N). A proportion can be expressed as a fraction of one hundred (percentage). In the example above, the proportion of men in the study is 20:100 or 20%.

$$f_i = \frac{n_i}{N}. \tag{4.1}$$

Rate describes the number of times n_i a particular value for a variable has been observed to occur (absolute frequency) in a defined population, over a specified period of time (Eq. 4.2). The rate measures how quickly an event of interest occurs and is always reported per some unit of time. For example, if 10 deaths are observed per 100 people included in a study and followed during 1 year, we can estimate an annual death rate of 10%.

$$f_i = \frac{n_i}{N} \times time. \tag{4.2}$$

4.2.1.1 Measures of Disease Frequency in Epidemiology (Incidence and Prevalence)

An important feature in the measurement of disease frequency in epidemiology is the concept of *population at risk*, which includes all the individuals who are susceptible to the disease being studied. In other words, the population at risk is the group of people, healthy or sick, who would be counted as cases if they had the disease being studied. For example, when estimating the frequency of prostate cancer, women are not included in the *population at risk*.

Prevalence measures the proportion of subjects with the disease/event in the population at risk, at a particular point in time or over a period of time (Eq. 4.3).

$$Prevalence = \frac{Number\ existing\ cases\ at\ a\ specified\ time}{Number\ people\ at\ risk\ at\ the\ specified\ time} \times (10^n). \qquad (4.3)$$

10^n is usually 100 (or n = 2) and prevalence is often expressed as a percentage.
The prevalence measures the probability of presenting the disease in a particular period of time being studied. It is often expressed as a percentage (number of cases per 100 people). The prevalence is a measure of disease burden in a population in a given location and at a particular time; it's also useful to compare disease burden across populations, locations, or time periods. For example, the prevalence of obesity was 36.5% among US adults during 2011–2014, higher in women (38.3%) than in men (34.3%) (Ogden et al. 2016).

Incidence There are two types of incidence measures, *cumulative incidence* and *incidence rate*.

Cumulative Incidence (Risk) measures the proportion of subjects who get the disease/event in the population at risk, over a period of time (Eq. 4.4). In this case the population at risk (susceptible of developing the disease) only includes people free of the disease at the beginning of the study period (prevalent/existing cases must be excluded).

$$Cumulative\ Incidence \frac{Number\ new\ cases\ in\ specified\ period}{Number\ at\ risk\ (disease-free)\ at\ start\ of\ period}$$
$$\times (10^n). \qquad (4.4)$$

10^n is usually 100 (or n = 2) and cumulative incidence is often expressed as a percentage.
The cumulative incidence measures the probability of developing the disease over the period of time being studied. It is a measure of the risk of getting the disease.
In an outbreak, the term ***attack rate*** is often used as a synonym for risk. It is the risk of getting the disease during a specified period, such as the duration of an outbreak.

Incidence rate (IR) or Incidence Density measures how rapidly new events occur in a population. The numerator is the number of people who get the disease/event in the population at risk over a period of time. The denominator is the sum of time periods during which each person is disease-free and thus "at risk" of developing the disease (*person-time*) (Eq. 4.5).

$$Incidence\ Rate = \frac{Number\ new\ cases\ in\ specified\ period}{\sum person-time\ at\ risk} \times (10^n). \qquad (4.5)$$

10^n is usually 100 (or $n = 2$) and incidence rate is often expressed as new cases per 100 person-time at risk.

Each person contributes one unit to the person-time denominator for each unit of time (month, year, etc.) of observation prior to developing the disease, becoming lost to follow-up or death (see Exercise 1). For example, one hundred people at risk for 6 months contribute the same amount of person-time as 50 people at risk for 1 year.

Exercise 1 *Suppose an investigator is conducting one observational study of the rate of stroke. He follows five people from baseline up to 4 years. The results are graphically displayed below, showing how many years each person remained in the study disease-free:*

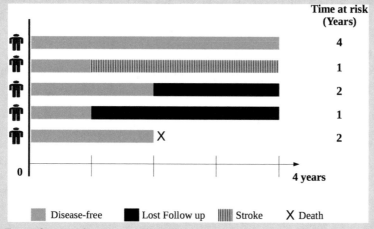

From this graph we can calculate:

- *Total person-years in the study = 4 + 1 + 2 + 1 + 2 = 10 person-years*
- *Incidence Rate of stroke = 2 cases per 10 person-years = 0.2 cases per person-year*
- *4-year cumulative incidence of stroke = 2/5 = 0.4 = 40%*

Relationship Between Prevalence and Incidence The prevalence of an event is dependent on both its *incidence rate* and its *average duration* (Eq. 4.6).

$$Prevalence = Incidence\ Rate \times Average\ Duration. \qquad (4.6)$$

For example, if the incidence of a disease is low but the duration of disease (i.e., until recovery or death) is long, the prevalence will be high relative to the incidence. This is the case of chronic diseases such as diabetes. On the other hand, if the incidence of a disease is high but the duration of disease is very short, the prevalence will be similar to the incidence. This is the case of acute conditions such as a common cold.

4.2.1.2   Other Commonly Used Measures of Disease Frequency in Epidemiology

Mortality or Crude Death Rate measures the risk or the probability of dying from any cause (or a specified cause) over the period of time being studied, usually 1 year. It includes the number of deaths in the numerator and in the denominator the number of persons at risk of dying during the study period (usually the size of the population at the middle of the study period) (Eq. 4.7).

$$Death\ Rate = \frac{Number\ deaths\ in\ a\ given\ period}{Number\ overall\ population\ in\ same\ period} \times 10^n. \qquad (4.7)$$

The death rates can be calculated for specific age groups of interest (age-specific death rate), and they can be adjusted for differences in the age distribution of two populations being compared (age-standardized death rate).

Case Fatality Rate (CFR) or Lethality measures the proportion of cases with a specified disease or condition who die over a period of time being studied (Eq. 4.8). It is a measure of the severity of the disease.

$$Fatality\ rate = \frac{Number\ deaths\ in\ a\ given\ period}{Number\ diagnosed\ cases\ in\ same\ period} \times 10^n. \qquad (4.8)$$

4.2.2   Association Measures

In epidemiological studies we can measure the strength of an association between a particular exposure and the subsequent occurrence of an event/disease. This requires the comparison of the disease frequency in two or more groups whose exposures have differed. These measures are often referred to as measures of effect and include the risk ratio (or relative risk, RR), incidence rate ratios (IRR), and odds ratios (OR), usually displayed in a contingency Table 4.2:

Risk Ratio (RR) compares the risk (cumulative incidence) of occurrence of a disease among individuals exposed (I_e) to that among those unexposed (I_o) (Eq. 4.9). It is the association measure used in cohort studies, from which incidences can be calculated.

$$RR = \frac{I_e}{I_o} = \frac{a/(a+b)}{c/(c+d)}. \qquad (4.9)$$

The RR can be used to quantify the strength of an association between a particular exposure and the subsequent occurrence of an event/disease. A RR > 1.0 indicates that the risk of disease is greater among those exposed compared with those

Table 4.2 Contingency table commonly used in epidemiology

	Present disease/event	Do not present disease/event	Total
Exposed	a	b	a + b
Unexposed	c	d	c + d
Total	a + c	b + d	a + b + c + d

unexposed (the exposure is a risk factor). For example, a RR of 1.2 means a 20% rise in the risk of the disease for those exposed compared to those who were unexposed. A RR < 1.0 (note that the RR cannot assume negative values) indicates a decreased risk of disease for the exposed (protective effect of the exposure) compared with those unexposed. Finally, a RR = 1 indicates that there is no association observed between the disease and the exposure, so the exposure has no effect on the risk of developing the disease.

The *incidence rate ratio* (IRR) is a similar measure, which compares incidence rates instead of cumulative incidences. Incidence *rate ratios* and *risk ratios* tend to be numerically similar for rare diseases.

Odds Ratio *Odds* are a transformation of the probability of an event. Let us imagine a situation where treatment A shows 20% of patients dead after 12 months. To transform this probability (20%) to *odds* let us first use proportions (rather than percentages) and the following equation:

$$Odds = \frac{p}{1-p}. \tag{4.10}$$

That is, the odds are defined as the probability of the event of interest happening (p) divided by the probability that the event does not happen ($1 - p$) (Eq. 4.10). In the example where 20% of patients are dead 12 months after exposure, the odds = 0.20/0.80 which is equal to 0.25. That is to say, the odds of the event of interest occurring are 0.25 to 1, or about 1:4 against.

When $p = 0.50$ (a 50/50 probability), the odds are equal to 1. This means the event is equally likely to occur or not to occur, that is, the odds are 1:1. When $p = 0.80$ (an 80% probability), the odds are 0.80/0.20, or 4.00. That means the odds are 4:1 in favor of the event happening, which makes sense because 0.80 is four times 0.20.

Odds ratios are usually used when comparing two groups on a dichotomous outcome. Here, the odds are calculated for both groups and then compared to each other as a ratio. Therefore,

$$Odds\ Ratio = \frac{Odds\ for\ Group\ 1}{Odds\ for\ Group\ 2}. \tag{4.11}$$

So if the odds are 0.50 in group 1 (e.g., 33% of patients are dead after 12 months in group 1) and 0.25 in group 2 (e.g., 20% of patients are dead), then the odds ratio is

0.50/0.25 or 2.00. The odds ratio (OR) of 2.00 means that the odds of the outcome in one group are twice the odds of the outcome in the other group.

Note that odds are not probabilities, and the OR is not a ratio of the probabilities involved (which is termed a risk ratio). A very useful feature is that the OR can be calculated from a case-control study, so it does not require knowledge of incidence rates. The formula (Eq. 4.12) can be derived from the contingency table presented above (Table 4.2).

$$OR = \frac{Odds_e}{Odds_o} = \frac{a/b}{c/d} = \frac{a*d}{b*c}. \tag{4.12}$$

When the disease is a rare event and the exposure is frequent in the population, we can assume that the OR is similar to the RR, if the cases and controls are representative of the general population with respect to exposure.

4.2.3 Measures of Potential Impact

The measures of disease impact estimate the health impact of a specific exposure on the occurrence of a disease in a particular population. These measures are useful to compare the potential impact of different public health strategies.

Attributable Risk (AR) or Risk Difference or Excess Risk is the incidence of the disease attributable to the exposure among the exposed group. It estimates the excess risk caused by the exposure in the exposed group, assuming causality. The AR is calculated as the difference between the incidence (risk) of the outcome among the exposed (I_e) and the incidence among the unexposed (I_o) (Eq. 4.13). Analogous to the risk difference, the rate difference is calculated by subtracting the incidence rate in the unexposed group from the incidence rate in the exposed group.

$$AR = I_e - I_o. \tag{4.13}$$

The AR is not often generalizable because it depends on the baseline risk in the unexposed, which often varies between populations. The AR can be expressed as a percentage of the incidence among the exposed, called *attributable fraction (% AR)* or *etiological fraction* (Eq. 4.14). The %AR is useful to estimate individual risks, e.g., to advise one exposed person of the expected reduction in the risk of the outcome if the exposure is eliminated (or reduced to the level of the comparison group) (see Exercise 2).

$$\%AR = \frac{(I_e - I_o)}{I_e} * 100 = \frac{(RR - 1)}{RR} * 100. \tag{4.14}$$

Exercise 2 *Suppose an investigator is conducting one observational study of the association between the exposure to X and the development of the disease Y. He follows 200 people during 1 year and observes that of the 100 exposed to X, 40 develop the disease Y; and of the other 100 unexposed to X, 20 develop the disease Y. These proportions are represented in the graph below:*

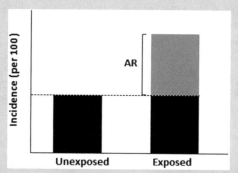

From the results of this study we can calculate RR = (40/100)/ (20/100) = 2.0

Being exposed to X increases the risk of developing the disease Y by 2 times:

AR = (40/100) − (20/100) = 20/100

For each 100 people exposed to X, 20 developed the disease Y due to the exposure X: %AR = AR/(40/100) = 50%

In the exposed group, 50% of the cases of disease can be attributed to the exposure X, i.e., would be prevented if the exposure was eliminated.

Population Attributable Risk (PAR) is the incidence of the disease attributable to the exposure among the entire population (not just among the exposed). It estimates the excess risk caused by the exposure in the entire population, assuming causality. The PAR is calculated as the difference between the incidence of the outcome among the entire population (I_t) and the incidence among the unexposed (I_o) (Eq. 4.15).

$$PAR = I_t - I_o. \tag{4.15}$$

The *PAR* can be expressed as a percentage of the incidence among the population, called *percentage of population attributable risk (%PAR)* (Eq. 4.16). The %PAR is relevant for public health decisions, since it measures the impact of exposure control measures in a population, i.e., the amount of the disease that could be reduced in the population if all the exposure is eliminated.

$$\%PAR = \frac{(I_t - I_o)}{I_t} * 100. \qquad (4.16)$$

Absolute Risk Reduction (ARR) It is a similar concept as the AR, but it measures the impact on the outcome when the exposure is protective (the incidence among the exposed (I_e) is lower than among the unexposed (I_0) (Eq. 4.17). It estimates the reduction in the rates of an undesirable outcome if the unexposed become exposed. It's a measure commonly used by pharmaceutical companies to express the benefits of using a particular medicine. For example, let's imagine that in an observational study comparing two treatments A and B to prevent stroke, the observed incidence of stroke was 0.3% in people taking drug A, compared with 0.6% in people taking drug B (the reference group). The ARR is 0.6–0.3% = 0.3%. That is, for each 1000 people taking drug A instead of B, there were 3 fewer stroke episodes.

$$ARR = I_o - I_e. \qquad (4.17)$$

The ARR can be expressed as a percentage of the baseline incidence (among the unexposed or reference group), called *Ppreventable fraction (PF)* or *relative risk reduction (RRR)* (Eq. 4.18). In the example above, the RRR is 0.3/0.6% = 50%, indicating that the risk of stroke was 50% lower in those taking drug A. Note that, although a 50% risk reduction sounds impressive when promoting treatment with drug A, the absolute risk difference is only 0.3%. Therefore, these two measures should be interpreted in conjuction. To be meaningful, the RRR needs to be set in the context of the baseline incidence of the event.

$$RRR = \frac{(I_o - I_e)}{I_o} * 100 = (1 - RR) * 100. \qquad (4.18)$$

> **Note** *These measures of impact cannot be calculated in case-control studies, as we are not measuring the incidence of the disease.*

4.3 Sources of Variability and Errors in Pharmacoepidemiology

Much of Pharmacoepidemiology is concerned with establishing associations between exposures and the risk of disease, which usually involves comparing representative groups of a population of interest that differ in exposure to a specific risk factor. In observational studies, however, often the groups being compared also share other characteristics that influence their risk of disease. In addition, observational studies are more prone to errors in the way the study sample is selected or during data collection and outcome measurement. Therefore, the association between an exposure and a disease may generally be due to (1) random errors, (2) systematic errors (*bias*), (3) confounding, or (4) causation. One wants to exclude/control the first three to be able to make causal inferences.

4.3.1   Errors (Random or Systematic)

In observational studies, a random error results in an estimate of effect being equally likely to be above or below the true value, as a result of chance. Random errors affect the precision of the study results, so they are usually quantified statistically and reduced to an acceptable level.

Systematic errors (called *bias*) result in an estimate of effect being more likely to be above or below the true value, resulting in a systematic deviation of inferences from the truth. *Bias* is often a consequence of errors during the design or conduct of an observational study. *Bias* should be avoided by careful study planning, since they cannot be controlled in the analysis; and if an association between an exposure and a disease results from *bias*, this simply means the finding is wrong.

The two major types of bias are known as *selection bias* and *information bias*.

Selection bias—results from the recruitment of patients (or retention in the study) in such a way that the sample being studied is systematically different from the target population to which the causal inference is to be made. For example, selection bias would result if heavy smokers are more likely to volunteer to participate in a study of the effect of smoking on the development of cardiovascular disease.

Information bias—results from systematic differences in the individual measurements or classification of the exposure or the disease being studied. For example, information bias would result if cases are more likely than controls to deny past exposure to a risk factor or if observers who know the exposure status systematically underestimate blood pressure measurements in the group of patients exposed to the treatment being studied.

4.3.2   Confounding

Confounding is a major issue in observational studies. Confounding occurs when the true estimate of the association between an exposure X and the outcome of interest Y is *hidden* or *distorted* by the effect of a third variable Z on the same outcome (Fig. 4.3). Failure to account for confounding can lead to the incorrect conclusion that the outcome Y is due to the exposure X.

For a variable to be a confounder, it must:

- Be associated with the exposure and be an independent risk factor of the outcome
- Be distributed unequally among the groups being compared

Fig. 4.3 Schematic illustration of a confounding in pharmacoepidemiology

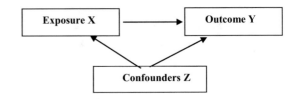

- Not be on the causal pathway between the exposure and the outcome of interest, that is, not be part of the chain of cause and effect that leads from the exposure to the outcome

4.3.2.1 How to Identify Confounding

Suppose the following results were obtained from an observational study of the association between drinking coffee and the risk of stroke:

	Stroke	
	Yes	No
Coffee drinkers	200	925
Coffee non-drinkers	90	960
	Estimated RR = 2.07	

The results of the study seem to indicate there is an association between drinking coffee and having a stroke (RR = 2.07). However, since it is known that people who drink coffee are more likely to smoke than people who don't drink coffee, the estimated association may actually reflect the association with tobacco use. In this study, smoking habits may be a confounder. To identify confounding we should stratify the results by the levels of the potential confounder:

	Group of smokers		Group of non-smokers	
	Stroke		Stroke	
	Yes	No	Yes	No
Coffee drinkers	100	650	38	337
Coffee non-drinkers	40	260	75	675
	Estimated RR = 1.00		*Estimated RR = 1.00*	

There is no statistical test to identify confounding. However, when we examine the measures of effect within each level (or strata) of the confounding variable, if they differ from the "crude" overall measure of effect (RR = 2.07), but are similar to each other (RR = 1.00), this is evidence of confounding. In this example, there is no association between drinking coffee and the risk of stroke (RR = 1), and smoking is a confounder variable in this study.

4.3.2.2   How to Deal with Confounding

Confounding is not an error but is concerned with alternative explanations for the effect being studied, so we should try to remove it to get nearer to the "true" effect of interest. Confounding can be handled in the statistical analysis using regression approaches, propensity score methods (see Sect. 4.4.2.1) or instrumental variables (see Sect. 4.4.2.2). When we use multivariate regression to deal with confounding, an "adjusted" estimate of effect is obtained as a weighted summary estimate of the results from the different strata of the confounding variable. We usually refer to this as "controlling" for a confounder. It is possible to control for several confounders simultaneously using multivariate statistical modeling.

If potential confounding remains even after the effect of many variables has been controlled for, we usually say we have *residual confounding*. This can happen for example when there are potential unmeasured confounders or when the confounders change over time.

4.3.3   Interaction (Effect Modification)

In observation studies, sometimes we are confronted with a situation where the effect of some exposure X on the outcome of interest Y is not merely confounded by another factor, but instead *it's modified by* another factor W. When an interaction is present, the effect of the exposure X differs according to each category of the effect modifier W.

4.3.3.1   How to Identify an Interaction

Suppose the following results were obtained from an observational study of the association between the use of combined oral contraception (COC) and the risk of venous thromboembolism (VTE):

	VTE	
	Yes	No
COC	353	54
Non-COC	253,000	73,000
	Estimated RR = 1.89	

It is known that smoking aggravates the risk of VTE in women using COC. To identify an interaction in this study, we stratified the results by the levels of the potential effect modifier:

	Group of smokers	Group of non-smokers
	VTE	VTE

(continued)

	Group of smokers		Group of non-smokers	
	VTE		VTE	
	Yes	No	Yes	No
	Yes	No	Yes	No
COC	329	133,671	86	119,000
Non-COC	32	39,000	22	34,000
	Estimated RR = 3.00		*Estimated RR = 1.07*	

When we examine the measures of effect within each level (or strata) of the effect modifier variable, if they differ from the "crude" overall measure of effect (RR = 1.89) *and* differ from each other (RR = 3.00 in the group of women who smoke vs. RR = 1.07 in the group of non-smokers), this is evidence of an interaction. Smoking is modifying the effect of COC on the development of VTE.

4.3.3.2   How to Deal with an Interaction

Interaction describes important relationships between two risk factors for the disease. So, while one tries to eliminate confounding, it is important to identify and describe an interaction by presenting the effect estimate stratified for each level of the effect modifier.

Interaction can be identified in the statistical analysis using regression approaches. When we use this approach, we create a special type of regression term called an interaction term by multiplying the two factors that we wish to test and then including the product in a multiple regression equation. A statistical test is then performed on the regression coefficient of the interaction term. If this test is statistically significant (usually at the 0.05 level), then effect modification is said to exist.

4.3.3.3   Stratification

Although the above procedure imagines testing an interaction term and controlling your error rate by using a statistical test to determine whether or not to stratify, there are times when one has planned to perform stratified analyses without a statistical test of an interaction term. This is perfectly legitimate when the desire is to examine the effect of the exposure separately in the two (or more) strata defined. As a method of statistical inquiry, it is best if this stratification is planned before any analysis begins. However, statisticians disagree on this point and some are much more permissive.

In addition to using stratification to examine heterogeneity of effects across strata, it is also possible to compute an overall estimate averaged across the strata to reduce bias or variability. The resulting averaged effect eliminates bias due to confounding by the stratification factor.

4.3.3.4 Three-Way, Four-Way, and More-Way Interactions

It is tempting to test three-way, four-way, and sometimes more than four-way interaction terms. One simple piece of advice is "don't," unless your data demand it. For example, an "exposure by effect modifier by time" interaction might be called for in a longitudinal study, where one is interested in whether the effect modification of the exposure varies over time. This might be a useful analysis to consider in longitudinal studies. However, as a general rule, the more terms added to an interaction, the more difficult the interpretation becomes.

The strength of the association between a predictor and an outcome variable may also be affected by a special case of confounding in the presence of mediator and moderator variables. These are introduced in Sect. 4.4.2.3 of the current chapter.

Key Concepts to Deal with Sources of Variability and Errors in Observational Studies

Random errors ➡ Quantify statistically	
Systematic errors (*bias*) ➡ Avoid	
Confounding ➡ Control	
Interaction ➡ Report	

4.4 Addressing Confounding/Interaction Analytically

4.4.1 Multivariate Analysis (OLS, Logistic, Cox, Others)

4.4.1.1 What It Is, When and Why to Use It

Often when dealing with scientific questions, we want to know if two things are associated. Is a new medication associated with better results for patients than an older medication? Is an increasing dose of diabetes medication associated with a larger decrease in HbA1c levels? How strongly are safety events associated with exposure to a medication?

When we try to answer these questions with data, one of the most powerful tools we have is regression. Simply put, regression is a method for quantifying the association of two (or more) variables. There are several types of regression, and the one to use has to do with the outcome and its distribution and the research question one is aiming at answering.

The different types of regressions are summarized below.

Ordinary Least Squares (OLS) Regression for Single and Multiple Predictors

For the analysis of continuous measures (blood pressure, HbA1c, quality of life measures), the preferred technique is called ordinary least squares (OLS) regression. The term ordinary is a misnomer, as although "ordinary," the OLS approach is a flexible and powerful way to answer many types of research questions. "Ordinary" refers to *linear* regression, as opposed to other types such as nonlinear regression and weighted regression.

OLS regression is usually introduced by describing its use as a prediction tool. If we want to assess the strength of association between two factors, one an exposure variable (e.g., to a new medication) and the other some outcome of interest (such as heart rate 60 min after exposure), we use a regression technique, and because the outcome in this case is a continuous measure, we use OLS regression.

To make our predictions, we gather data from a group of subjects on the dose of medication administered and their heart rate 60 min after administration. Using these data, we can derive an equation called a regression equation from the data. The mathematical values of this equation can be used to describe and assess the direction (positive or negative) and the magnitude (strength) of the association. Using this equation we can create predicted levels of the outcome for use with future patients. The equation we create based on our data can be simple or complex. The model equation for OLS regression is available in Table 4.3 at the end of Sect. 4.4.

If we use more than one predictor variable with an outcome, we have a multiple regression. An example of equations used for multiple regressions is provided in Table 4.3 and in the example below:

Example

Multiple regression equation	Interpretation
Returning to our medication and heart r example, suppose that we also know that age and sex have a role in predicting the heart rate of the patients: Heart rate $= \alpha + \beta 1 *$ Medication Dose $+ \beta 2 *$ Age $+ \beta 3 *$ Sex Heart rate $= 40.15 + 4.20 *$ Medication Dose $+ 0.14 *$ Age $+ 3.22 *$ Sex	This implies that we can get a predicted heart rate (beats per minute) by starting at 40.15 (the intercept), adding 4.20 for each gram of medication used, then adding 0.14 times age in years, and finally adding 3.22 times sex

Logistic Regression

When we have dichotomous (binary, or two category) outcome measures (dead or alive; recovered versus not recovered; treatment success versus treatment failure; etc.), we may want to model the probability of result A (e.g., dead) versus result B

Table 4.3 Types of modeling methods

Outcome	Modeling method	Equation	Interpretation
Continuous	OLS regression	$Y = \alpha + \beta X + e$	Y = outcome variable X = predictor variable α = intercept (on a graph, the intercept is the point at which the predicted value of y crosses the vertical axis) β = the "regression coefficient," slope of the line, the change in the predicted value of the outcome per each one unit change in the predictor e = "error," that is, the part of y we did not successfully predict
Continuous, multiple predictors	Multiple regression	$Y = \alpha + \beta 1 * X1 + \beta 2 * X2 + \beta 3 * X3 + e$	Y = outcome of interest $X1$, $X2$, and $X3$ = measured values of our predictors (of which there are now three) α = intercept $\beta 1$, $\beta 2$, and $\beta 3$ = regression coefficients e = error term, the unpredicted or unaccounted for variability in the outcome of interest
Dichotomous	Logistic regression	The probability $p_i = E(Y\vert X = x_i)$ is modeled by $\log(p_i/(1 - p_i)) = \alpha + \beta X$	Y = Y is 0 or 1 for each patient (say death) and each patients i has underlying even probability p_i of producing the outcome X = predictor variable $E(Y\vert X = x_i)$ = expected value of the outcome given the predictor variable X α = intercept β = the "regression coefficient"; to get the regression coefficient into the form of an odds ratio, we must counter-transform the regression coefficient β using exponentiation (or "anti-logging"), a transformation of the value from a logarithmic scale back to a normal arithmetic scale

(continued)

Table 4.3 (continued)

Outcome	Modeling method	Equation	Interpretation
Counts	Poisson regression	$\log[E(d_i\|x_i)] = \log[n_i] + \alpha + x_i\beta$	Let us assume we have two groups of people who have been exposed or not exposed to some risk factor of interest β = log relative risk for exposed patients compared with unexposed patients n_i = number of patients who are infected (i = 1) or are not infected (i = 0) d_i = number of deaths among people infected (i = 1) and uninfected (i = 0) x_i = 1 or 0 is a covariate that indicates patients who are (i = 1) or are not (i = 0) $E[(d_i\|x_i)]$: expected value of d_i given the covariate x_i values
Nested outcomes	Hierarchical level modeling	First level: $Y_{ij} = B_{0j} + B_{1j}X_{ij} + r_{ij}$ Second level: $\beta_{0j} = \gamma_{00} + \gamma_{01}G_j + U_{0j}$ $\beta_{1j} = \gamma_{10} + \gamma_{11}G_j + U_{1j}$ Combined Model: $Y_{ij} = \gamma_{00} + \gamma_{10}X_{ij} + \gamma_{01}G_j + \gamma_{11}GX_{ij} + U_{0j} + U_{1j}X_{ij} + r_{ij}$	Y_{ij} = dependent variable measured for ith level-1 unit nested within the jth level-2 unit X_{ij} = value on the level-1 predictor B_{0j} = intercept for the jth level-2 unit B_{1j} = regression coefficient associated with for the jth level-2 unit r_{ij} = random error In the level-2 models, the level-1 regression coefficients are used as outcome variables and are related to each of the level-2 predictors β_{0j} = intercept for the jth level-2 unit β_{1j} = slope for the jth level-2 unit G_j = value on the level-2 predictor γ_{00} = overall mean intercept adjusted for G γ_{10} = overall mean intercept adjusted for G γ_{01} = regression coefficient associated with G relative to level-1 intercept

			γ_{11} = regression coefficient associated with G relative to level-1 slope U_{0j} = random effects of the jth level-2 unit adjusted for G on the intercept U_{1j} = random effects of the jth level-2 unit adjusted for G on the slope
Survival analysis	Kaplan-Meier (product limit)—survival estimate	Probability of surviving t or more periods from entering the study is a product of the t observed survival rates for each period (i.e., the cumulative proportion surviving), given by the following: $S(k) = p_1 \times p_2 \times p_3 \times \dots \times p_t$ The proportion surviving period i having survived up to period i is given by: $p_i = (r_i - d_i)/r_i$	p_1 = the proportion surviving the first period p_2 = the proportion surviving beyond the second period conditional on having survived up to the second period and so on r_i = number alive at the beginning of the period d_i = number of deaths within the period
	Cox regression—hazard function estimate	The instantaneous rate of the event per unit of time, given that the individual has survived to that time: $h(t; xi) = h0(t)e^{x1B}, \quad t > 0$	Response variable = t_0, t, d Explanatory variable = x

(e.g., alive), using logistic regression. Like OLS, logistic regression can be used to establish the relationship between an exposure variable and the probability of an outcome. The exposure variable might be Treatment A versus Treatment B, and the outcome might be the probability of being dead or alive 12 months after exposure (a dichotomy).

The model equation for logistic regression looks very similar to that for OLS regression, but the dichotomous outcome is expressed in terms of log odds units (also known as "logits").

Other Types of Regression

Poisson Regression

In the examples above, regression was presented with a continuous (many levels) or a binary (two levels) outcome. Sometimes, the outcome may be completely different: the outcome could be counts of independent events.

Poisson regression may also be appropriate for rate data, where the rate is the count of events divided by the unit of observation. For example, a death rate is the count of deaths divided by person-years of observation. Poisson regression is a special case of the generalized linear model (GLM) for data that are not normally distributed; for Poisson regression, the generalized linear model assumes that the outcome variable has a Poisson distribution. If we consider, for instance, trying to predict the number of deaths resulting from flu virus infections in Norway, the Poisson distribution would assume that if d number of deaths (with a binomial distribution, dead or alive) from the flu are observed among n patients who contracted the flu virus, π is the probability that a person infected with the flu virus dies. The Poisson distribution is a simple way to make assumptions in the instance of count data, which simplifies the relation between the probability of an event in relation to the frequency of the observed event and the total sample size of the population.

The Poisson regression model is presented in Table 4.3. As observed in the Poisson regression model, the log (rate) parameter is modeled as the linear predictor of the outcome. Observed counts are assumed to be sampled from a Poisson distribution. Simple Poisson regression generalizes to multiple Poisson regression in the same way that simple logistic regression generalizes to multiple logistic regression.

Negative Binomial Regression

The negative binomial distribution can be used as an alternative to the Poisson distribution if there is an "overdispersed" count outcome variable. The main feature of the Poisson model is the assumption that the mean and variance of the count data are equal. However, this equal mean-variance relationship does not often occur in observational studies. In most cases, the observed variance is larger than the assumed variance, which is called "overdispersion." An example of overdispersion is that the number of observed deaths in an area is influenced by seasonal changes, such as the weather, air pollution, or a holiday. The underlying expected mean mortality count will change over time depending on these variables. For instance, in the flu example provided above, we can anticipate that deaths due to flu infections might be higher in winter than in the summer. Overdispersion results in underestimating the variance of the estimated parameter and thus produces a misleading conclusion if a Poisson distribution is assumed. Negative binomial regression can be considered a generalization of Poisson regression since it has the same mean structure as Poisson regression but has an extra parameter to handle overdispersion.

Hierarchical Linear Modeling

Hierarchical linear modeling (HLM), also called multilevel modeling, is a generalization of OLS regression with random effects that capture multilevel data. It is used to analyze variance in the outcome when the predictor variables are at varying hierarchical levels, for example, when patients in a given hospital share variance according to their common medical treatment team and common medical system. HLM accounts for situations where groups are clustered together, such as patients within the same hospital or geographical region. HLM simultaneously investigates relationships within and between hierarchical levels of grouped data, making it more efficient at accounting for variance among variables at different levels than other analyses.

In observational studies, there are an array of situations where HLM models can be used, for instance, for longitudinal data where observations are nested within individuals. Longitudinal HLM models, sometimes described as growth curve models, treat time in a flexible manner that allows the modeling of nonlinear change across time and accommodates uneven intervals between time points and unequal numbers of observations across individuals.

In addition to HLM's ability to assess cross-level data relationships and accurately disentangle the effects of between- and within-group variance, it is also a preferred method for nested data because it requires fewer assumptions than other statistical methods. HLM can accommodate non-independence of observations, missing data, small and/or discrepant group sample sizes, and heterogeneity of variance across repeated measures. A disadvantage of HLM is that it requires large sample sizes for adequate power. HLM equations used for a two-level model, the simplest form of HLM regression, are presented in Table 4.3.

Stepwise Regression

In an observational data set with many covariates, one possible goal of multiple variable regression is to identify a fitted model that provides reasonably precise estimates of the mean response using a parsimonious set of explanatory variables (covariates). If all models using a pool of covariates can be estimated, methods to choose the best models are available. Under some circumstances there may be considerable substantive knowledge about the phenomenon being observed that can offer guidance in selecting a limited number of covariates.

A large number of automated procedures exist to select a statistical model. Each has distinct criteria for optimal model selection. One popular class of model selection procedures, called stepwise selection, uses an automatic variable selection process that either adds (forward selection) or removes (backward elimination) individual covariates from a group of potential explanatory variables from the model at each step, thus the term "stepwise regression," Chapter 6 describes alternative and more powerful procedures for variable selection than those presented in this chapter.

The forward stepwise model starts with no covariates in the model. At each step, a predictor variable is added to the model in a sequential manner. Different model "goodness of fit" statistics coefficients help decide which variables are kept in the final model. The backward stepwise model starts with all covariates in the model; a covariate is removed from the model at each step. The algorithm includes a stopping rule based on a goodness of fit statistic that determines when no further covariates are removed from the model.

Properly used, the stepwise regression allows consideration of a large number of potential covariates and can be used to fine-tune model. A common example occurs when one tries to determine a set of potential genes from a sequenced genome that is related to a disease of interest. If there are no hypotheses as to which gene might be more likely to be associated with the disease a priori, stepwise regression could be a useful tool to identify a set of potentially responsible genes. It is also useful when the best possible prediction for individual patients is the goal and the association of variables in the overall model is of limited interest. However, there is no guarantee that the *best* model will be constructed from the available variables or even that a good model will be found by this procedure.

Residuals

When we make a regression line using a regression equation, we note that rarely do all the points of observed data fall exactly on our line. The regression line is the expected values, and *residuals* are the observable distance (error) between the expected values and the observed values. They can be viewed as a vertical distance from the line to each individual observed data point on a two-dimensional graph. The line that best fits the data is the line that is closest to the actual measured values. For mathematical reasons, residuals are squared to ensure that they don't cancel each other as some errors are positive and some negative. Hence the goal is choosing a line with the smallest total squared residuals or the "least squares." Residuals are therefore a sign that the model equation does not do a perfect job in explaining observed data. When residuals are too large however, several options exist to improve model prediction, including the addition of more explanatory variables as in multiple regression.

P-Values, Confidence Intervals, and Error

In practice the interpretation of the results of a regression analysis is more complex than simply looking at the regression coefficients themselves. Traditionally, statisticians used p-values—the proportion of replications of the study where a regression coefficient as large or larger than the one observed would arise by chance alone in a hypothetical population constructed under the null hypothesis that no actual relationship exists—as a basis for interpretation, and this trend continues.

When the p-value was less than 0.05, the result was deemed to be "statistically significant at the 0.05 level," meaning that less than 5 times out of 100 would we expect to get a result by chance alone that is as large or larger than the regression coefficient we estimated using our data and our statistical software.

More common now is to look at the 95% Confidence Interval, that is, the range of values that are compatible with the data we have. The 95% Confidence Interval is constructed mathematically using the variability of the data adjusted for the information the predictor variables share when predicting the outcome of interest. The details are complex and best left to computers and professional statisticians. It is enough to know that the 95% Confidence Interval gives us a range of values for the regression coefficient that are likely given the data collected and helps us to understand the degree of statistical uncertainty in the results our data give us.

Survival Analysis

Survival analysis concerns data collected in the form of time until an event of interest occurs and is also called time-to-event analysis. Historically the event of interest was death, but now survival analysis encompasses other events, such as time until diagnosis of a specific disease, time to experience an effect after initiating a treatment, etc.

In survival analysis, we analyze not only the **number** of people who experience the event of interest (a dichotomous variable of event status during the study observation period, e.g., 1 = event occurred or 0 = event did not occur) but also the **time** at which the event occurs for each individual.

The time-to-event is measured from time zero (the start of the study or the point from which the individual is considered to be at risk of experiencing the event of interest) until the first of the following:

1. The event occurs.
2. The participant is lost to follow-up.
3. Death [if not the event of interest].
4. The study ends.

These times to (2) and (3) are called censored times.

An important assumption in survival analysis is that the censoring is *non-informative*, i.e., people who are censored are representative of all people who remain at risk. Thus, censoring does not give us any information about the event being studied, and the information coming from patients lost to follow-up can be ignored.

In observational studies, patients often are lost to follow-up for reasons that can be associated with the study event. For example, patients whose disease is well controlled don't recognize the need to consult a doctor; or the most severe cases of a disease are lost to follow-up because patients change practice to seek additional medical advice. Several methods have been described to deal with the problem of informative censoring. These include imputation techniques for missing data, sensitivity analyses to mimic best and worst-case scenarios, and use of the dropout event as a study end-point.

Survival and Hazard

Survival data are generally described and modeled in terms of two related probabilities, namely, *survival* and *hazard*.

- The **survival probability** (also called the survivor function) $S(t)$ is the probability that an individual survives from the time zero to a specified future time t. Survival probabilities are then estimated for different values of t.
- The **hazard** is usually denoted by $h(t)$ or $\lambda(t)$ and is the probability that an individual who is at risk at time t has an event at that time. It represents the instantaneous rate of the event per unit of time, given that the individual has survived to that time.

In summary, the hazard relates to the incident event rate, while survival reflects cumulative non-occurrence of an event.

Kaplan-Meier (Product Limit): Survival Estimate

Survival curves usually plot time on the X-axis and survival (proportion of people at risk, i.e., free of the outcome of interest) on the Y-axis.

A number of methods can be used to model survival data, which differ in terms of the assumptions that are made about the distribution of survival times in the population. Some estimate the survival distribution by making parametric assumptions, including the exponential, Weibull, Gompertz, generalized gamma, log-logistic, and log-normal distributions (Rodríguez 2010). However, it is often hard to rely on any given parametric distribution to model times to event; hence we resort to more flexible non-parametric or semi-parametric modeling (Kaplan and Meier 1958).

Cox Regression: Hazard Estimates

The **hazard function** is the *probability that if an individual survives to t, he will experience the event in the next instant.* The hazard estimates the expected number of events per individual per unit of time. Suppose that the hazard at a particular time t is $k(t) = 0.5$ and that the unit of time is 1 year. This means that on average 0.5 events will occur per individual at risk 1 year. In a group of 20 individuals at risk during 2 years, we would expect to observe 20 events.

The aim of fitting a Cox model to time-to-event data is to estimate the effect of covariates on the baseline hazard function. The baseline hazard function is estimated non-parametrically. As a result, Cox regression models enable us to estimate a *hazard ratio* (HR) (see below for details on comparison of hazards). The Cox proportional hazards model is called a ***semi-parametric model***, because there are no assumptions about the shape of the baseline hazard function.

Comparing Survival Curves and Hazards

In observational studies, we are often interested in assessing whether there are differences in survival (or cumulative incidence of event) among different groups of participants.

Comparison of two survival curves can be done using a statistical hypothesis test called the *log rank* test. It is used to test the null hypothesis that there is no difference between the population survival curves (i.e., the probability of an event occurring at any time point is the same for each population). The *log rank test* for two groups computes the *chi-square* (X^2) test statistics that is based on summing up differences between the observed and expected number of events across all event times, where the expected number of events is computed under an assumption that the hazards for the two groups are equal at every event time.

Comparison of groups of participants with respect to their hazards can be done using the *Cox proportional hazard model*, which enables the difference between hazards of particular groups of patients to be tested while allowing for other factors. The Cox model estimates an HR, which gives a relative event rate between groups. An HR of 2.0 does not mean that the survival time in group A is twice the survival in group B. An HR of 2.0 means that a patient in group A who has not died at a certain time point has twice the probability of death by the next time point compared to a patient in group B.

In a Cox model it is assumed that the HR is constant over time, i.e., if the risk for dying at a particular point in time in group A is, for example, twice that in the risk in group B, then at any other time, it will still be twice that in the group B—this is known as the *proportional hazard assumption*.

The proportional hazard assumption is very important for the appropriate use of the *log rank test* and the *Cox proportional hazards regression model*. If this assumption does not hold, one approach is to stratify the data into subgroups within which the hazards are proportional and estimate different baseline hazards in each stratum.

Adjustment

Regression techniques can be used to create predicted values of outcome variables, which is a useful function; however, because more than one exposure (or predictor) variable can be used at a time, we can assess the relationship of variables in a much more complex situation. This approach is multiple regression as explained above, and it is the recommended way to handle adjustment, confounding, and effect modification.

The simplest way to use multiple regression approaches (whether OLS, logistic, Poisson, or proportional hazards models) is for the purpose of *adjustment*. For example, we may want to know what the average value of a sample of patients is for some variable (such as systolic blood pressure) "adjusted" for the effects of age.

Adjustment works by averaging out the effect of a separate factor (e.g., age) and often requires a regression approach. To do this sort of adjustment, simply add the adjustment factor to your regression equation.

4.4.2 Advanced Methods of Adjustment

4.4.2.1 Propensity Score

A major challenge in observational studies in Pharmacoepidemiology is that the treatment assignment is a deliberate choice made by physicians, patients, and/or the payer and is far from being random. So there may be multiple risk factors that are not balanced between comparison groups. As we described, model-based adjustments and stratification techniques are widely used in observational studies to deal with these confounders. However, these methods may not perform well when we have many confounders. In 1983, alternative methods for the control of confounding in observational studies based on propensity score were proposed (Rosenbaum and Rubin 1983).

The *propensity score* (PS) is the individual's probability of receiving a treatment conditional on observed baseline covariates. So, any two patients with the same PS have the same predicted probability of being exposed to treatment A rather than treatment B; and although they can have different values for specific covariates, overall the covariates included will be balanced. In other words, the multivariate distribution of the covariates used to estimate the PS differs only randomly between the two treatment groups. For this reason, PS are often said to mimic random treatment allocation in clinical trials, although they do so only with respect to confounders that have been measured.

Propensity Score Estimation

PS is most often estimated using a logistic regression model, in which treatment status is regressed on observed baseline characteristics. In observational studies, there are usually two possible treatments A and B. Each patient usually receives only one of the treatments and has one of the two potential outcomes, $Y(0)$ and $Y(1)$, the outcomes under the treatment A and the treatment B, respectively. The treatment effect is defined as $Y(1) - Y(0)$, and the average treatment effect is defined as $ATE = E (Y(1) - Y(0))$. Rosenbaum and Rubin (Rosenbaum and Rubin 1983; Rubin 1974, 1997) showed that unbiased estimates of ATE can be obtained by conditioning on the PS, where at each value of the PS the distribution of the covariates is the same in both treated groups. For this, Rosenbaum and Rubin defined two conditions that must be met:

- *Treatment assignment is independent of the potential outcomes conditional on the observed baseline covariates.* This condition is known as the "no unmeasured confounders" assumption: all variables that affect treatment assignment and outcome have been measured.
- *Every patient has a nonzero probability to receive either treatment.* This condition assumes that a patient with any covariate profile has a nonzero probability of treatment assignment. This means that if patients with certain covariate profiles have a zero probability of receiving either treatment, it is not possible to account for that in the PS modeling.

Variables Selection

A crucial issue when using PS methods is how to select the variables to include in the PS model. All the variables related to both the exposure and the outcome (the confounders) should be included in the PS model. Simulation studies suggest that variables that are unrelated to the exposure but related to the outcome should also be included in PS model. The inclusion of these variables will decrease the variance of an estimated exposure effect without increasing bias. In contrast, the inclusion of variables that are related to the exposure but not (or weakly related) to the outcome can increase the variance of the estimated effect without decreasing bias (Brookhart et al. 2006a). Recent research has shown that omitting covariate interactions that may be important for both predicting treatment assignment and/or outcome may result in a miss-specified PS model; therefore simplistic modeling strategies may be inadequate in these cases (Zagar et al. 2017).

During the process of fitting the PS model, it is important to check that covariates are balanced across exposure groups. We use a quantity similar to the effect size, known as the standardized bias, to quantify this balance. The standardized bias for continuous covariates is calculated by dividing the difference in means of the covariate between the treated group and the comparison group by the standard deviation. This process can be repeated until the balance no longer improves when adding terms to the PS model, or a decision criterion can be used, that, for example, considers a covariate balanced if the standardized bias is less than 0.25.

After estimating the PS, the next step is to evaluate the overlap of the PS distributions among the two exposure groups. This can be examined graphically (Fig. 4.4). It is common to observe non-overlap at the extremes of the PS distributions. If the non-overlap is small, the PS analysis can be restricted to the range of common PS, that is, excluding patients with a PS lower that the lowest PS observed

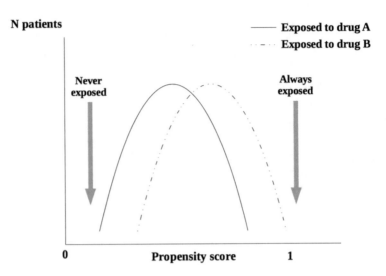

Fig. 4.4 Hypothetical distribution of propensity scores

in the comparison group and patients with the PS higher than the highest PS in the comparison group.

Once estimated, the PS is then a single "summarized" confounding covariate that can be used in various ways to control for confounding: *matching, stratification, and weighting strategies*. Adding the PS as a covariate to a regression model is also an option, although there is mixed evidence regarding its performance (Rubin 2004; Schafer and Kang 2008), and this is not recommended.

Matching

One strategy is to match each patient exposed to treatment A to one or more patients exposed to treatment B who share a similar value of the PS. A variety of matching methods are available that can include individual matching of patients with the closest propensity score (nearest neighbor matching) or selecting an equal number of patients in each exposed group within categories of PS (frequency matching). The matching can be done with or without replacement (each patient is uniquely matched to another patient).

Stratification

As an alternative to matching, we can include all the patients in the analysis and stratify them into subclasses based on their PS value, so that within the subclasses the propensity score is similar. We then estimate the *average treatment effect* (ATE) within each subclass as if assignment was completely random. To estimate the overall average treatment effect, we average the within-stratum estimated average treatment effects, weighted by the subclass sizes. Often we combine subclassification with further covariance adjustments.

Weighting Strategies

An alternative weighting technique may be used when the desired estimate is the ATE, the *inverse probability of treatment weighting* (IPTW) using the PS. With IPTW, each patient is weighted by the inverse probability of receiving the treatment.

A concern with IPTW may arise when some weights are very large and thus can bias the estimates of the treatment effect. To reduce the variability of the IPTW weights and give patients with extreme weights less influence, a technique referred to as *stabilization* is commonly used. Stabilization consists of multiplying the treatment and comparison weights (separately) by a constant, equal to the expected value of being in the treatment or comparison groups (Robins et al. 2000).

4.4.2.2 Instrumental Variables

In observational studies, the impact of confounders on the estimation of a causal treatment effect can be adjusted by methods such as propensity scores, regression, and matching. However, these methods only control for measured confounders. The instrumental variable (IV) method has been proposed to control for both measured and unmeasured confounders, although it should be emphasized that the causal analysis of observational data involves an untestable assumption about the IV (see details in "Assessing IV Validity and Strength" section). An instrumental variable (IV) is a variable that (see Fig. 4.5):

- Is associated with the exposure X
- Is independent of C (the association between the IV and X is not confounded by other variables)
- Is independent of outcome Y given X and C (there is no correlation between the IV and other variables explaining the outcome, except by the direct effect on X)

An appropriate IV can help address both measured and unmeasured confounding in observational studies, since it can realistically mimic the treatment allocation process of a randomized study.

Examples
An IV analysis can be most helpful in reducing unmeasured confounding by indication (i.e., when the indication for treatment is associated with the risk of

(continued)

the studied outcome). The "physician's prescribing preference" (PPP) for a given drug A over B can be used as a valid IV if the physician's preference is not associated with the outcome (physicians who frequently prescribe drug A are not more likely to co-prescribe drug C with an effect on the outcome of interest) nor to the patient-level confounders (physicians who prefer drug A are not systematically treating patients differently from physicians who prefer drug B) (Brookhart et al. 2006b; Uddin et al. 2016; Ionescu-Ittu et al. 2012; Smith and Ebrahim 2003). *The use of this preference-based IV is illustrated in a study comparing the effect of exposure to COX-2 inhibitors with non-selective, nonsteroidal anti-inflammatory medications on gastrointestinal complications* (Brookhart et al. 2006b).

Another example of the use of IV analysis that has become increasingly common is "Mendelian randomization"; in which genetic variants are IVs due to the random assortment of genes from parents to offspring, meaning that observational studies of genetic variants have similar properties to intention to treat analyses in randomized controlled trials (Bennett 2010; Smith 2006). *A classic example is a Mendelian dominant condition called "familial hyper-cholesterolemia," in which mutations of the low density lipoprotein (LDL) receptor gene lead to high circulating cholesterol concentrations (the exposure) and premature coronary heart disease (the outcome)* (Smith and Ebrahim 2005). *The inference to be made from this evidence (not susceptible to reverse causation or confounding) is that high blood cholesterol concentration is an important cause of coronary heart disease in the general population* (Smith and Ebrahim 2005).

Assessing IV Validity and Strength

Finding an appropriate IV can be challenging. It is important to evaluate whether the variable satisfies the assumptions needed to be a valid IV and if the association between the IV and the exposure is strong.

Not all of the assumptions of an IV can be tested. An F-test from a simple linear regression model can be used to assess whether an IV is associated with the exposure

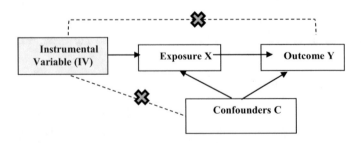

Fig. 4.5 Schematic illustration of the assumptions of an instrumental variable

X. However, there is no test to whether the IV is independent of unmeasured confounders and for the same reason the exclusion restriction (i.e., the IV only influences the outcome through its influence on the exposure under study) cannot be tested. Therefore, these assumptions need to be checked empirically based on the knowledge of the particular study subject. One way to assess whether these assumptions hold is to examine the association between the IV and the measured confounders (e.g., patient characteristics). If an IV is related to the measured confounders, then it's reasonable to expect that it is also related to the unmeasured confounders. Exploring the association between an IV and concomitant treatments can also help determine whether the exclusion restriction is violated. If the IV is associated with a concomitant treatment that affects the outcome, then the exclusion restriction is violated.

A second critical issue is the strength of the relationship between the IV and the exposure, with weaker instruments yielding less precise and more biased estimates, even if the IV is valid.

Estimation of Treatment Effect Using an IV

Klungel et al. (2015) published a good overview of the methods for the estimation of a treatment effect using an IV, indicating their possible advantages and limitations for epidemiological research (Klungel et al. 2015). In summary, if the exposure and outcome are both continuous variables and show a linear relation, the IV analysis generally uses the two-stage least squares method. In case of a nonlinear relation, a two-stage residual inclusion may be a suitable alternative. In time-to-event analysis using IVs, the two-stage method has been applied with a Cox proportional hazards model used as the second-stage model (Klungel et al. 2015).

In settings with binary outcomes as well as nonlinear relations between exposure and outcome, generalized method of moments (GMM), structural mean models (SMM), and bivariate probit models perform well, but GMM and SMM are generally more robust. The standard errors of the IV estimate can be calculated using a robust or bootstrap method (Klungel et al. 2015).

The interpretation of the IV effect estimates always needs to take into account the underlying assumptions of the estimation methods, the assumptions of the IV, and another assumption called the homogeneity/monotonicity assumption (Fang et al. 2012). Homogeneity assumes that the direction of the effect of IV on *X* is the same for everyone in the study sample (i.e., there is no effect modification). Under this assumption, the IV analysis estimates an average effect of the exposure. When the exposure effects are not homogeneous across IV levels, the IV estimates, usually called *local average treatment effect* (LATE), are only informative for a subset of the exposed population.

4.4.2.3 Mediator and Moderator Variables

Section 4.3 of this chapter introduced us to the concepts of confounding and effect modifiers. Mediator and moderator variables are other variables that could affect the strength of the association between predictors and outcomes in a model. An assumption of regression is that independent variables should not be correlated one with another. In health outcomes however, this is rarely the case, as a variable representing a biological factor such as an inflammatory marker, for instance, will likely affect the reporting of another variables such as fatigue, or pain, by a given patient.

Baron and Kenny (1986) introduced the concept of moderator and mediator variables to distinguish variables that could affect the strength of the association between an exposure/independent variable and an outcome/dependent variable (Baron and Kenny 1986).

A moderator variable is a variable that affects the direction and/or strength of the relation between an exposure and the outcome of interest. In other words, a moderator is a third variable that affects the correlation between two other variables (Fig. 4.6). In the more familiar analysis of variance (ANOVA) terms, a basic moderator effect can be represented as an interaction between an independent variable and a factor that specifies the appropriate conditions for its operation.

A variable may function as a mediator variable rather than a moderator to the extent that it accounts for the relation between the exposure and the outcome. A variable is a mediator when (1) there is a relationship between the independent and dependent variable, (2) there is a relationship between the independent and mediator variable, (3) there is a relationship between the mediator and the dependent variable, and (4) with the mediator added to the model, the relationship between the independent and dependent variables decreases and could become null if it is a complete mediation (Fig. 4.7). For example, when studying the association between socioeconomic status and the development of cardiovascular disease, the type of diet can be a mediator variable, since economic deprivation may influence diet, with consequences on the risk of cardiovascular disease.

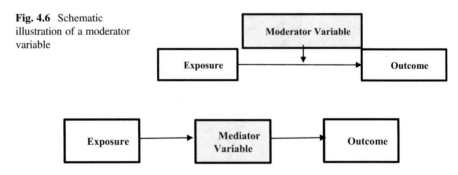

Fig. 4.6 Schematic illustration of a moderator variable

Fig. 4.7 Schematic illustration of a mediator variable

Whereas moderator variables specify when certain effects will hold, mediators speak to how or why such effects occur. Another way to think about this issue is that a moderator variable is one that influences the strength of a relationship between two other variables and a mediator variable is one that explains the relationship between the two other variables because it is on the causal pathway that connects the exposure to the outcome.

The general test for mediation is to examine the relation between the predictor and the outcome variable, the relation between the predictor and the mediator variables, and the relation between the mediator and outcome variables. All of these correlations should be high. The relation between predictor and outcomes should be reduced (to zero in the case of total mediation) after controlling the relation between the mediator and outcome variables. A regression model would model three independent variables: the predictor, the moderator, and an interaction term between the predictor and the moderator variable.

A confounding variable may appear similar to a mediator variable, except for the direction of the effect between them and the exposure variable. Mediators are additionally characterized as lying on the causal pathway between exposure and outcome. When adjusting for confounding in observational studies, care must be taken to not include mediator variables, to the extent that the effect of an exposure on an outcome goes through mediator variables, adjusting for those variables would wash away the effect of interest. Our main interest is to quantify whether and how much of the effect of the exposure on the outcome of interest is mediated by these variables and elucidate the relationship between the exposure and the outcome.

Structural Equation Modeling, Path Analysis, and the Assessment of Direct and Indirect Effects

Extending from the moderator model is path analysis and the analysis of simultaneous moderation analyses. When dealing with multidimensional relationships between and among constructs such as is the case in most Pharmacoepidemiological research, statistical approaches that go beyond univariate and multivariate linear regression where there is a single outcome variable and potentially multiple non-correlated exposure variables are often valuable. The optimal statistical environment for estimating these relationships is structural equation modeling (SEM) which is a sophisticated methodological approach that integrates concerns about measurement, statistics, and theory in one conceptual and analytic framework. Path analysis is the simplest form of SEM, as it can be thought of as a multiple regression focusing on causality.

Path analysis assesses the direct and indirect (through a mediator variable) effects between predictor and outcome variables. In path analysis models, mediator variables are both outcome variables for a direct path with a predictor variable situated at the beginning of the path (called an exogenous variable) and a predictor variable for an outcome variable situated further down the path (endogenous variable). The statistical significance of both direct and indirect paths can be obtained.

The structural model estimates the relationships between all variables assessed simultaneously and whether the effects among the different variables are direct or indirect (Kline 2005). These variables can influence one another unidirectionally (a recursive model) or reciprocally (a nonrecursive model) (Kline 2005). The data are tested to see how well they fit a specified model using a series of separate, but interdependent, multiple regression equations for each outcome variable simultaneously by specifying the structural model (Kline 2005). The strength of the influence of one factor on another is indicated by the *path coefficient* which is a standardized regression coefficient that also gives information about the directionality of the path. A variety of goodness of fit indexes exist to measure the discrepancy between the observed and the model implied covariance matrices, adjusted for the degrees of freedom of the model (Kline 2005).

References

Tascilar K, Dell'Aniello S, Hudson M, Suissa S. Statins and Risk of Rheumatoid Arthritis: A Nested Case-Control Study. Arthritis Rheumatol. 2016 Nov;68(11):2603-2611. doi: https://doi.org/10.1002/art.39774.

de Lacy E, Fletcher A, Hewitt G, Murphy S, Moore G. Cross-sectional study examining the prevalence, correlates and sequencing of electronic cigarette and tobacco use among 11-16-year olds in schools in Wales. BMJ Open. 2017 Feb 3;7(2):e012784. doi: https://doi.org/10.1136/bmjopen-2016-012784.

Ogden C.L., Carroll M.D., Fryar C.D., Flegal K.M. Prevalence of Obesity Among Adults and Youth: United States, 2011–2014. Available from https://www.cdc.gov/nchs/data/databriefs/db219.pdf. Accessed December 2016.

Rodríguez G. Parametric Survival Models. 2010. Available from http://data.princeton.edu/pop509/ParametricSurvival.pdf Accessed December 2016.

Kaplan EL, Meier P. Nonparametric estimation from incomplete observations. J Am Stat Assoc.1958;53:457–481.

Rosenbaum PR, Rubin DB. The central role of the propensity score in observational studies for causal effects. Biometrika. 1983;70:41–55.

Rubin D. Estimating causal effects of treatments in randomized and nonrandomized studies. Journal of Educational Psychology. 1974;66:688–701.

Rubin D.B. Estimating causal effects from large data sets using propensity scores. Annals of Internal Medicine. 1997;127:757–763.

Brookhart M.A., Schneeweiss S., Rothman K.J., Glynn R.J., Avorn J., Stürmer T. Variable selection for propensity score models. Am J Epidemiol. 2006a Jun 15;163(12):1149-56. Epub 2006 Apr 19.

Zagar AJ, Kadziola Z, Lipkovich I, Faries DE. Evaluating different strategies for estimating treatment effects in observational studies. J Biopharm Stat. 2017;27(3):535-553. doi: https://doi.org/10.1080/10543406.2017.1289953. . Epub 2017 Feb 7.

Rubin DB. On principles for modeling propensity scores in medical research. Pharmacoepidemiology and Drug Safety. 2004.

Schafer JL, Kang J. Average causal effects from nonrandomized studies: a practical guide and simulated example. Psychological Methods. 2008;13:279–313.

Robins JM, Hernan MA, Brumback B. Marginal structural models and causal inference in epidemiology. Epidemiology 2000;11:550–560.

Brookhart MA, Wang PS, Solomon DH, Schneeweiss S. Evaluating short-term drug effects using a physician-specific prescribing preference as an instrumental variable. Epidemiology. 2006b May; 17(3):268-75.

Uddin MJ, Groenwold RH, de Boer A, *et al*. Evaluating different physician's prescribing preference based instrumental variables in two primary care databases: a study of inhaled long-acting beta2-agonist use and the risk of myocardial infarction. Pharmacoepidemiol Drug Saf. 2016 Mar; 25 Suppl 1:132-41.

Ionescu-Ittu R., Abrahamowicz M., Pilote L. Treatment effect estimates varied depending on the definition of the provider prescribing preference-based instrumental variables. J Clin Epidemiol. 2012 Feb; 65(2):155-62.

Smith G.D., Ebrahim S. 'Mendelian randomization': can genetic epidemiology contribute to understanding environmental determinants of disease? Int J Epidemiol. 2003 Feb; 32(1):1-22.

Bennett D.A. An introduction to instrumental variables-part 2: Mendelian randomisation. Neuroepidemiology. 2010; 35(4):307-10.

Smith G.D. Randomised by (your) god: robust inference from an observational study design. J Epidemiol Community Health. 2006 May; 60(5):382-8.

Smith G.D., Ebrahim S. What can mendelian randomisation tell us about modifiable behavioural and environmental exposures? BMJ. 2005 May 7; 330(7499):1076-9.

Klungel O.H., Jamal Uddin M., de Boer A., Belitser S.V., Groenwold R.H., Roes K.C. Instrumental Variable Analysis in Epidemiologic Studies: An Overview of the Estimation Methods. Pharm Anal Acta 2015, 6:4. https://doi.org/10.4172/2153-2435.1000353

Fang G, Brooks JM, Chrischilles EA. Apples and oranges? Interpretations of risk adjustment and instrumental variable estimates of intended treatment effects using observational data. Am J Epidemiol. 2012 Jan 1; 175(1):60-5.

Baron, R. M., Kenny, D. A. The moderator-mediator variable distinction in social psychological research: Conceptual, strategic and statistical considerations. Journal of Personality and Social Psychology. 1986; 51: 1173-1182.

Kline RB. Introduction. Principles and Practice of Structural Equation Modeling. 2nd Ed. New York: The Guildford Press. 2005. 3-19.

Chapter 5
Causal Inference in Pharmacoepidemiology

Ashley Buchanan, Tianyu Sun, and Natallia V. Katenka

5.1   Introduction

The causal inference framework can be employed to quantify causal effects in both randomized and non-randomized settings. Often in pharmacoepidemiologic research, studies lack randomized interventions that allow for causal inference. There are important and meaningful causal questions to address for non-randomized interventions. Although causal inference in this setting can be more challenging, the exercise of identifying the assumptions, considerations in study design, and adjusting for sources of bias in analyses can result in studies that have meaningful designs and produce estimates of causal effects using methods with known limitations. Causal inference approaches can be employed in these settings to quantify the casual effects of medications on health outcomes.

> **Definition**   A *causal effect* means that an intervention, treatment, or exposure causes a subsequent health outcome.

A *causal effect* means that an intervention, treatment, or exposure, such as a prescription medication, causes a subsequent health outcome to occur. In contrast, an association means that the exposure meaningfully predicts the outcome. In order to ascertain causal effects, one can address sources of bias in study design, analysis, or both. The three sources of structural bias are confounding, selection bias, and measurement error. Approached in this way, we have a framework to distinguish

A. Buchanan (✉) · T. Sun
Department of Pharmacy Practice, University of Rhode Island, College of Pharmacy, Kingston, RI, USA
e-mail: buchanan@uri.edu

N. V. Katenka
Department of Computer Science and Statistics, University of Rhode Island, Kingston, RI, USA

© Springer Nature Switzerland AG 2020   181
O. V. Marchenko, N. V. Katenka (eds.), *Quantitative Methods in Pharmaceutical Research and Development*, https://doi.org/10.1007/978-3-030-48555-9_5

association from causation. Determining when association is causation can provide stronger evidence and the information needed to strengthen interventions and inform policy.

Counterfactuals, or potential outcomes, are a useful framework to improve the rigor of causal inference. For example, when a patient takes an aspirin, the patient attributes the resolution of their headache to the aspirin. The assumption is that without the aspirin, the headache would not have been relieved. Similarly, when a patient with high cholesterol takes statin, we assume the statin is what caused their cholesterol to lower to normal levels, such that without the statin, the levels would have remained harmfully elevated.

Many research questions in health outcomes research are ultimately concerned about causation to provide evidence for improvements in prescribing practices, inform black box warnings, and, ultimately, improve patient health. The field of causal inference methodology is broad, including a range of disciplines from computer scientists to epidemiologists, and its applications include such disciplines econometrics and implementation science. In this chapter, we provide an overview of the causal inference paradigm, review current methodology, and discuss applications of these concepts to strengthen and improve pharmacoepidemiologic research.

5.1.1 Challenges in Big Health Data

As compared to clinical trials and prospective cohort study, the greatest advantage of using administrative claims data and electronic health records (EHR) is convenience and large sample sizes, which can improve precision of the estimates. EHR data are typically generated from daily clinical practice of healthcare providers and aggregated to provide databases describing the health information of patients. These data sources often contain several of the following parts: demographic information; diagnostic information usually coded by the international classification of disease (ICD); current procedure terminology (CPT) codes; medication list; laboratory tests; and clinical documentation (Denny 2012). However, the scale and the structure of the EHR data bring unique challenges. EHR data can contain up to millions of patients who generate billions of inpatient/outpatient diagnosis and claims every year. Applying statistical models or simply creating descriptive tables often requires greater computational resources, time, and reliable software. In addition, some EHR data include clinical documentation, which might contain information about the severity of the disease and original hand-written diagnoses; however, the disease severity can be missing, which is often an important confounder when studying the effects of prescriptions on subsequent health outcomes (see Sect. 5.2.1 for a more complete discussion of confounding). Unlike structured information such as ICD codes, clinical documentation is an unstructured natural narrative variable, which can be challenging to extract specific information, such as diagnoses. Natural language processing offers some approaches to obtain accurate information from these records (Hripcsak et al. 1995).

Besides the unstructured information, the standardized measurement from the ICD or CPT code may not be accurately capturing the underlying exposure or health outcome of interest. This is an example of exposure or outcome misclassification. For example, one study reported that using expanded ICD-9 code to define the out-of-hospital sudden cardiac death had relatively high sensitivity (87%) and specificity (66%) (Iribarren et al. 1998). However, the agreement rate (as measured by the positive predictive value) between this method and physician diagnosis was low (27%). Furthermore, changes across versions of ICD could also raise concerns about comparability over time. The ICD-10 was implemented in 1999 for the death information in the USA. For example, the comparability ratio of ICD-10 over ICD-9 for the Alzheimer's disease (AD) was 1.55 indicating that ICD-10 would attribute 55% more death to AD than ICD-9 (Anderson et al. 2001).

Another major threat to conducting causal inference using EHR data is unmeasured confounding. For example, EHR data may not have information about the individual's lifestyle, such as smoking status, diet, and daily exercise. Without this information, the investigator may not be able to measure all necessary confounding variables in the analysis. This is a disadvantage of using EHR data to conduct pharmacoepidemiologic studies. To address this issue, if available, valid instrumental variables (IVs) could be employed, as described in Sect. 5.4.3. However, this approach requires additional assumptions, and, if they do not hold, the bias could be more extreme and unpredictable (Bound et al. 1995). For example, investigators defined an IV as combined physician preference and facility preference to evaluate the association between use of antipsychotic medications and death among elderly people in the Australia Veterans' Affairs database (Pratt et al. 2010). Although a candidate IV, there could be unknown or unmeasured common causes between the IV and the outcome. In this case, frequency of visits with a particular provider could be associated with the physician's preference and could also be associated with reducing the likelihood of the outcome death. Furthermore, patients may be more familiar with their frequently seen provider, which could improve treatment compliance and ultimately reduce the likelihood of death. This would violate the exclusion restriction assumption required for valid IVs. Approaches to evaluate the sensitivity of the IV to assumptions should be used, and new methods may be needed for some applications (Brookhart et al. 2006; Rassen et al. 2009).

The missing data in EHR data can lead to selection bias, which distorts the measure of association quantified in the study. For example, a study was conducted to assess the association between antidepressant medication and weight change among adults by using EHR data. However, only 24.8% of individuals (2408 out of 9704) had complete weight change information after 2 years of follow-up in the study (Haneuse and Daniels 2016). The missingness of the outcome could be associated with patient risk factors; patient behavior and disease conditions and approaches are needed to address the missing data in this setting. This presents yet another challenge for causal inference in EHR data. Fortunately, each of these challenges for conducting causal inference in EHR data can be conceptualized using a potential outcomes framework. We can then use this framework to determine appropriate estimands, assumptions, and methodology, improving inference in routinely-collected health data.

5.1.2 Causal Inference and Potential Outcomes

Causal inference can be framed using potential outcomes or counterfactuals. For the purposes of developing these concepts, we assume that the study population is near infinite, so we can ignore sampling error and focus on systematic biases due to confounding, selection, and measurement. We defer discussion of random variability to Sect. 5.3.

Let A be a dichotomous (i.e., binary) treatment that takes the value 0 when a patient is untreated and 1 when a patient is treated. Let Y be a dichotomous health outcome that takes the value 1 when the patient experiences the outcome of interest and 0, otherwise.

> **Definition** A *potential outcome* Y^a is the outcome that would have been observed if, possibly contrary to fact, treatment a was received.

A *potential outcome* $Y^{a=1}$ is the outcome that would have been observed if, possibly contrary to fact, treatment $a = 1$ was received. $Y^{a=0}$ is defined analogously. For example, A is an indicator that denotes if a patient received a prescription for a high-dose opioid medication (versus low-dose opioid medication (≤ 50 morphine milligram equivalents (MME))) following a surgery, and Y is an indicator for development of opioid dependence in the following year. Opioid dependence, known as opioid use disorder, is a documented history of opioid misuse or addiction. Table 5.1 displays the potential outcomes for 20 patients in the database. For example, patient 2 would have developed an opioid dependence if she/he received the opioid prescription after surgery, and she/he would have not developed opioid dependence if she/he did not receive the opioid prescription. Comparing the potential outcomes for any one patient is known as the *individual causal effect*. In practice, we only observe one of the two potential outcomes in practice. Requiring information on both potential outcomes while only observing one of the potential outcomes is known as the *fundamental problem of causal inference* (Holland 1986). Essentially, this could be viewed as a missing data problem, and thus many approaches from the missing data literature can be leveraged here. The potential outcomes framework was introduced by Neyman (1990), popularized by Rubin (1980), and is referred to as the "Neyman-Rubin" causal model. Subsequent work by Robins (2000) and Hernán et al. (2000) provided methodology for a time-varying exposure setting. In this chapter, we focus on estimation, as opposed to statistical testing, the more traditional focus of statistical literature.

Table 5.1 Developed opioid dependence potential outcomes Y^a with pain management intervention A among 20 patients who underwent surgery

Patient	$Y^{a=0}$	$Y^{a=1}$	A	Y
1	1	1	0	1
2	0	1	0	0
3	1	0	0	1
4	1	1	1	1
5	1	0	1	0
6	0	1	1	1
7	0	0	0	0
8	0	0	0	0
9	1	1	0	1
10	1	1	0	1
11	0	0	1	0
12	1	0	1	0
13	0	0	1	0
14	1	0	1	0
15	0	0	1	0
16	1	1	1	1
17	1	1	1	1
18	0	1	1	1
19	1	1	1	1
20	0	1	1	1

5.1.3 Definition of a Causal Effect

For each patient i in our database, with $i = 1, \ldots, n$, we can denote the potential outcomes by $Y_i^{a=1}$ and $Y_i^{a=0}$. Then, A has an effect on Y if (and only if) $Y_i^{a=1} \neq Y_i^{a=0}$. Similarly, A has no effect on Y for patient i if (and only if) $Y_i^{a=1} = Y_i^{a=0}$. In our data example (Table 5.1) for patient 2, A has a causal effect on Y because the patient developed opioid dependence if and only if she/he receives high-dose opioid prescription after surgery; whereas, for patient 7, A does not have a causal effect on Y because the patient does not develop opioid dependence during the study period regardless of receiving a high-dose opioid prescription or not. No effect for all individuals in the study is called the *sharp null hypothesis*.[1] Typically, the *individual causal effect* is defined as a contrast of the potential outcomes: $Y_i^{a=1} - Y_i^{a=0}$.

We now turn our attention to estimating average causal effects. The *average causal effect* in the population exists if $\Pr[Y^{a=1} = 1] \neq \Pr[Y^{a=1} = 1]$, or more generally, $E[Y^{a=1}] \neq E[Y^{a=1}]$ for any Y. There is no average causal effect in the population if

$$\Pr[Y^{a=1} = 1] = \Pr[Y^{a=0} = 1].$$

---

[1]This serves as the basis for many exact statistical tests and is beyond the scope of this chapter. We refer the reader to Imbens and Rubin (2015) for additional background on exact statistical tests for causal inference.

The sharp null hypothesis implies that there is no average causal effect in the population; however, no average causal effect in the population does not imply the sharp null. For example, high-dose opioid prescriptions may increase the risk of opioid dependence for some patients, but not on average across all patients.

Assumptions are required to estimate average causal effects in observational studies because only one of the two potential outcomes is actually observed. In addition, we use only these two potential outcomes to sufficiently represent all potential outcomes. These assumptions required for identifying causal effects are causal consistency, exchangeability, and positivity. Causal consistency[2] relates the observed outcome Y to the potential outcomes (Pearl 2010): $Y = Y^{a\,=\,1}A + Y^{a\,=\,0}(1 - A)$. Exchangeability implies that the potential outcomes are independent of the treatment assignment mechanism. Positivity means that the conditional probability of receiving every value of treatment is greater than zero.

Consistency is conceptually related to the *no multiple versions of treatment assumption*. This assumption means there is only one version of treatment and one version of control, or if there are multiple versions, they are irrelevant for the causal effect of interest, which is known as the *treatment variation irrelevance assumption* (Cole and Frangakis 2009; VanderWeele 2009; Pearl 2010). The no multiple versions of treatment assumption is part of a larger assumption, known as the *Stable Unit Treatment Value Assumption*, or SUTVA. SUTVA also includes the *no interference assumption*. That is, the treatment of one individual does not affect the potential outcomes of other individuals. Consistency and no interference comprise SUTVA because both assumptions play an important role in the two potential outcomes sufficiently representing all potential outcomes. In practice, the no interference assumption may not hold, such as in vaccine studies (Perez-Heydrich et al. 2014), educational intervention studies (Hong and Raudenbush 2006), or HIV prevention studies (Buchanan et al. 2018). In this setting, the potential outcomes can be indexed by each patient's exposure and the exposures of all other patients that could influence their outcome. When the no interference assumption is relaxed, estimation of causal effects is possible, and there is a rapidly developing literature to quantify effects in the presence of interference (Hudgens and Halloran 2008; Tchetgen and VanderWeele 2012; Benjamin-Chung et al. 2018; Buchanan et al. 2018.

Assumptions for Identifying Causal Effects
1. Exchangeability (unconditional or conditional)
2. Treatment variation irrelevance
3. Positivity

In the causal inference literature, we consider measures that are important in epidemiologic studies: risk difference (*RD*), risk ratio (*RR*), and odds ratio (*OR*).

---

[2]This is not the same concept as statistical consistency of statistical estimators (i.e., convergence in probability).

These measures describe the causal effect of treatment and are referred to as *effects* or *effect measures*. The *causal risk difference (RD)* is defined as

$$RD = \Pr\left[Y^{a=1} = 1\right] - \Pr\left[Y^{a=0} = 1\right] = E\left[Y^{a=1}\right] - E\left[Y^{a=0}\right].$$

The *causal risk ratio (RR)* is defined as

$$RR = \frac{\Pr\left[Y^{a=1} = 1\right]}{\Pr\left[Y^{a=0} = 1\right]}.$$

The *causal odds ratio* (OR) is defined as

$$OR = \frac{\Pr\left[Y^{a=1} = 1\right] / \Pr\left[Y^{a=1} = 0\right]}{\Pr\left[Y^{a=0} = 1\right] / \Pr\left[Y^{a=0} = 0\right]}.$$

Note that under the null hypothesis of no causal effect of A on Y, the causal $RD = 0$, the causal $RR = 1$, and the causal $OR = 1$, respectively. We compare these to expressions for the measures of association. The *associational risk difference (RD)* is

$$RD = \Pr[Y = 1|A = 1] - \Pr[Y = 1|A = 0]$$
$$= E[Y|A = 1] - E[Y|A = 0].$$

In turn, the *associational risk ratio (RR)* and the *associational odds ratio (OR)* are defined as

$$RR = \frac{\Pr[Y = 1|A = 1]}{\Pr[Y = 1|A = 0]},$$

and

$$OR = \frac{\dfrac{\Pr[Y = 1|A = 1]}{\Pr[Y = 0|A = 1]}}{\dfrac{\Pr[Y = 1|A = 0]}{\Pr[Y = 0|A = 0]}}.$$

These associational measures are unadjusted and may be non-null even if no effect exists due to confounding. Confounding arises when treatment A and outcome Y share a common cause. See Sect. 5.2.1 for a complete discussion of confounding. If $A \perp Y$ (i.e., A is independent of Y), then the associational RD is 0, and associational RR and OR are both 1. To identify average causal effects in the absence of confounding (e.g., a randomized controlled trial), determining when the

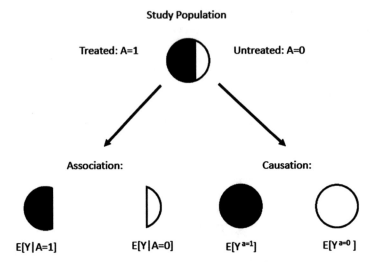

Fig. 5.1 Diagram of the components for a causal contrast (right) versus an associational contrast (left)

associational measure equals the causal measure can inform the assumptions needed to identify causal effects. In the absence of selection bias and measurement error, the associational measure will equal the causal measure in a randomized study. For analysis of observational data without randomization, the exercise is determining if and when the conditional associational measure equals the causal measure. Based on Fig. 5.1, we need to identify the assumptions required for the partial circles on the left to inform the full circles on the right. That is, we need to determine when the outcomes observed among those treated and untreated can provide information about potential outcomes as if the entire study population was treated and untreated, respectively.

5.1.4   A Short Introduction to Causal Directed Acyclic Graphs

Performing a causal inference analysis requires determining the assumptions and requires input from substantive area experts. In more complex settings, determining these assumptions can be challenging. *Directed acyclic graphs* (DAGs) can be used to better understand causal mechanisms and clarify assumptions. Communication between analysts and investigators can be facilitated with DAGs, and, most importantly, assumptions can be made explicit prior to analyses and conclusions.

DAGs contain nodes representing random variables, such as Y for an outcome, L for a covariate, and A for a treatment or exposure. As often structured, time flows from left to right between the random variables; thus, a temporal sequence is established between the random variables on the graph. Consider Fig. 5.2 displays

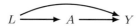

Fig. 5.2 Example of a simple directed acyclic graph with three nodes L, A, Y and arrows denote a causal effect

a DAG, where, for example, A is an indicator for receipt of an opioid prescription after surgery, L is an indicator for previous history of uncontrolled pain, and Y is an indicator for subsequent opioid dependence in the year following surgery. Let $A \rightarrow Y$ indicate there is a *direct causal effect* (i.e., not mediated through any other variables on the graph) for at least one patient in the study. A lack of an arrow in the DAG indicates that A has no direct causal effect on Y for any patient.

DAGs are directed, which means that $L \rightarrow A$ means that L causes A, but not vice versa. Acyclic means there are no cycles in the graph; that is, a variable cannot cause itself either directly or through other variables. A *causal DAG* is a DAG where common causes of any pair of variables on the graph are also on the graph.

We now familiarize the reader with graph theory notation for a DAG. Define a DAG G as a graph whose nodes (i.e., vertices) are random variables $V = (V_1, \ldots, V_m)$ with directed edges (i.e., arrows) and no non-directed edges. Two vertices joined by an edge are called *adjacent*. A *path* between two nodes consists of a sequence of vertices that are adjacent. A *directed cycle* is a directed path of the form $V_j \rightarrow V_k \rightarrow V_j$ for $k \neq j$. *Parents of a node* are the set of nodes from which there is a directed arrow into that node, and this is denoted by *PA*. In Fig. 5.2, $PA_Y = \{L, A\}$. Thus, V_m is a descent of V_j (and V_j is an ancestor of V_m) if there is a directed path $V_j \rightarrow V_m$. We now have the concepts to define a causal DAG. A graph G is a causal DAG if:

1. The lack of an arrow between nodes can be interpreted as the absence of a direct causal effect.
2. All common causes, even if unmeasured, of any pair of variables on the graph are themselves on the graph.
3. Any variable is a cause of its descendants.

To link a DAG to observable random variables, we can invoke the *causal Markov assumption*: Conditional on its direct causes, a variable V_j is independent of any variable for which it is not a cause. When developing and evaluating DAGs, we can make assumptions and condition on variables to block all paths that are not the causal path of interest (i.e., backdoor paths). A *backdoor path* is a non-causal pathway from A to Y. In a DAG, when a variable is conditioned on, a box is placed around the random variable. For example, in Fig. 5.2, let A denote a pain management intervention, Y denote subsequent opioid use disorder, and L denote history of any substance use disorder. By conditioning on any history of substance use disorder, we block the backdoor path from $A \leftarrow L \rightarrow Y$. Blocking all backdoor paths is achieved by conditioning on any variables that are not colliders or not conditioning on colliders (or descendants of colliders). L is a *collider* on the path in Fig. 5.3 because two arrowheads point to this node. L is a common effect of Y and A, and note that the concept of a collider is path specific. In general, colliders block the

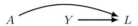

Fig. 5.3 Example of a simple directed acyclic graph (DAG) with collider node L

flow of association along the path in which they lie. For example, if we condition our analysis to only include patients with subsequent overdose, we are possibly conditioning on a collider of high-dose opioid exposure and the outcome opioid dependence and could be inducing an association between A and Y that may not be the causal effect of A on Y.

We now explain how DAGs can be used to determine the exchangeability assumption required to identify causal effects. A path is *open* or *closed* according to the following rules:

1. If there are no variables being conditioned on, a path is blocked (closed) if and only if it contains a collider.
2. A path which contains non-colliders that are conditioned on is blocked.
3. A collider that has been conditioned on does not block a path.
4. A collider that has a descent that has been conditioned on does not block a path.

A path is blocked if and only if it contains a non-collider that has been conditioned on or it contains a collider, which has not been conditioned on and has no descents that have been conditioned on. Two variables are *d-separated* if all paths between them are blocked. Otherwise, two variables are *d-connected*. If two variables are d-separated given some other variable L, then the two variables are conditionally independent given the third variable. That is, A is independent of Y conditional on L. This is important because conditional exchangeability is required to identify causal effects.

To summarize, two variables are *unconditionally* or *marginally associated* if (1) one causes the other or (2) they share common causes; otherwise, they will be marginally independent. We refer the interested reader to Greenland et al. (1999a), Pearl (1995), and Pearl (2003) for a complete discussion of causal DAGs. Below, we employ DAGs to examine structural biases. There are also single-world intervention graphs (SWIGs) available to identify causal effects, but they are beyond the scope of this chapter (for more details see Richardson and Robins 2013).

5.1.5 Randomized Experiments

Although pharmacoepidemiology often involves retrospective observational studies, we dedicate some discussion in this chapter to randomized experiments. Observational studies conceptualized as an ideal randomized trial is a powerful tool (see Hernán and Robins 2016). Frequently, randomized trials are unethical or not feasible, and thus observational studies are an available study design to study certain medications and medical devices. Simply analyzing all available data can leave our analyses fraught with biases, including selection bias due to conditioning on variables after the baseline period of the study. Without consideration of the causal mechanism, models may lack important confounding variables. Identifying the target trial and emulating that in observational data provides an opportunity to design and analyze studies to minimize the impact of these biases on our study results.

Consider a randomized experiment in which patients are assigned treatment $a = 1$ and $a = 0$ randomly in the entire study with 65% of the patients randomized to treatment. That is, the treatment assignment mechanism is independent of their potential outcomes. This design is a *marginally randomized experiment*. In this setting, we have *marginal exchangeability* $Y^a \perp A$ for $a = 0, 1$. The potential outcomes are independent of the treatment. It is important to note that this does not mean that the observed outcome Y is independent of the treatment. We can relax this assumption and assume *mean exchangeability* $E[Y^a | A = 1]=E[Y^a|A = 0]$ for $a = 0, 1$.

> **Exchangeability** The potential outcomes are independent of the treatment assignment mechanism.

If this assumption of exchangeability holds, then $E[Y^a = 1]=E[Y^{a\,=\,1}| A = 1]= E[Y | A = 1]$. The first equality holds by mean exchangeability, and the second equality holds by causal consistency. The right side of the equation is identifiable from the observed data. A causal parameter is *identifiable* if it can be estimated using the observed data. Similarly, $E[Y^a = 0]=E[Y | A = 0]$. When mean exchangeability and causal consistency hold, the causal effects are identifiable in the observed data.

In randomized experiments assuming no measurement bias and no selection bias, association is causation (see Sect. 5.2). However, if the data did not arise from a marginally randomized experiment, marginal exchangeability does not necessarily hold. In Table 5.2, the data arises from a conditionally randomized trial in which 71% of the participants are randomly assigned if $L = 0$ and 50% are randomly assigned if $L = 1$. Thus, $E[Y | A = 1] = 7/13$ and $E[Y | A = 0] = 4/7$, so the associational $RD = -0.03$ (i.e., protective). However, $E[Y^a = 1] = 11/20$ and $E[Y^a = 0] = 11/20$, so the causal $RD = 0$. There is a protective association and a null causal effect, so we note an example where association is not causation because marginal exchangeability does not hold. If marginal exchangeability does not hold, we may be willing to assume exchangeability conditional on measured covariate(s).

Consider a randomized experiment in which 50% of the participants are randomly assigned if $L = 0$ and 71% are randomly assigned if $L=1$ (Table 5.2), where L denotes a history of opioid use disorder. That is, patients with a history of opioid use disorder have a lower chance of being prescribed high-dose opioids. The design is a *conditionally randomized experiment*. In this design, marginal exchangeability may not hold. For example, individuals with a history of opioid use disorder are less likely to receive opioids than those without a documented opioid use disorder. If these individuals with opioid use disorder are more likely to develop opioid

Patient	$Y^{a=0}$	$Y^{a=1}$	A	L	Y
Table 5.2 Opioid dependence potential outcomes Y^a with pain management intervention A and history of opioid use disorder L among 20 patients who underwent surgery					
1	1	1	0	1	1
2	0	1	0	1	0
3	1	0	0	1	1
4	1	1	1	1	1
5	1	0	1	1	0
6	0	1	1	1	1
7	0	0	0	0	0
8	0	0	0	0	0
9	1	1	0	0	1
10	1	1	0	0	1
11	0	0	1	0	0
12	1	0	1	0	0
13	0	0	1	0	0
14	1	0	1	0	0
15	0	0	1	0	0
16	1	1	1	0	1
17	1	1	1	0	1
18	0	1	1	0	1
19	1	1	1	0	1
20	0	1	1	0	1

dependence if prescribed opioids, then $\Pr\left[Y^{a=1} = 1 | L = 0\right] = \frac{7}{14} < \frac{4}{6} = \Pr\left[Y^{a=1} = 1 | L = 1\right]$, so $Y^{a=1}$ is not independent of A. We can consider conditionally randomized experiments as two separate marginal experiments. Therefore, conditional exchangeability holds, which implies the potential outcomes are independent of the treatment conditional on the measured covariate L, that is, $Y^a \perp A \,|\, L = l$ for a, l = 0, 1. For those familiar with the missing data literature, the potential outcomes are missing completely at random (MCAR) in a marginally randomized experiment and missing at random (MAR) in a conditionally randomized experiment.

In a conditionally randomized experiment,

$$E[Y^a] = \sum_l E[Y^a \,|\, L = l] \Pr[L = l] = \sum_l E[Y^a \,|\, A = a, L = l] \Pr[L = l],$$

where the second equality holds by conditional exchangeability. Then, by causal consistency,

$$E[Y^a] = \sum_l E[Y \,|\, A = a, L = l] \Pr[L = l].$$

We now have an expression written entirely in terms of the observed random variables (L, A, Y), and the causal effect is identifiable; that is, we can estimate the causal effect using the observed data. Under conditional exchangeability, the standardized mean equals the counterfactual mean had all individuals in population received treatment a. For example, the causal RR is

$$\frac{\Pr\left[Y^{a=1}=1\right]}{\Pr\left[Y^{a=0}=1\right]} = \frac{\sum_l E[Y=1\mid A=1, L=l]\Pr[L=l]}{\sum_l E[Y=1\mid A=0, L=l]\Pr[L=l]}.$$

Considering sampling variability, an unbiased (in large samples) estimator of the causal *RR* is

$$\widehat{RR} = \frac{\sum_l \widehat{\Pr}[Y=1\mid A=1, L=l]\,\widehat{\Pr}[L=l]}{\sum_l \widehat{\Pr}[Y=1\mid A=0, L=l]\,\widehat{\Pr}[L=l]},$$

where each of the probabilities is estimated by plugging in observed proportions. Analogous expressions can be defined for the causal *RD* and *OR*.

Alternatively, inverse probability weighting (IPW) can be employed to estimate causal effects. IPW estimators inverse weight each observation by the probability of the exposure actually received conditional on variables L, creating a pseudopopulation in which there is no association between L and A (Lunceford and Davidian 2004). Consider the following Horvitz-Thompson-type IPW estimator of $E[Y^a]$:

$$\frac{1}{n}\sum_{i=1}^{n}\frac{I(A_i=a)Y_i}{\Pr[A_i=a\mid L_i]},$$

where the indicator function $I(A_i=a)=1$ if $A_i=a$ and $I(A_i=a)=0$, otherwise. The estimator is unbiased when the denominator is known for all a, l in a conditionally randomized study and conditional exchangeability holds. The quantity $\Pr[A=1\mid L=l]$ is known as the *propensity score* (Imai and Van Dyk 2004; Rosenbaum and Rubin 1983). A key result about propensity scores is if $Y^a \perp A \mid L$, then $Y^a \perp A \mid \Pr(A=1\mid L=l)$. This implies that we can identify causal effects within stratum of the propensity score; however, this may perform poorly in finite samples (Lunceford and Davidian 2004).

For the data example in Table 5.2, $\Pr[Y^{a=1}=1] - \Pr[Y^{a=0}=1] = 0$, so the causal parameter $RD = 0$. The estimates based on the standardized estimator are

$$\widehat{\Pr}\left[Y^{a=1}=1\right] = \frac{5}{10}\times\frac{14}{20}+\frac{2}{3}\times\frac{6}{20}=0.55,$$

$$\widehat{\Pr}\left[Y^{a=0}=1\right] = \frac{2}{4}\times\frac{14}{20}+\frac{2}{3}\times\frac{6}{20} = 0.55.$$

Similarly, the estimates based on the IPW estimator are

$$\widehat{\Pr}\left[Y^{a=1}=1\right] = \frac{1}{20}\left[\frac{2}{\left(\frac{3}{6}\right)}+\frac{5}{\left(\frac{10}{14}\right)}\right] = 0.55,$$

$$\widehat{\Pr}\left[Y^{a=0}=1\right] = \frac{1}{20}\left[\frac{2}{\left(\frac{3}{6}\right)}+\frac{2}{\left(\frac{4}{14}\right)}\right] = 0.55.$$

Therefore, $\widehat{\Pr}\left[Y^{a=1}=1\right] - \widehat{\Pr}\left[Y^{a=0}=1\right] = 0$ when either nonparametric estimator (standardized or IPW) is employed.

5.1.6 Observational Studies

An observational study can be conceptualized as a conditionally randomized experiment under three conditions:

1. The values of treatment under comparison correspond to well-defined interventions.
2. The conditional probability of receiving every value of treatment, though not decided by investigators, depends only on the measured variables.
3. The conditional probability of receiving every value of treatment is greater than zero, i.e., positive.

In an observational study, when the treatment or exposure is not randomized, marginal exchangeability $Y^a \perp A$ is questionable. However, investigators may be willing to assume that exchangeability holds conditional on variables L, that is, $Y^a \perp A \mid L$. For example, suppose that patients with unmanaged pain are more likely to receive opioids and also at an increased risk for opioid dependence. We may not be willing to assume $Y^0 \perp A$; however, we may be willing to assume $Y^0 \perp A \mid L$, that is, conditional on the variable unmanaged pain.

Unfortunately, it is not possible to verify $Y^a \perp A \mid L$ because Y^a is never observed for those with $A \neq a$. Thus, causal inference in observational studies relies on expert knowledge to select L to ensure the conditional exchangeability assumption is plausible. In Sect. 5.1.3, we introduced causal graphs, which can be employed with expert knowledge to determine the set of variables L. The conditional exchangeability assumption will not hold if there are unmeasured confounders U; thus, this assumption is often referred to as the *no unmeasured confounders assumption*. We may collect more variables to include in L; however, the existence of unmeasured confounders may remain. Furthermore, it is possible that the inclusion of additional measured variables can introduce bias (Cole and Hernán 2008). The addition of a variable that is not a confounder may introduce selection bias due to *collider stratification* (i.e., conditioning on a collider). For the example of pain management intervention after surgery, opioid overdose after surgery is a possible collider, and if measured, conditioning on this variable may introduce bias. In light of this, we can rely on expert knowledge to assess the plausibility of conditional exchangeability. Machine learning techniques with substantive expert knowledge could be employed (see Westreich et al. 2010). We can assess the existence of U and conduct sensitivity analysis (Robins et al. 2000a). We could also derive bounds for the parameters of interest (Cheng and Small 2006).

The *positivity assumption* is required for causal inference in observational data. Specifically, $\Pr[A = a \mid L = l] > 0$ for all L such that $\Pr[L = l] > 0$. In Table 5.2, positivity holds because there are individuals at both levels of treatment for each level of the covariate L. Positivity would not hold, for example, if all patients with unmanaged pain could never be prescribed opioids. Positivity can sometimes be empirically verified.

> **Positivity** There is a probability greater than zero of being assigned to each of the treatment levels for all values of the covariate L.

The well-defined interventions assumption is also required to identify causal effects. Until now, we have assumed that there are only two versions of the treatment, $a = 0$ and $a = 1$, and, thus, two potential outcomes. However, there may be different versions of treatment $a = 1$. For example, opioid prescriptions have different doses, quantity supplied, and formulations. These different aspects of treatment could result in different potential outcomes (Pearl 2010). The no multiple versions of treatment assumption can be relaxed by defining more treatment levels and corresponding additional potential outcomes (VanderWeele 2009; Cole and Frangakis 2009).

Causal inference requires well-defined interventions. Conceptualizing an ideal randomized experiment to emulate with observational data can greatly improve the results obtained from observational studies. In addition, describing the policy to implement can further sharpen the scope of an observational study. When treatments are not well-defined, issues of multiple versions of treatment and positivity violations can occur. There is also the well-known adage "no causation without manipulation." That is, we will only consider treatments A that are manipulable. In pharmacoepidemiology research, most interventions are manipulable, as they are part of healthcare delivery. However, in the social epidemiology literature, much debate remains about estimation of causal effects of social constructs, such as race and gender (Glymour and Spiegelman 2017; Howe et al. 2017; Hernán 2016). If we are not willing or able to assume positivity, conditional exchangeability, and/or well-defined interventions, prediction (or association) can be evaluated. From a public health perspective, we will often want to make claims beyond associations and prediction to understand why associations exist and inform the development of future interventions and policy.

5.1.7 Using Big Data to Emulate a Target Trial

We discuss how to employ administrative claims and electronic health records (EHR) to emulate a target trial when data from a randomized trial is not available (Hernán and Robins 2016). Suppose we have a large database of healthcare claims to emulate a trial of high-dose versus low-dose opioid therapy among patients who recently had surgery on the risk of opioid dependence. Because the investigators did not design this study, the available data may not contain all the necessary information, so consultation with those providing the data and validation studies are required. For this discussion, we assume that adequate validation studies were performed for the measures of interest in the database. With this framework that makes the target trial explicit, causal inference methods can be employed to address structural biases in this setting.

> **Using Big Data to Emulate a Target Trial**
> 1. Eligibility criteria
> 2. Treatment strategies
> 3. Assignment procedures
> 4. Study period
> 5. Outcome
> 6. Causal contrast
> 7. Statistical analysis plan

There are six elements that should be considered in study design and analysis in this setting of administrative claims and EHR data: (1) eligibility criteria; who to include in our analysis; (2) treatment strategies, the medical intervention we want to investigate and how to measure it; (3) assignment procedures, how the participants will be assigned and blinded; (4) study period, the start and end of baseline and follow-up period; (5) outcome, the endpoint of the study and variables in the EHR data to ascertain this; and (6) causal contrasts, intention-to-treat (ITT) effect or per-protocol effect. (7) Statistical analysis plan: model to be implemented and covariates that should be included in the model, which are specified prior to analysis work (Hernán and Robins 2016).

Eligibility Criteria. The observational analyst should employ the same eligibility criteria that would have been applied in the target trial. Furthermore, the chosen population must be "eligible" for each level of treatment considered; that is, equipoise must hold for the research question. In our example at baseline, we would only include recent surgery patients who had no evidence of existing opioid use disorder for 1 year, which means they had to be included in the database for at least 1 year and experience surgery early enough (in the calendar time of the observed data) to also possibly contribute 1 year of follow-up. Importantly, we cannot exclude patients based on post-baseline events, as this could introduce selection bias.

Treatment Strategies. We first need to determine the parameter(s) of interest (e.g., causal risk difference comparing the average potential outcomes as if everyone was exposed to if no one was exposed in our study population). Then, we will need to identify those who have baseline data consistent with the strategies of interest. In our example, we will need to identify those who were opioid-free for 1 year prior to surgery and then classify patients according to their pain management regimen (high-dose opioids vs. low-dose opioid) during the baseline period. This comparison of exposures can help to avoid problems of comparing prevalent and incident exposure cases. Furthermore, we should also make our comparison group well-defined. For example, we could consider those who received opioids at high versus low doses based on a morphine milliequivalent (MME) threshold of 50 MME/day during the baseline period.

Assignment Procedures. To emulate comparisons of treatment strategies with randomized treatment strategies, we must ensure conditional exchangeability holds, where the groups are defined by the treatment strategies, perhaps by employing a DAG. Then, the choice of our methodology depends on whether treatment strategies are defined at baseline or changing over time (see Sect. 5.4.2 for a discussion of time-varying exposures) and the choice of the target parameter. Adjustment for baseline confounders can be performed using matching, stratification or regression, standardization or inverse probability weighting, g-estimation, or doubly robust estimators. To note, standardization or inverse probability weighting quantifies a parameter in the entire study population, while matching quantifies a parameter in the matched study sample. If the observational database does not have sufficient information on baseline or time-dependent confounders, emulating the randomized trial will not be possible. However, approaches such as outcome controls (Lipsitch et al. 2010) and new methods to extract additional information from administrative data sets may offer a solution when information on confounders is limited (Hripcsak et al. 1995).

Study Period. To determine the study period, we define when the follow-up of patients begins (typically at "randomization") and then follow patients until the event of interest, death, loss to follow-up, or the administrative end of the study. The duration of follow-up can be informed by the disease or condition and practical constraints such as the length of follow-up among patients in the database.

Outcome. We could use the database to identify those who had an opioid dependence within 1 year after surgery. Validation studies of the health outcomes are often needed to ensure that medical codes are capturing the outcome of interest. Often, doctors will be aware of the treatment, so outcome ascertainment will not be blinded, except if the outcome is obtained from an external data source, such as death, which is typically ascertained from a death registry.

Causal Contrast. Two common causal effects of interest are the intention-to-treat effect and the per-protocol effect. The intention-to-treat effect compares the effect of being assigned to the treatment strategies at baseline, regardless of compliance after baseline. The per-protocol effect compares the effect of following the treatments as specified in the study protocol. Both of these could be estimated in the observational data. In observational data, to quantify the intention-to-treat effect, we compare the initiators of different treatment strategies, assuming exchangeability conditional on baseline covariates. To quantify the per protocol effect, we need to adjust for both baseline and time-varying confounding, as patients continue the strategies after baseline, and, therefore, adjustment for time-varying confounding is needed. Furthermore, there may be selection bias due to loss to follow-up. In that case, adjustment for time-varying variables is required to identify both the intention-to-treat and per-protocol effects. As discussed earlier in this chapter, when time-varying variables are affected by treatment strategies, g-methods are typically required.

Statistical Analysis Plan. A baseline period must be defined. Eligibility must be met by the end of the baseline period, and study outcomes must be counted after the end of the baseline period. In our target trial, the start of follow-up is when the treatment strategy is assigned. With an observational exposure, we can emulate baseline as the time when an eligible individual initiates a treatment strategy. Patients can meet eligibility at a single time point, which may vary across individuals, or at multiple times. For the latter case, there are two unbiased choices: use a single eligible time (e.g., the first eligible) and all eligible times or a subset of all eligible times. Grace periods can be specified for initiation of therapy, which more closely emulates what is typically done in medical practice. However, these grace periods allow for an individual's observational exposure to follow more than one strategy, which becomes particularly unclear for those who have events during the grace period. The target trial provides an approach aligned with the potential outcomes framework for causal inference. This approach can allow for identification of assumptions and limitations, leading to stronger inference based on administrative claims and EHR data.

5.1.8   Effect Modification and Interaction

In this section, we clarify the distinction between effect modification and interaction because these concepts are often conflated. This distinction defines the goal of the analysis and better informs the approach. The terms effect modification and interaction are sometimes used interchangeably. In this section, we describe interaction as a causal concept related to, but different from, effect modification.

Effect Modification. We may be interested in causal effects in the whole population or only a subset of the population. For example, we may be implementing a hepatitis A vaccination program that will reach all individuals in the population. Alternatively, we may be interested in a hepatitis C testing and, if needed, treatment targeted only to people who inject drugs who are at high risk for disease progression.

Define M to be a baseline covariate (and not affected by treatment A) taking values 0 and 1. Effect modification is scale dependent and sometimes called effect measure modification. *Additive effect modification* exists if

$$E[Y^{a=1} - Y^{a=0}|M = 1] \neq E[Y^{a=1} - Y^{a=0}|M = 0].$$

There is *multiplicative effect modification* if

$$\frac{E[Y^{a=1}|M = 1]}{E[Y^{a=0}|M = 1]} \neq \frac{E[Y^{a=1}|M = 0]}{E[Y^{a=0}|M = 0]}.$$

There is qualitative effect modification if the effects are in opposite directions. There is qualitative, additive effect modification if and only if there is qualitative, multiplicative effect modification. Otherwise, there may exist effect modification on the additive scale, but not on the multiplicative scale, and vice versa.

For example, suppose $\Pr[Y^a = {}^1 = 1|M = 1] = 0.9$, $\Pr[Y^a = {}^1 = 1|M = 0] = 0.2$, $\Pr[Y^a = {}^0 = 1|M = 1] = 0.8$, and $\Pr[Y^a = {}^0 = 1|M = 0] = 0.1$. There is no additive effect modification because

$$E[Y^{a=1} - Y^{a=0}|M = 1] = 0.1 = E[Y^{a=1} - Y^{a=0}|M = 0].$$

However, there is multiplicative effect modification because

$$\frac{E[Y^{a=1}|M = 1]}{E[Y^{a=0}|M = 1]} = \frac{0.9}{0.8} \neq \frac{0.2}{0.1} = \frac{E[Y^{a=1}|M = 0]}{E[Y^{a=0}|M = 0]}.$$

For a dichotomous (or binary) M, the stratified causal RDs are

$$E[Y^{a=1}|M = m] - E[Y^{a=0}|M = m].$$

For this to be identifiable with randomization of A, exchangeability (conditional or unconditional) must hold within levels of M, that is, $Y^a \perp A \mid M$. This would hold in a randomized experiment regardless of stratification by M. In the absence of randomization, we may be willing to assume conditional exchangeability $Y^a \perp A \mid \{L, M\}$. Importantly, effect modification by M does not imply that M has a causal effect on Y. For example, suppose M is surgery type and there is effect modification by M. There are more high-dose opioid prescriptions for those with more invasive surgeries. The surgery itself does not impact the outcome opioid use disorder, but rather the pain management modality has a different causal effect depending on surgery type. We could describe effect modification as heterogeneity of causal effects across strata of M.

Effect modification can be of interest for three reasons. First, if M modifies the effect of treatment A on the outcome Y, then the average causal effect will differ between populations with different prevalences of M. Thus, the average causal effect is not transportable or generalizable to other populations and lacks external validity (Cole and Stuart 2010). Second, evaluating the presence of effect modification is helpful to identify the groups of patients that would benefit most from the intervention. Third, identification of effect modification may improve understanding of the mechanisms that lead to the outcome.

To identify effect modification by variables M, we stratify by M, assume conditional exchangeability $Y^a \perp A \mid \{L, M\}$, and then adjust for L within strata defined by levels of M. For the prescription opioid example, we stratify by surgery type before adjusting for unmanaged pain L to determine if the average causal effect of the pain management strategy after surgery differed by use of high-dose opioids (vs. low-dose opioids). Standardization or IP weighting that conditions on M can be used to adjust for L, and stratification is used to identify effect modification by M.

Interaction. Interaction requires a joint intervention. For example, A is high-dose opioid prescription, and E is a physical therapy regimen. Each individual now has four potential outcomes $Y^{a,e}$ for a, $e = 0$, 1. There is interaction between two treatments A and E if the causal effect of A on Y after a joint intervention that sets E to 1 differs from the causal effect of A on Y after a joint intervention that sets E to 0. There is an interaction between A and E on the additive scale if

$$E\left[Y^{a=1,e=1} - Y^{a=0,e=1}\right] \neq E\left[Y^{a=1,e=0} - Y^{a=0,e=0}\right].$$

In other words, the effect of high-dose opioid prescriptions is different if everyone also had physical therapy, compared to if no one had physical therapy. Equivalently, there is interaction on the additive scale if

$$E\left[Y^{a=1,e=1} - Y^{a=1,e=0}\right] \neq E\left[Y^{a=0,e=1} - Y^{a=0,e=0}\right].$$

Note that the potential outcomes for interaction are indexed $Y^{a,e}$, while the potential outcomes for effect modification are indexed Y^a. For interaction, one must be able to manipulate both E and A to consider causal contrasts. To identify interaction effects, exchangeability, positivity, and well-defined interventions are required for both treatments, either marginally $Y^{a,e} \perp A$, E or conditionally $Y^{a,e} \perp A, E \mid L$. Consider the following marginal structural model (MSM):

$$E[Y^{a,e}] = \beta_0 + \beta_1 a + \beta_2 e + \beta_3 a e.$$

We discuss MSMs in more detail in Sect. 5.3.3. In this model, there is additive interaction if and only if $\beta_3 \neq 0$. If there is confounding, a generalized propensity score can be constructed, where the exposure weights conditional on covariates are estimated for each intervention and then multiplied together to obtain a single weight.

5.2 Important Sources of Bias in Pharmacoepidemiology

One of the most important objectives of pharmacoepidemiology is to evaluate the effectiveness and safety of medication in real-world settings. However, there are many factors that could affect patient health outcomes that are challenging to address by observational study designs alone. For example, besides the use of prescription medication, patients' smoking status could affect their health outcomes, such as lung disease. Without randomization, we cannot simply assume the experimental group and control group are comparable with respect to smoking status. In other words, unconditional exchangeability might not hold in this situation. To accurately esti-mate the causal relationship between the exposure and the outcome, we need to better understand these factors that differ by exposure group and also impact the outcomes, which can lead to biases if left unaddressed. In general, biases can be grouped into three categories: confounding, selection bias, and measurement error. In pharmacoepidemiology, a confounder is usually related to the pathological or physiological phenomenon, which contributes to the progress of outcome and may also be associated with the treatment; selection bias is the distortion due to how patients are included in our analysis, e.g., missing data and loss to follow-up; measurement error arises with inaccuracy of ascertainment and measurement of outcomes, exposures, or confounders (Strom 2006).

5.2.1 Confounding

Confounding occurs when treatment A and outcome Y share common cause L. The cause or factor L is also called a *confounder*. In most cases, L is a vector of multiple variables.

> **Confounding** When treatment A and outcome Y share common cause L.

The following causal diagram (Fig. 5.4) shows the simplest structure of confounding. Besides the direct causal pathway $A \rightarrow Y$, there is another open backdoor path from treatment to outcome: $A \leftarrow L \rightarrow Y$. For instance, investigators want to evaluate the effect of treatment A (e.g., anti-hypertension drug) on the outcome Y (e.g., myocardial fraction). In this setting, other comorbidities such as severity of hypertension could affect the probability that subject received antihyper-tensive medication from physicians and also affect the risk of myocardial fraction. To be more specific, adjustment for L, in this case would be addressing confounding

$$L \longrightarrow A \longrightarrow Y$$

Fig. 5.4 Causal diagram for the simplest confounding structure

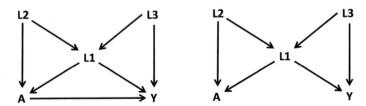

Fig. 5.5 Example causal diagram for confounding with original graph (left) and graph with direct effect of treatment removed (right)

by indication for a prescription (Strom 2006). This is a straightforward structure of confounding. There are more complicated cases when L has an indirect effect on Y or it has an indirect effect on A. For example, in Fig. 5.5 left panel, $L1$, $L2$ and $L3$ are all cofounders for treatment A and outcome Y.

With the definition and the basic structure of confounding, we could use a two-step approach to identify confounding from a causal diagram: (1) Delete all arrows from treatment A to another variable to create a new graph. In other words, remove the direct causal effects of A; (2) In the revised graph, see whether there are still unblocked paths. If there is no open path after all treatment effects were removed, then there is no confounding, and exchangeability holds (Greenland et al. 1999a). Otherwise, there is confounding and exchangeability does not hold. To accurately assess the causal relationship between treatment A and outcome Y in the presence of a confounder L, we would need to block all the backdoor paths (24). To achieve this goal, there are two more questions that needed to be considered: (1) Can we block all the backdoor paths? (2) What is the minimum subset of L to block all the backdoor paths? Now, we apply these approaches to the causal diagram above (Fig. 5.5).

On the left panel of Fig. 5.5, the original graph is displayed. After removing the direct effect of treatment, the modified graph is displayed on the right side. There are three open backdoor paths: $A \leftarrow L_2 \rightarrow L_1 \rightarrow Y$; $A \leftarrow L_1 \leftarrow L_3 \rightarrow Y$; and $A \leftarrow L_1 \rightarrow Y$. If we only condition on L_1, then three paths are blocked. However, we simultaneously open another path: $A \leftarrow L_2 \rightarrow \boxed{L_1} \leftarrow L_3 \rightarrow Y$. To block all paths, we need to condition on the set $\{L1, L2\}$ or $\{L1, L3\}$.

The causal structural definition of confounding and the traditional definition differ. The traditional definition requires confounders to be variables that meet the following criteria: (1) not on the direct causal pathway between treatment and outcome; (2) associated with treatment; and (3) associated with the outcome (Greenland et al. 1999a). In some cases, this traditional definition would suggest to condition on certain variables that would open a previously blocked backdoor path. In the following causal diagram (Fig. 5.6), L would be categorized as a confounder based on traditional criterions. However, once we conditioned on L (denoted by a box on the corresponding variable in the causal DAG), a backdoor path $A \leftarrow U_1 \rightarrow \boxed{L} \leftarrow U_2 \rightarrow Y$ now be an open path because L is a collider (on that path). In the next section, we provided a more complete discussion of colliders.

Fig. 5.6 Example causal diagram that meets the traditional definition of confounding

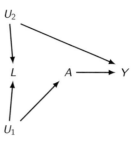

5.2.2   Selection Bias

Selection bias arises when the distribution of certain variable(s) in the sample is different from the distribution in the study population. For example, patients with prior history of significant opioid use may be more willing to seek surgery. Thus, it is challenging to determine if high-dose opioids actually increase the risk of opioid dependence, or rather individuals already using high-dose opioids are more likely to seek surgery, resulting in more identified cases of opioid dependence. In general, under the null (i.e., no causal effect between the exposure and the outcome), selection bias can be defined as the bias resulting from conditioning on the common effect of two variables, one of which is either the treatment or associated with the treatment and the other is either the outcome or associated with the outcome. For example, selection bias can occur by opening a backdoor path between treatment A and outcome Y by conditioning on a *collider C* (i.e., a node where two arrowheads meet), and this is known as *collider stratification*. However, collider stratification is not required for selection bias to occur when there is a causal effect of the exposure on the outcome (Hernán 2017).

> **Selection bias** Bias that arises when the parameter of interest in a population differs from the parameter in the subset of individuals from the population that is available for analysis.

The following causal diagram shows the simplest structure of selection bias (Fig. 5.7). Besides the direct causal effect of treatment A on outcome Y, there is another open path $A \rightarrow C \leftarrow Y$ because we conditioned on the collider C. For example, we are interested in the causal relationship between nonsteroidal anti-inflammatory drugs (NSAIDs) ($A = 1$) and peptic ulcer ($Y = 1$) in the adult population (Strom 2006). However, we only included patients who come to the hospital for an upper endoscopy check ($C = 1$). Patients who have peptic ulcer and experience abdominal pain would more likely receive this test. Meanwhile, a peptic ulcer is a known side effect of NSAIDs. Thus, people who are on this medication with adnominal pain would be more likely to take this test. As a consequence, the measured result is distorted, and it becomes difficult to determine whether the NSAIDs actually increase the risk of a peptic ulcer, or rather individuals using

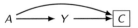

Fig. 5.7 Causal diagram for the simplest selection bias structure conditioning on C

Fig. 5.8 A causal diagram
in which both confounder
and selection bias exist

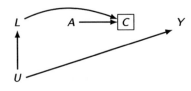

Fig. 5.9 A causal diagram
in which both confounder
and selection bias exist

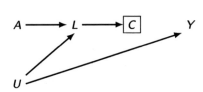

NSAIDs have a higher chance to receive the diagnostic test resulting in more identified cases of peptic ulcer.

This is an example of self-selection bias or volunteer bias. There are several other types of selection bias. For example, differential loss to follow-up occurs when participants drop out from the study is associated with the outcome Y (Hernán and Robins 2020). Furthermore, a study could be prone to both confounding and selection bias, as shown in the following causal diagram (Fig. 5.8). In this hypothetical study, we are interested in the causal relationship between the use of statin medications A and 5-year all-cause mortality Y among patients with diabetes. C is dropout prior to the end of the study (e.g., last visit attended was more than 1 year prior to end of study). L is the measured socioeconomic status, and U includes unmeasured variables, such as reliable transportation to medical visits. Lack of transportation could result in the patient to no longer attend study visits and eventually drop out of the study. Furthermore, lack of transportation could also be associated with an increased risk of mortality. To identify the causal effect of A on Y in this example, we could condition on L to block the backdoor path.

In general, there are situations where simply conditioning on L would not account for selection bias (Fig. 5.9). In this example, C still indicates the dropout, and L is an adverse effect of treatment A which could lead to dropout. U is the unmeasured concomitant over-the-counter (OTC) medication, which might have similar effects as our study medication of interest (e.g., OTC medications are typically not captured in administrative claims data). If we condition on L, the backdoor path is open because conditioning on collider or its descendant could not block the path. In this example, we would need to use inverse probability censoring weighting because, once we condition on both L and A, Y is independent from C. Therefore, we can estimate unconditional measures in the weighted population, rather than within levels of L. We will discuss this estimator further in Sect. 5.3.3.

5.2.3   Measurement Error

Until now, we have assumed an ideal study where all variables (A, Y, L, C) are measured accurately. However, this is usually not the case, especially in pharmacoepidemiology. For example, in an observational study, the treatment A can be measured using prescription claims records in an administrative claims database. We are able to determine if the patient received the prescription from the pharmacy; however, we have no information about the actual adherence to treatment A. Furthermore, we do not know if the patient even initiated the treatment. In this situation, we could not assume that the observed data accurately represents an individual's exposure and this treatment misclassification could potentially impact our estimation of the true relationship between treatment A and outcome Y. In summary, *measurement bias/error* arises when the observed association between A and Y is changed as a result of the process by which the study data are measured.

> **Measurement Error** When the observed association between A and Y is changed due as a result of the process by which the study data are measured.

In the following causal diagram (Fig. 5.10), we display the basic structure of measurement error where measurement error exists for both treatment A and outcome Y. In this figure, A and Y are the true treatment and outcome; A^* and Y^* are the measured treatment and outcome; U_A and U_Y are the measurement errors for treatment and outcome.

Consider a hypothetical cohort study (Fig. 5.11) where we plan to assess the effect of over-the-counter nonsteroidal anti-inflammatory drugs (OTC NSAIDs) among patients with coronary heart disease (CHD). The outcome is measured by

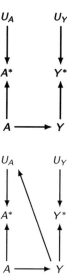

Fig. 5.10 The structure of measurement error (U_A and U_Y)

Fig. 5.11 The structure of misclassification and recall bias existing at the same time

patient recall of their medical history. Here, U_Y is the misclassification of the outcome ($Y^* + U_Y = Y$). Because the outcome has already happened, subjects with CHD tend to have a better memory of their medication history than those who do not have the condition. This is U_A, the recall bias, of the exposure history.

Measurement error has four different casual structures and could be classified according to two separate properties: dependence and differential. The measurement bias is *independent* when U_A and U_Y are independent; it is *nondifferential* when both U_A and Y and U_A and U_Y are independent. In our first example (Fig. 5.10), there is no open path between U_A and Y, U_A and U_Y, and U_Y and A. We could say that the measurement error is independent and nondifferential (Hernán and Robins 2020). In the second example (Fig. 5.11), the recall bias is independent but differential because the outcome Y could affect U_A. The particular structure of the measurement error can help to determine which methods are appropriate. However, these methods are beyond the scope of this chapter. There are many methods existing in the literature particularly for measurement error that is independent and nondifferential. These methods often rely on modeling assumptions and validation samples (i.e., samples in which there is no measurement error). Readers could find the suitable method based on the causal structure for their study (VanderWeele and Hernán 2012; Ogburn and VanderWeele 2012; Dosemeci et al. 1990).

Confounding, selection bias, and measurement error are almost inevitable in pharmacoepidemiologic studies. Investigators should consider biases in their own study design and analyses, employ causal DAGs as a powerful and reliable tool to identify them, and minimize biases by improving study design and applying proper statistical methods. For instance, investigators could employ certain study designs to avoid selection bias, collect adequate data to adjust for confounding, and choose a valid and consistent instrument to obtain measurements. During the data analysis, investigators should use appropriate statistical methods to reduce bias, such as inverse probability weighting (IPW), which was introduced in Sect. 5.1.4, and have a complete understanding of the assumptions and limitations of the methodology for their study design.

5.3   Causal Modeling in Pharmacoepidemiology

Until this section, we considered estimating causal effects in study populations of near infinite size, so we could ignore random fluctuations and focus on the structural biases of confounding, selection, and measurement error. We now introduce causal modeling for pharmacoepidemiology. As part of the modeling, we also consider random variability introduced by selecting the sample from an infinite target population. Herein, we discuss marginal structural models as an approach to quantify causal effects. For baseline exposures, outcome model-based approaches can be used, which yield *conditional* causal effects. In some cases, such as a linear model, the conditional causal effect equals the marginal causal effect, but this is not always the case (Greenland et al. 1999b). If marginal effects are of interest, we can standardize over the distribution of covariates L. The g-formula and g-estimation of structural nested models approaches are related but beyond the scope of this chapter (Hernán and Robins 2020). Marginal structural models can be fit using inverse probability weights, whereas a g-formula approach uses standardization. Both approaches can be used to estimate causal effects in observational data and require the same identifiability assumptions but are based on different modeling assumptions (i.e., correct specification of the exposure model or outcome model, respectively). Doubly robust or augmented estimators are also available, which provide a consistent estimator if either the exposure or outcome model is correctly specified (Bang and Robins 2005). On the other hand, structural nested models require the inclusion of effect modifiers, if they exist, for valid inference (Robins et al. 1992).

An alternative approach employed in causal inference is matching. There are many forms of propensity score matching. The basic idea is to form a matched population in which the treated and untreated are exchangeable because they have the same distribution of the propensity score $\Pr[A = a| L = l]$. For example, one can match the treated to the untreated patients. The subset of the original study population comprised of treated and untreated pairs is the matched population. Under exchangeability and positivity given by the propensity score, the unconditional, associational estimators in general will be consistent for causal effects in the *matched* population. If there are individuals that cannot be matched on their propensity score, the target population may differ from the matched population. Full coverage of matching is beyond the scope of this chapter, and we refer interested readers to Sekhon (2011) and (Stuart 2010).

5.3.1 Random Variability

We employ a frequentist framework; that is, we assume the sample (i.e., study population) is a random sample from an infinite super-population (Casella and Berger 2002). In other words, we observe n independent and identically distributed copies of (A_i, Y_i). We make a distinction between identification versus estimation. Identification involves determining the assumptions necessary to identify parameters. Estimation is the process of using the observed data to quantify causal parameters. The characteristics of the super-population are referred to as *parameters* or *estimands*. For example, $\Pr[Y = 1| A = 1]$ and $P[Y^a = 1]$ are two examples of parameters. We construct *estimators* from the observed study data. For example,

$$\widehat{\Pr}[Y = 1|A = 1] = \sum_{i=1}^{n} Y_i I[A_i = 1] / \sum_{i=1}^{n} I[A_i = 1]$$

is an estimator. The numerical value of an estimator for a particular data set is an estimate, e.g., $\widehat{\Pr}[Y = 1|A = 1] = 5/10$. The parameters are denoted by Greek letters, e.g., θ, with the corresponding estimator denoted by $\widehat{\theta}_n$. The estimator depends on the sample size denoted subscript n. An estimator is unbiased if $E\left[\widehat{\theta}_n\right] = \theta$, where E is notation for the expectation. That is, the expected value of the estimator equals the true parameter. An estimator is consistent if $\widehat{\theta}_n \xrightarrow{p} \theta$. That is, an estimator converges to the true value as the number of samples increases. Assuming exchangeability, such as in a randomized trial, the unconditional risk differences, risk ratios, and odds ratios are consistent estimators of the causal risk differences, risk ratios, and odds ratios, respectively.

5.3.2 Motivation for Modeling

If we have a small study with a limited number of categorical variables, modeling approaches may not be needed. For example, we could employ estimators of the mean that are simply averages. Extending to multiple exposure groups, estimators of the mean in each group could be used. However, once we have a continuous exposure A, we can no longer use a nonparametric (i.e., distribution free) estimator of the mean. In fact, we require a model in this setting. If exposure A is continuous, we could consider a linear mean model $E(Y | A) = \theta_0 + \theta_1 A$. Using either maximum likelihood estimation (MLE) or ordinary least squares (OLS) regression, we can obtain consistent estimators of the parameters and calculate the predicted means (Ali et al. 2005).

A *model* is defined as an a priori restriction on the distribution of the data. For example, a linear model assumes the curve is a straight line. A parametric model is akin to adding information that is not in the data to compensate for a lack of sufficient information in the data. Parametric models allow for consistent estimation that may not be possible otherwise. However, parametric models allow for correct inference only if the restrictions captured by the model are correct. Causal inference based on models is only valid if there is *no model misspecification*. However, nonparametric estimators typically make no a priori restrictions on the distribution of the data. Methods described in this chapter prior to this section are based on nonparametric estimators.

In a setting with two treatment options, model-based estimates are identical to parametric estimators when the model is saturated; that is, when the number of parameters in the model matches the number of population quantities that can be estimated in the model. For example, a model for two population means includes two parameters, θ_0 and θ_1. This is considered saturated because the model cannot estimate any additional terms. If exposure A is non-binary, more flexible regression models can be specified by including nonlinear terms, up to model saturation. As the number of parameters decreases, stronger assumptions are made about how "smooth" the data distribution is. Increasing the number of parameters in the models often comes at a cost. For example, the model with three parameters will be consistent if the model with fewer parameters is consistent; however, the model with more parameters will be less precise (i.e., have larger standard errors). This is known as the *bias-variance tradeoff* (Cole and Hernán 2008). Analysts using models need to decide if more protection against bias is worth the cost in the variance. In the following sections, we assume the models are correctly specified. In any data analysis, causal or not, the validity of models and fit should be evaluated using diagnostics, and sensitivity analyses regarding the model specification should be performed.

5.3.3 Marginal Structural Models

One way to quantify causal effects is through a *marginal structural model* (MSM), which is a model for mean counterfactual outcomes. "Structural" refers to the modeling of the expectation of the counterfactual outcome. In addition, this is a "marginal" model because we are modeling the marginal distribution of the counterfactual rather than the joint or conditional distribution (Hernán et al. 2000; Robins et al. 2000b) or because it may not include any covariates (Hernan and Robins 2020; Hernán et al. 2002). One method for fitting marginal structural models is inverse probability (IP) weighting.

As in the earlier part of this chapter, the goal of the analysis is to estimate the causal effect of a high-dose opioid prescription A after surgery (a binary exposure) on subsequent risk of developing opioid dependence during the following year Y. Our causal estimand of interest is $\Pr[Y^{a=1} = 1] - \Pr[Y^{a=1} = 1]$. This is the difference in the proportion with opioid dependence that would have been observed if all patients were prescribed high-dose opioids after surgery, compared to the proportion with opioid dependence if all individuals in the population were prescribed low-dose opioids. Because the exposure A is not randomly assigned, there may be confounding, so we are only willing to assume conditional exchangeability. In our example, we could assume conditional exchangeability on L, where L includes sex, age, race, education, prior history of unmanaged pain, a comorbidity index, prior history of heavy alcohol use, and surgery type. Assuming conditional exchangeability $Y^{a} \perp A \mid L$, i.e., that covariates L are sufficient to block all backdoor paths, we can use IP weighting to estimate the causal contrast of interest. In a conditionally randomized trial, the exposure weights are a known function of the covariates L. However, in an observational setting, the treatment assignment mechanism $\Pr[A = a \mid L = l]$ is unknown and needs to be estimated.

If L is low dimensional, $\Pr[A = a \mid L = l]$ could be estimated nonparametrically based on sample means. However, in our example, L is an eight-dimensional covariate and includes continuous and categorical covariates, so a model is required. A logistic regression of $\Pr[A = 1 \mid L = l]$ on all eight covariates could be used and can be more flexible with the inclusion of nonlinear terms for continuous variables and interaction terms (Howe et al. 2011). Based on the fitted model, we compute the probabilities for each level of the exposure and then weight each observation by the conditional probability of the exposure actually received. The inverse weighting creates a pseudo-population in which we fit the linear model (using either MLE or OLS), specifically $E[Y|A] = \theta_0 + \theta_1 A$. If A is binary, this method estimates the parameters of the saturated marginal structural model $E[Y^a] = \beta_0 + \beta_1 a$. The outcome variable in the model is a potential outcome.

Stabilized weights defined as $\Pr[A = a]/\Pr[A = a|L]$ can be employed. When the IPW model is not saturated (i.e., has more population parameters than parameters in the model), the stabilized weights will tend to yield narrower 95% confidence intervals. The estimator with unstabilized weights is akin to a Horvitz-Thompson estimator in the survey sampling literature, while the estimator with stabilized weights is akin to a Hajék-type estimator (Horvitz and Thompson 1952; Binder 1983). If the models are correctly specified, the stabilized weights are expected to have a mean of one. Otherwise, there may be model misspecification or violations of positivity.

Marginal structural models can be extended to allow for continuous exposure A. There is a distribution of A, rather than a probability. For example, we might assume the usual linear model $A = \alpha L + \epsilon$, where $\epsilon \sim N(0, \sigma^2)$ in order to estimate $f(A|L)$ and $f(A)$ to compute the stabilized weights $f(A)/f(A|L)$, where $f(x)$ is the continuous distribution of the random variable X (i.e., probability density function). Based on the estimated stabilized weights, each observation is weighted to create a pseudo-population, and the outcome model is fit in the pseudo-population, for example, $E[Y|A = a] = \theta_0 + \theta_1 a + \theta_2 a^2$. If the outcome is dichotomous/binary, the outcome model can be fit as a logistic regression model for a marginal structural logistic model.

In MSMs, covariates can be included to assess effect modification. For example, let prior unmanaged pain be V (yes vs. no), and consider the MSM

$$E[Y^a|V] = \beta_0 + \beta_1 a + \beta_2 Va + \beta_3 V.$$

There is additive effect modification if $\beta_2 \neq 0$. The parameters of the MSM can be consistently estimated by fitting $E[Y|A, V] = \beta_0 + \beta_1 A + \beta_2 VA + \beta_3 V$ via weighted least squares. The weights based on the covariates L must also include V in addition to all other variables sufficient to ensure exchangeability within levels of V. The numerator of the stabilized weight can also include V.

In addition to inverse probability of exposure weights, one could consider censoring weights. In the case that there is a large number of participants missing the outcome, selecting only those with non-missing outcome values may introduce selection bias (Sect. 5.2.2). Let $C = 1$ if the opioid dependence outcome was missing (e.g., no medical visit during the year following surgery) and $C = 0$ otherwise. The unstabilized weights are now defined as

$$\frac{A(1 - C)}{\Pr[C = 0|A, L]\Pr[A = 1|L]} + \frac{(1 - A)(1 - C)}{\Pr[C = 0|A, L]\Pr[A = 0|L]}.$$

5.4 Advanced Topics

In this section, we discuss time-to-event or survival data, which is common in the evaluation of health outcomes. Often a binary/dichotomous event does not provide sufficient information about a patient's health outcome, and estimators based on this type of outcome may be biased due to censoring or loss to follow-up. Time-to-event analyses can offer a more accurate representation of patient outcomes over time (e.g., mortality), as a delay in the time to certain health outcomes can be clinically meaningful. Often in pharmacoepidemiology, exposures, such as prescription medications, are varying over time and are also subject to time-varying confounding. By including these time-varying variables that are confounders in the outcome model, one is also conditioning on a possible intermediary variable (i.e., collider). Therefore, standard methods are not appropriate in this setting, and a g-formula approach (e.g., MSM) or g-estimation is required to ensure valid inference (Hernán and Robins 2020). In addition to challenges in evaluation of biomedical data, the employment of administrative data or electronic health data offers unique challenges, including unmeasured confounding and misclassification. We present instrumental variables as one approach that may be possible in some settings to address unmeasured confounding in large healthcare databases; however, there are other approaches in the literature (Lipsitch et al. 2010; VanderWeele and Ding 2017).

5.4.1 Causal Survival Analysis

Survival analysis can be used in pharmacoepidemiologic research to compare the time to occurrence of clinical events between treatment or exposure groups (Cole and Hudgens 2010). The outcome of interest is time to an event, such as death. T is the time to an event of interest (e.g., death, cancer, flu infection) after the start of study follow-up. Administrative censoring occurs at some fixed or known time point after the start of follow-up (e.g., 1 year after surgery). Left censoring is when the outcome occurs before the study period (e.g., opioid dependence prior to the start of the study).

The survival time T is known only for individuals whose events were observed. For those who were censored, we only know that T is greater than the censoring time. The survival probability $\Pr(T > k)$ is defined as the probability that the survival time is greater than or equal to t. The survival curve starts at $\Pr(T > 0) = 1$ for $k = 0$ and decreases monotonically as time k increases. The *risk* (or cumulative distribution function) is $\Pr(T \leq k) = 1 - \Pr(T > k)$. The hazard is defined as the instantaneous probability of the event occurring at time k among those who had not developed it before time k and is denoted by $\Pr(T = k \mid T = k - 1)$. Note that the hazard and risk are different measures.

In our example, rather than considering the overdose event as a binary variable (yes vs. no) by the end of 1 year of follow-up, we can analyze time to the first overdose after surgery and denote this by T and denote the counterfactual survival times by T^0 and T^1 (i.e., survival time, if contrary to fact, a patient was not exposed and survival time, if contrary to fact, a patient was exposed). Randomized trials are the gold standard to estimate exposure effects on survival time, but are not always ethical or feasible. Although observational studies may provide estimates of effects when trial data are unavailable, the validity of these estimators is often threatened by confounding (Greenland and Morgenstern 2001). As in the single binary outcome case, confounding occurs when the exposure and outcome share a common cause. Furthermore, studies with follow-up can be prone to selection bias due to informative dropout. This type of selection bias occurs when the mechanism of dropout is associated with exposure and covariates. The Cox proportional hazards regression model (Cox 1972), the standard approach in survival analysis, can account for multiple measured confounders. Unfortunately, the Cox model provides only a single summary measure (i.e., hazard ratio), which can be difficult to interpret (Hernán 2010). In addition, this model requires the proportional hazards assumption in the exposure groups.

As an alternative to the standard Cox model, we discuss a method that uses inverse probability (IP) weights to estimate the effect of an exposure that is fixed at study entry. Under certain assumptions, this method can be used to mimic a randomized trial when only observational data are available. In particular, unlike the standard Cox model, this approach allows for estimation of marginal effects which compare the distribution of outcomes when the entire population is exposed versus when the entire population is unexposed (Kaufman 2010). This IP-weighted approach naturally leads to Kaplan-Meier (Kaplan and Meier 1958) type survival curve estimates that account for confounding by multiple covariates (Cole and Hernán 2004, 2008; Xie and Liu 2005; Sato and Matsuyama 2003).

Researchers are often interested in estimating effects of an exposure fixed at study entry. IP-weighted Cox models are a method to compare the timing of clinical events under two different exposures, mimicking results in randomized trials. The Cox proportional hazard model can be written as $h_i(t|\bar{a}(t)) = \exp(\beta \bar{a}(t))h_0(t)$, where $h(t)$ denotes the hazard function at time t and $\bar{a}(t)$ denotes the treatment history up to time t. An IP-weighted Cox model is fit by maximizing a weighted partial likelihood, where participant i who died or was diagnosed with AIDS at time t from baseline contributes the term $\left\{ \dfrac{\exp(\beta A_i)}{\sum_{R_{j(t)}} w_j(t) \exp(\beta A_j)} \right\}^{w_i(t)}$, where $R(t)$ is the risk set at time t and $\exp(\beta)$ is the hazard ratio for a unit difference in exposure A_i accounting for confounding measured by covariates through the estimated IP weight w_i (discussed below) (Robins et al. 2000, b). Slight modification of the likelihood is needed in the presence of tied survival times. The robust variance estimator (Lin and Wei 1989) can be employed to account for the fact that the IP weights are estimated (Westreich et al. 2010). For readers interested in a review of the standard Cox model, see Collett (2015).

As defined below, the estimated IP weight $\widehat{w}_i(t)$ is the product of an estimated time-fixed IP exposure weight $\widehat{w}_{1i}$ and an estimated time-varying IP censoring weight $\widehat{w}_{2i}(t)$ for each participant i at each survival time t (defined below). The time-fixed IP exposure weights are constructed to account for confounding by covariates measured at baseline. Different versions of these weights have been proposed. We recommend the stabilized IP exposure weight w_{1i} defined as the ratio of the marginal probability of having the exposure that participant i had, formally $\Pr(A_i = a_i)$, to the covariate-conditional probability of having the exposure that participant i had, formally $P(A_i = a_i \mid L_i)$, where L_i are the measured covariates for participant i assumed sufficient to adjust for confounding. If we do not appropriately adjust for confounding, the estimated association between the exposure and study outcome may be far from the truth (i.e., biased). Because these IP weights are unknown, the probabilities of exposure are estimated using the observed data.

The time-varying IP censoring weights are constructed to account for possible selection bias due to dropout (Robins et al. 2000, b). In our example, patients last observed alive and without diagnosed opioid dependence more than 3 months prior to the administrative end of the study (i.e., 1 year after surgery) were considered censored (i.e., lost to follow-up). Participants received a time-varying weight that corresponds to their probability of remaining uncensored. This stabilized IP weight $w_{2i}(t)$ is defined as the ratio of the marginal probability of remaining in the study (i.e., uncensored), formally $\Pr(D_i > t \mid A_i)$, where D_i is the time from the start of the study (i.e., baseline) to dropout for participant i, to the covariate-conditional probability of remaining in the study, formally $\Pr(D_i > t \mid Z_i, Z_i(t), A_i)$, where Z_i and $Z_i(t)$ are the measured common causes of dropout and the study outcome for participant i up to time t. (Note the covariates in the dropout weight model can be different than the covariates in the exposure weight model.) If we do not appropriately adjust for the common (time-varying) causes of dropout and study outcome, the estimated association between the exposure and outcome may be biased due to dropout. Again, because these IP dropout weights are unknown, the probabilities of remaining free of dropout are estimated using the observed data.

Standardized survival curve estimates $\widehat{\Pr}(T^1 > k)$ and $\widehat{\Pr}(T^1 > k)$ can be obtained by fitting an IP-weighted Cox model stratified by exposure with no covariates and then using a Kaplan-Meier-type estimator, nonparametrically estimating the baseline survival functions for the two strata (Cole and Hernán 2004). In the absence of weighting, these survival curve estimates will be (asymptotically) equivalent to Kaplan-Meier estimates obtained separately for each of the exposure strata (Collett 2015).

We only discussed exposure groups defined at baseline thus far in this chapter. When interest focuses on exposures that change over time, methods must be adapted accordingly. When a time-varying variable is a risk factor for the outcome, predicts later exposure, and is affected by prior exposure, standard statistical methods (e.g., Cox models with time-varying covariates) are biased and fail to provide consistent estimators of effects (Hernán et al. 2000, 2013; Robins et al. 2000, b; Cole et al. 2003). IP weighting can be generalized to account for time-varying confounders

(Robins et al. 2000, b). For example, among patients who had surgery, starting a new medication for anxiety (e.g., benzodiazepines) during the follow-up period is a risk factor for opioid dependence, predicts subsequent treatment with opioids, and is affected by prior treatment; thus, the IP-weighted Cox model is appropriate for studying the effect of time-varying opioid therapy on opioid dependence while adjusting for time-varying current use of medication for anxiety.

The hazard ratio can be problematic for two reasons (58). First, because the hazards vary over time, the hazard ratio also varies over time. The hazard ratio at time k may be different from time $k + 1$. In many published papers that report survival analyses, a single hazard ratio is reported, which is the weighted average of the time-specific hazard ratios, and is often hard to interpret. In contrast, survival and risks are always presented at a specific time during follow-up. Second, even if we present the time-specific hazard ratios, their causal interpretation is not straightforward. The hazard ratio at time $k + 1$ conditions on having survived to time k. This can be conceptualized as an example of selection bias induced by conditioning on a post-treatment variable that is affected by treatment.

Due to these limitations, we briefly describe an approach to estimate survival/ risks. Our interest is in estimating the survival function, and one approach for this is estimating the hazard at each time m and then cumulatively multiplying up to the survival time of interest at time k. We can estimate the hazard for treatment A at each discrete time either nonparametrically or with a parametric logistic regression model (Hernán and Robins 2020).

5.4.2 Time-Varying Exposures

Consider a binary time-varying treatment or exposure, and denote this by A_k, which can take the values 0 for unexposed and 1 for exposed at each time k, $k = 0, \ldots, K$. The health outcome of interest Y is measured at time $K + 1$ from study entry. If the outcome only depends on the exposure at the prior time, we denote the potential outcome at time $K + 1$ by Y^{a_k}. We denote the exposure history as $\bar{A}_k = \{A_0, A_1, \ldots, A_k\}$ and the covariate history up to time k as $\bar{L}_k = \{L_0, L_1, \ldots, L_k\}$ denote. Assume L_k is measured prior to A_k at time k. If we are interested in the parameter at a particular time k defined as $E[Y^{a_k}] - E[Y^{a_k}]$, we can simply apply techniques discussed earlier in this chapter. There are many possible treatment regimens or plans, and let $\bar{a} = \{a(0), a(1), \ldots, a(K)\}$ denote a possible treatment regimen. For example, this could be always exposed $\bar{a} = \{1, 1, \ldots, 1\}$ or never exposed $\bar{a} = \{0, 0, \ldots, 0\}$. We define $Y^{\bar{a}}$ as the potential outcome at time $K + 1$ for regime $\bar{a}$. Thus, each individual has $2^{\{K+1\}}$ potential outcomes. The time-varying treatment A_k has a causal effect on the average value of Y if $E[Y^{\bar{a}}] - E[Y^{\bar{a}'}] \neq 0$ for at least two regimens $\bar{a}$ and $\bar{a}'$.

> **Definition** The time-varying treatment A_k has a causal effect on the average value of Y if $E[Y^{\bar{a}}] - E[Y^{\bar{a}'}] \neq 0$ for at least two regimens $\bar{a}$ and $\bar{a}'$.

Dynamic treatment strategies are when the treatment strategy $\bar{a}_k$ at time k depends on an individual's time-varying covariate(s) $\bar{L}_k$. For example, patients living with HIV historically initiated HIV treatment only after their CD4 cell counts declined below a certain threshold. In this case, the time-varying HIV treatment depends on the patient's history of CD4 cell counts. *Static treatment strategies* are strategies $\bar{a}$ for which treatment does not depend on covariates.

The g-formula, IPTW, and g-estimation can provide consistent estimators of counterfactual quantities such as $E[Y^{\bar{a}}]$ under more general versions of causal consistency, conditional exchangeability, and positivity. By consistency, if $\bar{A} = \bar{a}$, then $Y^{\bar{a}} = Y$. The extension to conditional exchangeability is $Y^{\bar{a}} \perp\!\!\!\perp A_k | \{\bar{A}_{k-1}, \bar{L}_k\}$. Similarly, the positivity assumption is $\Pr[A_k = a_k | \bar{A}_{k-1} = \bar{a}_{k-1}, \bar{L}_k = \bar{l}_k] > 0$ if $\Pr[\bar{A}_{k-1} = \bar{a}_{k-1}, \bar{L}_k = \bar{l}_k] > 0$. If $\bar{L}_k$ has a continuous component, then this probability is always zero, and, in that case, we can replace the probability expression with the probability distribution function denoted by $f\{A_k | \bar{A}_{(k-1)}, L_k\}$.

As in the simpler setting of an exposure at a single time point, we can consider an idealized randomized experiment for this setting. These three conditions will in general hold in a sequentially randomized experiment with full compliance. A sequentially randomized experiment is a randomized experiment in which the exposure value at each successive visit k is randomly assigned with known randomization probabilities that, by design, may depend on a patient's past exposure $\bar{A}_{k-1}$ and covariate history $\bar{L}_k$. The assumption of conditional exchangeability is sometimes referred to as the *assumption of sequential randomization* or the *assumption of no unmeasured confounders*.

In this time-varying exposure setting, a causal parameter $E[Y^{\bar{a}}]$ may not be identifiable under all treatment strategies. For example, for static strategies at each time k, all backdoor paths into A_k that do not go through any future treatment must be blocked. This is known as the *generalized backdoor criterion*.

We define *time-varying confounders* as time-varying covariates $\bar{L}_k$ that are sufficient together in this setting with the treatment history $\bar{A}_{k-1}$ to block all backdoor paths between subsequent treatment A_k and outcome Y. As mentioned earlier in this chapter, most standard methods of confounder adjustment in this setting will be biased even if all confounders are measured.

To illustrate this, consider a hypothetical study that assesses the effect of buprenorphine/naloxone as part of medication-assisted therapy for opioid use disorder on subsequent overdose, measured at the end of follow-up among 25,000 patients with opioid use disorder. The outcome at time $K + 1$ is a function of measured comorbidities, history of incarceration, and education level, as well as unmeasured employment status. We are interested in the parameter $E[Y^{\bar{a}=\bar{1}}] - E[Y^{\bar{a}=\bar{0}}]$, that is, ever exposed versus never exposed. Let A_0 and A_1

Table 5.3 Opioid overdose potential outcomes Y^a with buprenorphine/naloxone therapy exposure A and employment status L among patients with opioid use disorder

$A(0)$	$L(1)$	$A(1)$	N	$Y(1)$	$E\{Y|A(0), L(1), A(1)\}$
0	0	0	1700	900	0.53
0	0	1	4200	1600	0.38
0	1	0	5100	3050	0.60
0	1	1	1000	420	0.42
1	0	0	3700	1250	0.34
1	0	1	2900	700	0.24
1	1	0	4000	1550	0.39
1	1	1	14,000	5000	0.36

Variables are indexed by time t

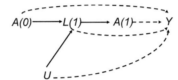

Fig. 5.12 Causal diagram for our hypothetical study of opioid overdose caused by buprenorphine therapy exposure A, employment status L among patients with opioid use disorder, and U is unmeasured baseline education status

equal 1 if the subject received buprenorphine at times $t = 0$ and $t = 1$, respectively, and 0 otherwise. The binary covariate L_1 is temporally prior to A_1 and takes the value 1 if the patient has employment at time $t = 1$ and 0 otherwise. Assuming no sampling variability, the data from our study are displayed in Table 5.3. We assume the data arose from a sequentially randomized experiment where treatment A_1 was randomly assigned based on covariate L_1 and A_0 was marginally randomized.

The causal DAG for our hypothetical study can be represented by Fig. 5.12, where U is the subject's baseline education status, an unmeasured variable. The dotted arrows indicate that we do not know, based on prior subject-matter knowledge, whether these causal arrows are present. The goal is to assess whether the arrows are present or not using the observed study data. Our target parameter is $E\left[Y^{\bar{a}=\bar{1}}\right] - E\left[Y^{\bar{a}=\bar{0}}\right]$.

First, consider the edge from A_0 to L_1. In Fig. 5.12, one or both of the A_0 to Y and L_1 to Y arrows may be present, but we cannot conclude anything beyond this. L_1 is both a confounder and a collider on the causal path between A and Y. Thus, we need to adjust for the possible confounding of L_1 to draw inference about the effect of A_1 on Y. However, if we adjust for L_1 using standard methods, we cannot consistently estimate the effect of A_0 on Y due to possible selection bias induced by conditioning on L_1. Because this standard approach is not valid, we might consider standardization; however, this also conditions on L_1, which is a collider on the non-causal path $A_0 \rightarrow \boxed{L_1} \leftarrow U \rightarrow Y$. Alternatively, inverse probability of treatment weighted estimators can be constructed as in the point exposure setting, where now the weights are defined as $\Pr\left[A_k = a_k \mid \overline{A}_{k-1} = \overline{a}_{k-1}, \overline{L}_k = \overline{l}_k\right]$ at each time k. A nonparametric estimator can be constructed as

$$\frac{1}{n}\sum_i W_i Y_i I\left[\overline{A}_i = \overline{a}\right] \quad \text{or} \quad \frac{\sum_i W_i Y_i I\left[\overline{A}_i = \overline{a}\right]}{\sum_i W_i\, I\left[\overline{A}_i = \overline{a}\right]},$$

where W_i denotes unstabilized treatment weights:

$$W_i = \prod_{k=0}^{K} \frac{1}{f\left\{A_{ik}\mid A_{i(k-1)}, L_{ik}\right\}}.$$

We use f to denote the exposure weight that allow for both continuous and binary exposures.

A consistent estimator of the weights is known in a sequentially randomized experiment; therefore, the IPTW estimator is consistent in a sequentially randomized experiment. In an observational study, the IPTW is consistent if the estimated weights are based on correctly specified parametric models. In practice, if there are a large number of time periods, the product in the denominator of the weights can become small for some subjects who receive inordinately large weights. Employing a stabilized weight may be more efficient (i.e., have a smaller variance) in this setting, and this can be written as

$$SW_i = \prod_{k=0}^{K} \frac{f\left\{A_{ik}\mid A_{i(k-1)}\right\}}{f\left\{A_{ik}\mid A_{i(k-1)}, L_{ik}\right\}}.$$

Due to the large number of potential outcomes 2^{K+1} relative to the sample size n, the approach may require modeling even in a sequentially randomized trial. We could consider a continuous response Y and that it is hypothesized that the mean outcome increases linearly as a function of the cumulative exposure $\overline{a}$. That is,

$$E[Y^a] = \eta_0 + \eta_1 \operatorname{cum}(\overline{a}),$$

where $\operatorname{cum}(\overline{a}) = \sum_{k=0}^{K} a(k)$. This model is not saturated because there are $2^{\{K+1\}}$ unknown counterfactual means versus two model parameters. Because any unsaturated model may be misspecified, the evaluation of model fit is important. This MSM with a time-varying exposure can be fit via inverse probability treatment weights. A weighted ordinary least squares regression model, $E[Y|\overline{A}] = \gamma_0 + \gamma_1 \operatorname{cum}(\overline{A})$, can be fit in the weighted data using stabilized or unstabilized weights. In an observational study, the weights must be estimated, typically using a logistic model. We can obtain a conservative estimator of the variance using a robust (i.e., empirical sandwich) estimator of the variance. Typically, inference is more precise using a stabilized weight. One way to test if an MSM is misspecified is to fit a more flexible parametric model by, for example, including a quadratic term or cumulative exposure up to a certain visit, and compare the fit of this model to the more parsimonious one using an appropriate statistical test. In addition, the mean of the stabilized weights should be one, and deviations from this indicate possible model misspecification or positivity violations. As in the point exposure setting, these models can be extended to evaluate effect modification by adding the effect modifier and interaction with the effect modifier to the outcome model. For the stabilized weights, the effect modifier can also be included as a covariate in the numerator (Talbot et al. 2015). MSMs are easy to implement using standard software, and we strongly encourage readers to employ these methods, particularly in the setting of a time-varying exposure with time-varying confounding.

5.4.3   Instrumental Variables

Accurate assessment of the causal relationship between treatment and outcome requires adjustment for confounding, elimination of selection bias, and minimization of measurement error. However, there still could be bias remaining in our analysis due to unknown or unmeasured variables. In Sect. 5.2, we discussed how randomization ensures balance of all measured and unmeasured covariates. Due to ethical or financial limits, investigators often employ retrospective observational study designs in pharmacoepidemiologic research. In this setting, instrumental variables (IVs) can be used to distinguish the causal effect of treatment on outcome from residual confounding bias. Often, there are policy and program changes that impact a patient's eligibility for treatment, which can be used to emulate a conditional randomization procedure with the observed data. However, IVs require alternative assumptions, which, if violated, can produce biases that are unpredictable, and determining an IV in the absence of randomization can be challenging.

The following causal DAG (Fig. 5.13) shows the basic structure of IVs. Z represents the instrument, and U represents confounding caused by unmeasured covariates. The definition of IV contains three conditions:

1. Z and A are associated.
2. Z could only affect Y through A.
3. Z does not share same causes with Y.

Fig. 5.13 The basic structure of a instrumental variable

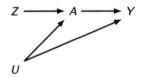

The second condition is also known as exclusion restriction. For example, in a pharmacoepidemiologic study, treatment A is the use of medical marijuana for pain management, outcome Y is opioid use disorder, and Z is policy/availability of medical marijuana in different states. Here, Z could not directly cause Y, but Z could affect Y through A. A few more common examples of IVs in pharmacoepidemiology include genetic factors, physician preference, and access to a certain clinical center or hospital (Hernan and Robins 2010).

Before addressing IVs in an observational setting, we will develop the concepts in the setting of a randomized trial in which there was sub-optimal patient adherence with the treatment regimen despite efforts to maximize treatment compliance. Let Z be the randomized intervention, A be a measure of adherence, and Y be the primary outcome. Because Z is randomized, we could assess the intent-to-treat (ITT) effect (i.e., the effect of being assigned the treatment strategy Z on Y). The ITT does not require for confounder adjustment because the intervention Z was randomized. For example, the causal relative risk is defined as

$$RR = \frac{\Pr\left(Y^{z=1} = 1\right)}{\Pr\left(Y^{z=0} = 1\right)}.$$

A valid estimator of the ITT causal relative risk can be obtained using the approach described in Sect. 5.1.4. If treatment adherence is perfect in the study, the ITT effect equals the true treatment effect of A on Y. If treatment adherence was sub-optimal, investigators may be interested in the causal effect among those who would have adhered under both assigned interventions at baseline (or "always compliers"). This is known as the *complier average causal effect* (CACE). If treatment adherence is perfect in the study, the CACE equals the ITT effect. In this example of a randomized trial, Z is a valid IV. If we make addition assumption of monotonicity or no defiers (i.e., those who always take the treatment other than assigned one ($A^{z=1} >= A^{z=0}$) do not exist), we could identify CACE.

$$CACE = \frac{E(Y|Z = 1) - E(Y|Z = 0)}{\Pr(A = 1|Z = 1) - \Pr(A = 1|Z = 0)}.$$

We now return to our example of medical marijuana policy as the instrumental variable. Although observational studies lack randomization, it may be possible to employ changes in policies or programs that give rise to "natural experiments." Here, treatment A is medical marijuana for pain management, outcome Y is opioid use disorder, and Z is policy/availability of medical marijuana in different states. The target parameter is the complier average causal effect. Before computing the estimator of this effect, we first must evaluate the plausibility of the assumptions. The policy for medical marijuana certainly affects the access to medical marijuana for pain management. Furthermore, this policy likely only affects opioid use disorder through the use of medical marijuana for pain, specifically by substituting this for opioid medications. The assumption that medical marijuana policy in a state and an individual's risk for opioid use disorder do not share common causes is plausible. The fourth assumption (i.e., no defiers) means that those patients residing in states without a medicinal marijuana program would not use medical marijuana. After careful consideration of these assumptions, the complier average causal effect can be estimated using appropriate models extending the approach described above.

5.5 Concluding Remarks

As we enter the era of big data in health research, it is advantageous for the medical research field to leverage large administrative claims databases and electronic health records. Although pharmacoepidemiology as a field has been using these databases to evaluate associations and predictions, we now have the tools to move toward causal inference in pharmacoepidemiology. This framework can allow for identification of sources of biases resulting improved inference, methods development, and future studies to improve information obtained from these large databases. By making the target trial explicit in analyses, we are more rigorous in the design and analysis of observational data. For implementation of causal inference methodologies in SAS (SAS Institute Inc., Cary, NC, USA), we recommend using standard procedures in combination to estimate causal effects. Sample code can be found in Buchanan et al. (2014), Buchanan et al. (2018), and Hernán et al. (2000). Alternatively in SAS, we recommend employing PROC CAUSALTRT (SAS Institute Inc. 2016). For matching analyses, we recommend PROC PSMATCH (SAS Institute Inc. 2016). Through both methods development and high-impact applications, causal inference in pharmacoepidemiology provides the tools to go beyond predicting future health outcomes to change health outcomes and inform health policy and, ultimately, improve patient health.

Acknowledgments The authors thank Dr. Stephen Kogut and Dr. Mireille Schnitzer for their comments that greatly improved this chapter. Dr. Ashley Buchanan and Tianyu Sun are partially supported by Institutional Development Award Number U54GM115677 from the National Institute of General Medical Sciences of the National Institutes of Health, which funds Advance Clinical and Translational Research (Advance-CTR). Drs. Ashley Buchanan and Natallia Katenka are partially supported by Avenir Award Program for Research on Substance Abuse and HIV/AIDS (DP2) 1DP2DA046856-01 from the National Institute on Drug Abuse of the National Institutes of Health. The content is solely the responsibility of the authors and does not necessarily represent the official views of the National Institutes of Health.

References

Ali M, Emch M, Von Seidlein L, Yunus M, Sack DA, Rao M, Holmgren J, Clemens JD. Herd immunity conferred by killed oral cholera vaccines in Bangladesh: a reanalysis. *The Lancet.* 2005;366(9479):44-9.

Anderson RN, Miniño AM, Hoyert DL, Rosenberg HM. Comparability of cause of death between ICD-9 and ICD-10: preliminary estimates. *National Vital Statistics Reports.* 2001;49(2):1-32.

Bang H, Robins JM. Doubly robust estimation in missing data and causal inference models. *Biometrics.* 2005;61(4):962-73.

Benjamin-Chung J, Arnold B. F., Berger D., Luby S. P., Miguel E., Colford JrJ. M., & Hubbard A. E. Spillover effects in epidemiology: parameters, study designs and methodological considerations. *International Journal of Epidemiology.* 2018;47(1):332–347.

Binder DA. On the variances of asymptotically normal estimators from complex surveys. *International Statistical Review/Revue Internationale de Statistique.* 1983;51(3):279–92.

Bound J, Jaeger DA, Baker RM. Problems with instrumental variables estimation when the correlation between the instruments and the endogenous explanatory variable is weak. *Journal of the American Statistical Association.* 1995;90(430):443-50.

Brookhart MA, Wang P, Solomon DH, Schneeweiss SJ Evaluating short-term drug effects using a physician-specific prescribing preference as an instrumental variable. *Epidemiology.* 2006;17 (3):268.

Buchanan AL, Vermund SH, Friedman SR, Spiegelman D. Assessing Individual and Disseminated Effects in Network-Randomized Studies. *American Journal of Epidmeiology.* 2018; 187(11): 2449-2459.

Buchanan AL, Hudgens MG, Cole SR, Lau B, Adimora AA, Women's Interagency HIV Study. Worth the weight: using inverse probability weighted Cox models in AIDS research. *AIDS Research and Human Retroviruses.* 2014;30(12):1170-7.

Casella G, Berger RL. *Statistical Inference*: Duxbury Pacific Grove, CA; 2002.

Cheng J, Small DS. Bounds on causal effects in three-arm trials with non-compliance. *Journal of the Royal Statistical Society (Series B).* 2006;68(5):815-36.

Cole SR, Frangakis CE. The consistency statement in causal inference: a definition or an assumption? *Epidemiology.* 2009;20(1):3-5.

Cole SR, Hernán MA. Constructing inverse probability weights for marginal structural models. *American Journal of Epidemiology.* 2008;168(6):656-64.

Cole SR, Hudgens MG. Survival analysis in infectious disease research: describing events in time. *AIDS.* 2010;24(16):2423.

Cole SR, Hernán MA. Adjusted survival curves with inverse probability weights. *Statistical Methods in Medical Research.* 2004;75(1):45-9.

Cole SR, Hernán MA, Robins JM, Anastos K, Chmiel J, Detels R, Ervin C, Feldman J, Greenblatt R, Kingsley LJ. Effect of highly active antiretroviral therapy on time to acquired immunodeficiency syndrome or death using marginal structural models. *American Journal of Epidemiology.* 2003;158(7):687-94.

Cole SR, Stuart EA. Generalizing evidence from randomized clinical trials to target populations: the ACTG 320 trial. *American Journal of Epidemiology.* 2010; 72(1): 107–115.

Collett D. *Modelling Survival Data in Medical Research.* (2015) Boca Raton: Chapman and Hall/CRC.

Cox DR. Regression models and life-tables. *Journal of the Royal Statistical Society*: Series B (Methodological).* 1972;34(2):187–202.

Denny JC. Mining electronic health records in the genomics era. *PLoS computational biology.* 2012;8(12):e1002823.

Dosemeci M, Wacholder S, Lubin JH. Does nondifferential misclassification of exposure always bias a true effect toward the null value? *American Journal of Epidemiology.* 1990;132(4):746-8.

Glymour MM, Spiegelman D. Evaluating public health interventions: 5. Causal inference in public health research—do sex, race, and biological factors cause health outcomes? *American Journal of Public Health.* 2017;107(1):81-5.

Greenland S, Pearl J, Robins JM. Causal diagrams for epidemiologic research. *Epidemiology.* 1999a;(10):37-48.

Greenland S, Robins JM, & Pearl J. Confounding and collapsibility in causal inference. *Statistical Science.* 1999b;14(1):29-46.

Greenland S, Morgenstern H. Confounding in health research. *Ann Rev of Public Health*. 2001;22 (1):189–212.

Haneuse S, Daniels M. A general framework for considering selection bias in EHR-based studies: what data are observed and why? *eGEMS*. 2016;4(1):1203.

Hernán MA. Invited commentary: selection bias without colliders. *American Journal of Epidemiology*. 2017;*185*(11), 1048–1050.

Hernán MA, Brumback BA, Robins JM. Estimating the causal effect of zidovudine on CD4 count with a marginal structural model for repeated measures. *Statistics in Medicine*. 2002;21(12): 1689–1709.

Hernán MÁ, Brumback B, Robins JM. Marginal structural models to estimate the causal effect of zidovudine on the survival of HIV-positive men. *Epidemiology*. 2000;11(5):561–70.

Hernán MA, Robins JM. *Causal Inference*: What If. Boca Raton: Chapman & Hall/CRC. 2020

Hernán MA, Robins JM. Using big data to emulate a target trial when a randomized trial is not available. *American Journal of Epidemiology*. 2016;183(8):758–64.

Hernán MA. Does water kill? A call for less casual causal inferences. *Annals of Epidemiology*. 2016;26(10):674-80.

Hernán MA. The hazards of hazard ratios. *Epidemiology*. 2010;21(1):13.

Hernán MA, Hernández-Díaz S, Robins JM. Randomized trials analyzed as observational studies. *Annals of Internal Medicine*. 2013;159(8):560-2.

Holland P. Statistics and causal inference. *Journal of the American Statistical Association*. 1986;81 (396):945-60.

Hong G, Raudenbush SW. Evaluating kindergarten retention policy: A case study of causal inference for multilevel observational data. *Journal of the American Statistical Association*. 2006;101(475):901-10.

Horvitz DG, Thompson DJ. A generalization of sampling without replacement from a finite universe. *Journal of the American statistical Association*. 1952;47(260):663-85.

Howe CJ, Dulin-Keita A, Cole SR, Hogan JW, Lau B, Moore RD, Mathews WC, Crane HM, Drozd DR, Geng EJ. Evaluating the Population Impact on Racial/Ethnic Disparities in HIV in Adulthood of Intervening on Specific Targets: A Conceptual and Methodological Framework. *American Journal of Epidemiology*. 2017;187(2):316-25.

Howe CJ, Cole SR, Westreich DJ, Greenland S, Napravnik S, Eron Jr JJ. Splines for trend analysis and continuous confounder control. *Epidemiology*. 2011;22(6):874.

Hripcsak G, Friedman C, Alderson PO, DuMouchel W, Johnson SB, Clayton PD. Unlocking clinical data from narrative reports: a study of natural language processing. *Annals of Internal Medicine*.1995;122(9):681-8.

Hudgens MG, Halloran ME. Toward causal inference with interference. *Journal of the American Statistical Association*. 2008;103(482):832-42.

Imai K, Van Dyk DA. Causal inference with general treatment regimes: Generalizing the propensity score. *Journal of the American Statistical Association*. 2004;99(467):854-66.

Imbens, G. W., and Rubin, D. B. (2015). Causal inference in statistics, social, and biomedical sciences. New York: Cambridge University Press.

Iribarren C, Crow R, Mstat PH, Jacobs Jr D, Luepker R. Validation of death certificate diagnosis of out-of-hospital sudden cardiac death. *The American Journal of Cardiology*. 1998;82(1):50-3.

Kaplan EL, Meier PJ. Nonparametric estimation from incomplete observations. *Journal of the American Statistical Association*. 1958;53(282):457-81.

Kaufman JSJE. Marginalia: Comparing adjusted effect measures. *Epidemiology*. 2010;21(4):490-3.

Lipsitch, M., Tchetgen, E. T., & Cohen, T. (2010). Negative controls: a tool for detecting confounding and bias in observational studies. *Epidemiology*, 21(3), 383

Lin DY, Wei LJ. The robust inference for the Cox proportional hazards model. *Journal of the American Statistical Association*. 1989;84(408):1074-8.

Lunceford JK, Davidian M. Stratification and weighting via the propensity score in estimation of causal treatment effects: a comparative study. *Statistics in Medicine*. 2004;23(19):2937-60.

Neyman JS. On the Application of Probability Theory to Agricultural Experiments. Essay on Principles. Section 9. (Translated and edited by DM Dabrowska and TP Speed, *Statistical Science* (1990), 5, 465–480)1923;10:1–51.
Ogburn EL, VanderWeele TJ. On the nondifferential misclassification of a binary confounder. *Epidemiology.* 2012;23(3):433.
Pearl J. Brief Report: On the Consistency Rule in Causal Inference: "Axiom, Definition, Assumption, or Theorem?". *Epidemiology.* 2010:872-5.
Pearl J. Causal diagrams for empirical research. *Biometrika.* 1995;82(4):669-88.
Pearl J. Causality: models, reasoning, and inference. *Econometric Theory.* 2003;19(675–685):46.
Perez-Heydrich C, Hudgens MG, Halloran ME, Clemens JD, Ali M, Emch ME. Assessing effects of cholera vaccination in the presence of interference. *Biometrics.* 2014;70(3):731-41.
Pratt N, Roughead EE, Ryan P, Salter A. Antipsychotics and the risk of death in the elderly: an instrumental variable analysis using two preference based instruments. *Pharmacoepidemiology and Drug Safety.* 2010;19(7):699-707.
Rassen JA, Brookhart MA, Glynn RJ, Mittleman MA, Schneeweiss SJ. Instrumental variables I: instrumental variables exploit natural variation in nonexperimental data to estimate causal relationships. *Journal of Clinical Epidemiology.* 2009;62(12):1226-32.
Richardson TS, Robins JM. Single world intervention graphs (SWIGs): A unification of the counterfactual and graphical approaches to causality. Center for the Statistics and the Social Sciences, University of Washington Series Working Paper. 2013;128(30):2013.
Robins JM. (2000) Marginal structural models versus structural nested models as tools for causal inference. *Statistical Models in Epidemiology, the Environment, and Clinical Trials.* New York: Springer, 95–133.
Robins, JM, Blevins D, Ritter G, Wulfsohn M. (1992). G-estimation of the effect of prophylaxis therapy for Pneumocystis carinii pneumonia on the survival of AIDS patients. Epidemiology, 319-336.
Robins JM, Rotnitzky A, Scharfstein DO. (2000a) Sensitivity analysis for selection bias and unmeasured confounding in missing data and causal inference models. *Statistical Models in Epidemiology, the Environment, and Clinical Trials.* New York: Springer, p. 1–94.
Robins JM, Hernan MA, Brumback B. Marginal structural models and causal inference in epidemiology. Epidemiology. 2000b;11(5): 550–560.
Rosenbaum PR, Rubin DB. The central role of the propensity score in observational studies for causal effects. *Biometrika.* 1983;70(1):41-55.
Rubin DB. Randomization analysis of experimental data: The Fisher randomization test comment. *Journal of the American Statistical Association.* 1980;75(371):591-3.
SAS Institute Inc. 2016. SAS/STAT® 14.2 User's Guide. Cary, NC: SAS Institute Inc
Sekhon JS (2011). *Matching*: Multivariate and propensity score matching software with automated balance optimization: the matching package for R. version 4.9–7.
Sato T, Matsuyama YJE. Marginal structural models as a tool for standardization. *Epidemiology.* 2003:680–6.
Strom BL (2006). Pharmacoepidemiology. West Sussex, UK: John Wiley & Sons.
Stuart EA. Matching methods for causal inference: A review and a look forward. *Statistical science.* 2010;25(1):1–21.
Talbot D, Atherton J, Rossi AM, Bacon SL, Lefebvre G. A cautionary note concerning the use of stabilized weights in marginal structural models. *Statistics in Medicine.* 2015;34(5):812-23.
Tchetgen EJT, VanderWeele TJ. On causal inference in the presence of interference. *Statistical Methods in Medical Research.* 2012;21(1):55-75.
VanderWeele TJ. Concerning the consistency assumption in causal inference. *Epidemiology.* 2009;20(6):880-3.
VanderWeele TJ, Ding P. Sensitivity analysis in observational research: introducing the E-value. *Annals of Internal Medicine,* 2017;167(4):268–274.

VanderWeele TJ, Hernán MA. Results on differential and dependent measurement error of the exposure and the outcome using signed directed acyclic graphs. *American Journal of Epidemiology*. 2012;175(12):1303–10.

Westreich D, Lessler J, Funk MJ. Propensity score estimation: neural networks, support vector machines, decision trees (CART), and meta-classifiers as alternatives to logistic regression. *Journal of Clinical Epidemiology*. 2010;63(8):826-33.

Xie J, Liu C Adjusted Kaplan–Meier estimator and log-rank test with inverse probability of treatment weighting for survival data. *Statistics in Medicine*. 2005;24(20):3089-110

Chapter 6
Statistical Data Mining of Clinical Data

Ilya Lipkovich, Bohdana Ratitch, and Cristina Ivanescu

6.1 Introduction

6.1.1 What Is Data Mining?

Data mining is understood broadly as a set of analytical tools and methods for extracting nontrivial information from the data so that it can be transformed into useful knowledge and practical tools. Data mining has been evolving and applied in multidisciplinary contexts, and its definitions vary depending on the viewpoint. The following definition reflects the view of the Knowledge Discovery in Databases (KDD):

- Data mining is the nontrivial extraction of implicit, previously unknown, and potentially useful information from large data sets or databases.

  A typical statistician's view of data mining expressed succinctly in a textbook by Hand et al. (2001) places more emphasis on the interpretability of discovered "relationships" for decision-makers:

- "Data mining is the analysis of (often large) observational data sets to find unsuspected relationships and to summarize the data in novel ways that are both understandable and useful to the data owner."

I. Lipkovich (✉)
Eli Lilly and Company, Indianapolis, IN, USA
e-mail: ilya.lipkovich@lilly.com

B. Ratitch
Bayer Inc., Montreal, Quebec, Canada

C. Ivanescu
IQVIA, Amsterdam, Netherlands

© Springer Nature Switzerland AG 2020
O. V. Marchenko, N. V. Katenka (eds.), *Quantitative Methods in Pharmaceutical Research and Development*, https://doi.org/10.1007/978-3-030-48555-9_6

In Pharma there is no established definition of what data mining is; however, summarizing our experience and observations of the current practices across the industry, we can formulate it broadly as any post hoc analyses:

- "Data mining is any post-hoc analysis of existing clinical data to provide answers to relevant scientific, clinical, and business questions to internal and external stakeholders."

In this review chapter, we take a broad view on data mining in clinical settings as a valuable and principled element in a large cycle of knowledge discovery and confirmation from healthcare data that facilitates a full and efficient use of vast amounts of available data. It is a type of data analytics for problems that have the following common features:

- A large amount of available data in terms of the number of records (patients) and/or the number of features (variables) that has at least some of the following properties:

  - Typically arising from observational studies, or representing "observational elements" embedded within randomized trials
  - Collected for a different purpose than the intended "data mining" analyses
  - Dispersed over different databases

- The relationships that need to be learned from the data may be obscured by

  - Both random and systematic errors
  - Various inconsistencies in data collection and variable construction
  - Missing data (likely "not completely at random")
  - The presence of irrelevant data (noise features) that need to be filtered out
  - Redundancy in relevant data ("overlapping" variables)
  - Time-dependent causal mechanisms with unknown lags
  - The presence of both short-lived and long-term time effects
  - Dynamic dependencies between variables that may change over time
  - Unknown causal relationships among variables
  - Unmeasured confounders and spurious associations between variables

This chapter is organized as follows. In the rest of the introduction section, we present the framework for data mining and machine learning (DMML) and try to connect it with important tasks in drug development. Section 6.2 lays out the key concepts of DMML. Section 6.3 contains a brief overview of selected methods with more emphasis on those that will be featured in our case studies. Section 6.4 summarizes the principles of data mining with clinical data and suggests some elements of the statistical plans for DM. Section 6.5 contains three case studies. Finally, in Sect. 6.6, we provide a brief discussion of the key points of the chapter.

6.1.2   *Machine Learning and Data Mining Framework*

The fields of data mining and machine learning emerged as a combination of computer science and statistics methods with some additional unique objectives and emphases. As in computer science, one goal of machine learning is to build algorithmic solutions and machines to solve problems; as in statistics, another goal is to do reliable inference from data. The unique objectives of machine learning include the emphasis on how computers can "program themselves" (learning) and how to most effectively capture, store, and retrieve patterns and regularities in data. Data mining is a closely related field, which employs many machine learning and statistics methods. Data mining activities are typically focused on discovering new insights from databases that are often big, heterogeneous, and/or unstructured and which are presumed to contain interesting patterns not known or not sufficiently understood a priori. To name just a few sources, excellent introductions and textbooks in machine learning and data mining are provided by Mitchell (1997), Hand et al. (2001), Hastie et al. (2009), Clarke et al. (2009), Witten et al. (2011), Domingos (2012), and Goodfellow et al. (2016).

Although statistical modeling and machine learning have been developing as separate disciplines, the similarities between the two abound, and they can be used in synergetic ways (Friedman 1997; Hand 1998; Vapnik 2006). Statistical modeling approaches often formulate some assumptions regarding the data distribution and the relationship between the dependent and independent variables and place emphasis on the interpretability of the model and the ability to do inference about the underlying data generation mechanism including the effect of individual predictors on the response.

Somewhat simplifying matters, we can describe classical statistical modeling as largely focusing on estimating a model from which the data arose: $Y = f(X) + \varepsilon$, where ε represents a random error induced either by an experimental procedure, random sampling, or other sources of uncertainty. The error term is modeled with some parametric family of distributions, often with a common assumption that the random errors have the expected value of zero, $E(\varepsilon) = 0$, and is independent of X. In statistics, it is common to refer to X as a set of independent or predictor variables and to Y as a response, outcome, or dependent variable. For a continuous outcome variable Y, $f(X)$ is the conditional mean $f(x) = E(Y|X = x)$ and is referred to as a regression function. For a categorical outcome $Y = \{j : j = 1, .., k\}$, the same representation gives rise to a classification function, where $E(Y = j|X = x)$ models the probability of group membership.

For example, in clinical studies, one of the central objectives is to assess whether treatment has a statistically significant effect on a response variable and to estimate the magnitude of the treatment effect. This is often done by estimating a fairly simple statistical model with treatment represented by one of the independent variables and then performing statistical tests about the treatment effect and estimating mean treatment effect based on that model. For example, in the context of continuous outcome variable, it is the mean difference in response under the experimental treatment versus control, possibly adjusted for other independent (pretreatment) variables included in the model, such as baseline patient characteristics. In this case, the goal is to do inference from the data collected so far, without a further objective of predicting responses for future individual patients. As can be further illustrated with this and other applications in healthcare, the classical view focuses on hypothesis testing applied to a single test or a small number of pre-specified tests with clearly defined multiplicity adjustment strategy.

This framework can be contrasted with that of data mining and machine learning (DMML) where the "learning" aspect refers to the ability of a computational system to acquire new knowledge from its environment and data or to organize existing knowledge in a way that facilitates its use. The "machine" aspect emphasizes the automated and algorithmic fashion of the learning, not involving "human intervention." In machine learning, often there is also an objective of creating a "machine" (computational system or tool), which, once trained, can be deployed for future use with new data. This is reflected in a ubiquitous use of the term "training data set" or "training sample" in DMML to designate the data that are available at the learning stage and implying that there will be more data to come.

The differences between classical statistics and machine learning have been a subject of lively debates (see, e.g., Breiman 2001a, b on two modeling cultures within statistics). Unlike classical statistics, DMML methods tend to rely less on formal distributional assumptions and often work with "black box" representations of the target unknown function $f(x)$, where the interpretability of the effect of the individual input variables on the output may be limited and not of primary interest and the emphasis is rather on the quality of prediction for future cases.

Classical examples of machine learning for prediction is speech and character (e.g., handwriting) recognition and (more recently) email spam detection where arguably the interpretability of the prediction rules does not play a key role (see, e.g., email spam Example 1 in Hastie et al. 2009). However, the situation is quite different in applications of machine learning in the healthcare such as automated diagnosis of patients where both healthcare providers and patients are not only interested in accurate prediction but would also like to know which features are primarily responsible for discriminating the "events" from "non-events." Here relying on pure "black box" solutions may be less desirable: although a black box model may be entertained as the prediction tool, it then should be followed by various visualizations facilitating the interpretability, such as a decision tree, a variable importance graph, a partial dependence plot, or a low-dimensional projection. This shift from a "black box" to a more transparent and interpretable data mining, reminding us of the exploratory data analysis (EDA, Tukey 1977) with its emphasis on "looking at the data," differentiates the outlook of modern "data miners" from that of "machine learners."

Another distinction can be made between the role of modeling assumptions and model selection in the classical statistics and DMML. In the former, analysis often relies on "standard assumptions" and pre-specified models, while in practical situations the analyst is discouraged from "looking at the data" (even for validating the analysis assumptions) in fear of data dredging, as multiple "looks" may arguably inflate the false positive rates. This outlook is at odds with the discovery nature of the statistical science. Sometimes analysts may act under implicit assumptions that "pre-specified" means "valid," resulting in suboptimal models entertained at "confirmatory stage." While these are not examples of the best application of classical statistics, they often occur in practice, especially in the healthcare settings where pre-specification of analyses required by regulatory agencies played a key role and became a part of the culture. Data visualizations historically did not play an important role in this "traditional" view of data analysis, perhaps because of the fear of "looking at the data" when implementing pre-specified confirmatory analyses. Nevertheless, things are gradually changing, and most large pharmaceutical companies have been creating data mining and visualization groups to facilitate data analysis and presentation in all phases of drug development.

DMML by its nature relies on model selection using data-driven methods with an emphasis on discovery rather than confirmatory analysis. Unlike classical statistics, the emphasis in DMML is not on hypotheses testing but on generating plausible hypotheses that are data-driven ("random"), rather than pre-specified. On the other hand, data-driven model selection inherent in data mining methods may often occur "behind the scenes," and the statistical uncertainty associated with model selection is left unaccounted for in the final analyses and decision-making based on these analyses. Again, perhaps reflecting not the best practices of data mining, the final inference is sometimes based on the findings of a last stage of a complex multistage data mining procedure ignoring the uncertainty associated with all the previous stages. Model validation and incorporation of the uncertainty associated with the entire DMML strategy in the prediction and inference is extremely important for generating useful insights and tools but may be very challenging to implement. Like EDA, data mining (somewhat in contrast with machine learning, having an emphasis on fully automated analysis strategies) encourages various graphical displays and low-dimensional data representations facilitating model selection and interpretability.

Table 6.1 summarizes the above discussion points on the differences and commonalties between data mining/machine learning and traditional statistics.

We conclude this discussion by observing that the distinctions made may oversimplify and overdramatize the situation, and a trend has been emerging for convergence between the "classical" statistics and DMML under a unifying framework where both elements are considered from a common modeling perspective of "statistical learning" emphasizing some general principles such as achieving a trade-off between bias and variance (see Hastie et al. 2009). Many ideas and approaches developed in the two disciplines independently and use different terminologies but share similar concepts and properties. One indication of convergence between the two domains is an increasing interest in developing "classical" inferential procedures for machine learning techniques, such as for inference "after model selection." For example, see Wager et al. (2014) on bagging and random forest, and (Meinshausen et al. 2009, Lockhart et al. 2014, Tian et al. 2016) on post-selection inference in the context of L1 (lasso) penalized regression and related methods. Another example of such blending is procedures that combine classical

Table 6.1 Data mining/machine learning versus "classical" statistics

Classical statistics	Data mining/machine learning
Typically uses relatively small data sets collected from designed experiments or by sampling from well-defined populations	Large and often dispersed and heterogeneous data sets, often collected for (business) purposes other than the data mining
Assumes a data generation mechanism: $y = f(X) + \varepsilon$, where $f(X)$ has relatively simple structure (e.g., a linear model) and the error term(s) are represented by parametric distributions	Often poses its task as recovering unknown function $f(X)$ which may be a "black box" (i.e., fairly complex nonlinear relationship) while the presence of statistical uncertainty (noise) is often ignored
The objective is to estimate parameters for the entire population from available sample(s)	The objective is to obtain predictions for new (future) cases or extract useful features that reveal underlying (unknown) structure. The analysis data often represent the entire population
Focus on hypothesis testing applied to a single test or a small number of pre-specified tests with clearly defined multiplicity adjustment strategy	Hypothesis generation (knowledge discovery) rather than formal hypothesis testing, less emphasis on statistical significance (often rather focusing on controlling the false discovery rate)
Interpretability is an important element of modeling culture where the structure of $f(X)$ is driven by few pre-selected variables, mainly based on existing domain knowledge or factors of a designed experiment	The "black box" modeling makes interpretability neither important nor easily attainable; however, in data mining applications, the decision-makers often desire to have the decision rules expressed in interpretable form
Modeling relies on "standard assumptions," often discouraging "looking at the data" in fear of data dredging. Underutilizes the discovery element of statistical science	Relies on model selection using data-driven methods with emphasis on discovery rather than confirmatory analysis; incorporation of uncertainty associated with model selection however may be challenging to implement for multistage data mining strategies
Visualization does not play important role, perhaps because of the fear of data dredging when implementing pre-specified confirmatory analyses	Data mining (like EDA and in contrast with machine learning) encourages graphical displays facilitating model selection and interpretability

multiplicity control in hypothesis testing with model averaging for design and analysis of dose-finding studies introduced in (Bretz et al. 2005) and implemented in R package **MCPMod** (Bornkamp et al. 2009).

6.1.3 Machine Learning Tasks for Solving Clinical Problems

For decades, healthcare data have traditionally been analyzed using statistical methods, but the applications of machine learning and data mining have been constantly growing in all areas of health informatics, from molecular biology and genetics, to clinical research, to epidemiology. There are a few major areas in health informatics (Herland et al. 2014): bioinformatics typically focuses on the molecular-level data; neuro-informatics concentrates on analysis of brain imaging data; clinical informatics involves analysis of patient data; public health informatics applies data mining and analytics to population-level data; and translational bioinformatics is an interdisciplinary field that develops techniques for integrating biological and clinical data. In this chapter, we focus on clinical informatics.

Traditional view of the scope of data mining and machine learning in drug development is that its place is primarily in preclinical and early-phase drug discovery (e.g., using machine learning for gene expression analysis). Using data mining in later stages of drug development (Phases 3, 4) is often considered with suspicion as a euphemism of data dredging that sponsors may use to promote favorable views of their products and make unsubstantiated claims (e.g., of enhanced efficacy in sub-populations identified through data mining). Many consider complete pre-specification of analyses in late stages of drug development as the necessary condition of their validity. However, learning from data is a continuous process that does not stop at the beginning of Phase 3. Clearly, not everything is known at the time of new study design, and so not all meaningful analyses can be preplanned; therefore, extracting as much evidence from data as possible, even post hoc, maximizes good use of patient data and resources allocated to a clinical trial. There is indeed a striking contrast between the vast amount of patient-level data (on efficacy and safety) collected in the course of a clinical trial and reporting trial results with a few summaries (ultimately, a single P-value for the primary analysis), which suggests large amounts of data collected may be underutilized in the drug development process.

Contrary to this view, we believe that data mining is an integral part on all stages of the drug development process. However, we promote *principled* data mining (as opposed to "data dredging") and to this end outline some principles and good practices of clinical data mining.

In our review of data mining methodologies, we focus on methods most useful for clinical trial data analysis; however, most of the methodologies equally apply to observational studies where treatment assignments are driven by prescribers' decisions and not by chance. In fact, as we argue, observational studies and randomized clinical trials (RCTs) have much in common, and this is exactly why data mining (and model selection as its integral element) is needed in both. Often, we can consider clinical trial data as observational study embedded in an RCT. Even in the perfectly designed and conducted RCT, post-randomization events, such as dropouts, effectively break the randomization and make comparison of simple summaries by treatment arm biased and therefore require model-based analysis, even for the assessment of treatment effect under the intention-to-treat (ITT) principle.

Here, we list some general analytic tasks that arise with clinical data (whether originated from a randomized trial or not) that lend themselves to applications of data mining methods, and we group these tasks under more traditional headings of supervised, semi-supervised, or unsupervised learning. Specific examples for some of these tasks will be provided in Sect. 6.5 using case studies.

6.1.3.1 Supervised Learning

Supervised learning occurs when the DMML system is provided both the input and the correct output for a set of training cases and is tasked with learning a function that maps input to output, with the goal of being able to predict the output for future, unlabeled input instances. The initial, labeled set (x_i, y_i), $i = 1, \ldots, N$, of inputs x_i (a p-dimentional vector) and outputs y_i is referred to as a training set, and the learning algorithm adapts its internal representation of the input-output relationship $\widehat{f}(x_i)$ to minimize some measure of differences between the observed and predicted outputs: y_i and $\widehat{f}(x_i)$, e.g., residual sum of squares $RSS = \sum_{i=1}^{N} \left(y_i - \widehat{f}(x_i) \right)^2$. Supervised learning problems are further grouped into classification when the output variable is a category (e.g., mild, moderate, severe) and regression when the output variable is a real value (e.g., blood pressure or weight).

Some common tasks in the healthcare setting include:

Patient diagnostics. Applications of building diagnostic models informed by various patient-level covariates (symptoms) started to appear decades ago, for example, a simple diagnostic tool was constructed using tree-based decision rules that allowed clinicians of an emergency unit to make a quick assessment whether a patient with non-traumatic chest pain can be diagnosed with a myocardial infraction using ECG and other available markers (Mair et al. 1995). An example of increasing use of diagnostic tools incorporating AI algorithms is a recent approval by FDA of *OsteoDetect*, an image processing device that "analyzes wrist radiographs using machine learning techniques to identify and highlight distal radius fractures during the review of posterior-anterior (PA) and lateral (LAT) radiographs of adult wrists" (FDA 2018).

Building predictive models for patients' future outcomes. Models may be built to predict safety or efficacy outcomes, informed by assigned treatment, biomarkers available prior to treatment initiation, and evolving (early) patient outcomes. Examples of such clinical applications of supervised learning are predicting mortality and readmission after a discharge from an intensive care unit in order to avoid premature discharges from the unit for future patients (Ouanes et al. 2012) and predicting cancer susceptibility, cancer recurrence, and cancer survival (Konstantina et al. 2015).

Modeling intermediate outcomes as part of a treatment evaluation strategy. Supervised learning often arises in clinical applications not as a goal in itself but rather as an intermediate step for obtaining more accurate estimates of treatment effects. This is especially true for evaluating treatment effect in observational trials but also applies to RCTs. For example, to account for missing data, methods of inverse probability weighting can be employed that require modeling the probability of a patient remaining in the trial through specific time. Here the goal is not to predict patient's dropout as such but rather to correct for selection bias in the primary analyses caused by the fact the dropouts may have occurred not completely at random but were associated with patients' covariates and early outcomes. As another example, imputation methods are often used for the same purpose of accounting for selection bias due to dropouts. Constructing an imputation model or a model for inverse probability weighting can often be successfully done using "black box" methods of supervised learning that have an advantage over simple regression methods in that they utilize all available data and do not require preselection of key predictor variables nor assume any specific form of their relationship with the probability of dropout which are typically unknown to the investigators. See Tang and Ishwaran (2017) for comparison of various strategies for imputing missing data via random forest algorithms. In our case study in Sect. 6.5, we will provide an example of using machine learning method to estimate treatment effect under informative treatment switching via inverse probability weighting.

6.1.3.2 Unsupervised Learning

In unsupervised learning, the DMML system is not provided with any "correct answer" such as a training sample where all cases are correctly labeled into target categories or values but rather is designed to discover and model the underlying structure and patterns in the data with the goal of acquiring a better understanding of the data. Unsupervised learning problems are broadly grouped into clustering, where the objective is to discover inherent groupings of similar units described by data (e.g., groups of patients with similar treatment outcomes), and association, where the goal is to discover interesting relations between variables (e.g., co-occurrence of certain diseases or events) which can be also thought of as clustering, although in the variable/feature space.

Some common tasks and examples include:

Clustering to identify patients with similar efficacy outcomes in the absence of a definite single outcome measure determining patient's response to treatment. This is especially relevant for diseases where the patients' well-being is described by a set of variables representing complementary and sometimes conflicting clinical criteria and scales, which is often the case in neuroscience and some other areas. Example of this is clustering patients in treatment of fibromyalgia, as such patients often show great variability in symptoms domains for which a given treatment may be beneficial (Lipkovich et al. 2014; Abtroun et al. 2016). Clustering of patients in the multivariate space of disease symptoms may lead to construction of better criteria for clinical response as well as understating what patient characteristics are driving response in different domains of symptoms.

Identifying patients with distinct response profiles (or trajectories) over time. Response profiles may represent different types of patients, e.g., "early responders who later fail," "relapsers," "gradual responders," "sustained responders," etc. Clustering can be done using traditional statistical methods of analysis of growth curves via finite mixture random effects with categorical latent variables representing class membership (Muthén et al. 2002), as well as by application of multivariate clustering methods, e.g., Lipkovich et al. (2008).

Use of methods for association learning. This objective has been explored in pharmacovigilance to uncover drug-adverse event relationships and drug-drug interactions in spontaneous reporting systems and large healthcare databases such as electronic health records and administrative claims (Harpaz et al. 2012).

Detecting outliers and unusual patterns, often in the context of fraudulent assessment of outcomes. See, e.g., O'Kelly (2004) for a case study illustrating the use of statistical multivariate techniques to identify fraudulent clinical data.

6.1.3.3 Semi-supervised Learning

Note that in many situations learning may need to proceed in an unsupervised manner even in a prediction setting for regression or classification problem where the target variable is entirely missing in the observed (training) data. An interesting case that falls somewhere in between the supervised and unsupervised learning is predicting differences in outcomes for a patient under different treatment regimes (treatment effects) given his/her characteristics. This is not a supervised learning problem because in a typical parallel arm clinical trial, a patient is assigned only to one treatment (experimental or control), and therefore the patient-level treatment differences are unobserved, similar to class labels in the clustering problem. However, because one of the treatment outcomes is observed for every patient, these hypothetical differences can be predicted using methods of traditional supervised learning as building blocks. Here we provide examples of such tasks under the heading of semi-supervised learning:

Subgroup identification. Heterogeneity of treatment effect has been recognized in many therapeutic areas leading to a growing interest in precision medicine (also referred to as personalized medicine) so that therapies can be tailored to characteristics of the patients as well as their environment and lifestyle (Ashley 2015). Much research has been dedicated to identifying genetic traits that are responsible for variations in disease susceptibility and response to treatments, but subgroup identification also extends to other demographic and clinical characteristics that may be predictive of the treatment effect (often referred to as biomarkers). In this setting, the researchers may be presented with a large set of potential biomarkers, and the objective is to determine a small subset that can be used to reliably describe patient profiles with the most beneficial treatment effect or a favorable benefit-risk balance (see Lipkovich et al. 2017). We provide a review of various methods for subgroup identification in Sect. 6.3.3 and illustrate with a case study in Sect. 6.5.1.

Estimating optimal treatment regimes. Another clinical problem closely related to precision medicine which also falls under the semi-supervised learning framework is construction of optimal dynamic treatment regimes (DTRs) utilizing information on patient's characteristics and accumulated patient's outcomes at each decision point. In many health disorders, especially chronic conditions, sequential decision-making is necessary to adapt treatment over time in response to the evolving health status of the patient. This is especially important if there is a high degree of heterogeneity in individual long-term responses to treatment and when treatment may need to be adjusted as a result of emerging side effects. DTRs thus extend the concept of precision medicine to time-varying treatment regimes where therapy (type, dose, and/or timing) may be adjusted over time based on the up-to-date patient information and may be influenced by earlier treatment choices (Murphy 2003, 2005; Chakraborty and Murphy 2014). Development of evidence-based dynamic treatment regimes, just like evidence-based recommendations for the initial choice of treatment, is part of building clinical decision support systems for the entire treatment cycle. Several methods for estimation of optimal DTRs, e.g., Q-learning and A-learning, originate in a subfield of machine learning known as reinforcement learning (Sutton and Barto 1998) where the focus is on decision-making in stochastic dynamic environments. We review the problem and methods of estimation of optimal DTRs in Sect. 6.3.3 and present a case study in Sect. 6.5.2. Although the problem of identifying optimal regimes is a semi-supervised learning problem (in absence of explicit information of what is the optimal regime in training data), it often uses supervised learning approaches as integral components. For example, methods of outcome-weighted learning construct DTRs by casting it in as a series of classification problems (Zhao et al. 2015).

6.1.3.4 Feature Selection and Dimensionality Reduction

A cornerstone of machine learning and data mining methods (whether supervised or unsupervised) is feature selection and dimensionality reduction. Databases often contain a multitude of variables which are potentially related to the problem at hand, but it may not be known in advance which attributes are in fact useful and which are irrelevant or redundant given other attributes. The challenge is compounded by the fact that machine learning often starts with "feature expansion" resulting in transforming the initial set of covariates into a broader set of "features" (e.g., adding variables capturing information on two- and three-way covariate interactions or using feature expansion via radial basis functions). Given this enriched set of features, the DMML system needs to extract useful information to reduce model complexity, improve accuracy, and facilitate interpretation. Feature selection refers to an automatic selection of data attributes that are most useful and relevant for predictive modeling (supervised learning) or identifying patterns in data (unsupervised learning). Examples of such methods for supervised learning range from traditional stepwise model selection techniques to more sophisticated methods of penalized estimation (e.g., lasso method a.k.a. L_1 penalty) and ensemble learning (see Sects. 6.2 and 6.3 for more details). Often feature expansion and selection can be done within a single analytic strategy (e.g., as in support vector machines (SVMs) with a kernel-based feature expansion and an L_1 penalty).

Dimensionality reduction also aims at reducing the number of attributes in a data set, but unlike feature selection, it does so by creating new, fewer combinations of attributes that nevertheless capture the key information in the data (e.g., using methods based on principal components and singular value decomposition). These methods can be used in the context of both supervised and unsupervised learning.

In this chapter we will provide case studies covering some of the above tasks. Clearly, it would be impossible to cover all applications of data mining in clinical research in a single chapter. While we provide some reference to a broader set of applications, we would like to explicitly mention some areas that will not be covered here: applications of data mining/machine learning in molecular biology, genomics, proteomics, microarray data, and medical imaging. While some of case studies will use methods that are applicable to analysis of epidemiological studies and real-world databases (such as claims/electronic medical records), we will not have specific examples here.

6.2 Overview of Key Concepts

The power of machine learning algorithms is in their ability to provide solutions to difficult problems by generalizing from a limited set of examples observed in real life (a training set). This is not unlike statistical inference where, in order for the results to be of practical utility, the inference performed from a finite set of data samples must be generalizable to a population of interest (e.g., finite population as in survey sampling or hypothetical population as in making inference for "future" patients). Therefore, good accuracy/performance on the training data set is typically not the ultimate goal, and performance on new data not included in the training set is of greater importance. In supervised learning, it is a common practice to divide the available data into a training set and a test set so that the solution can be developed on the training set and its performance evaluated on the test set, representing new data not used for learning. In this context, the performance metric applied to the training set while the learning is taking place (e.g., the R-square) often serves as a surrogate for the ultimate performance measure—generalization ability. However, focusing on this surrogate measure, especially when fitting complex models (i.e., with a large number of parameters), may lead to overfitting, so that the model "describes" the random error (noise) in the training data rather than the underlying relationship. Avoiding overfitting and improving generalization performance requires careful consideration, which we review in this section.

6.2.1 Bias-Variance Trade-Off

One important aspect of a machine learning algorithm's performance is the bias-variance trade-off. The generalization error can be decomposed into two main components: bias and variance. For example, as discussed in the previous section, in supervised learning (for continuous outcome), the objective is to find a mapping for the input-output relationship $\widehat{f}(x)$ which minimizes the expected prediction error $E\left(y - \widehat{f}(x)\right)^2$ which can be decomposed as

$$E\left(y - \widehat{f}(x)\right)^2 = \left(Bias\left[\widehat{f}(x)\right]\right)^2 + Variance\left[\widehat{f}(x)\right] + \sigma^2,$$

where σ^2 is an irreducible error (e.g., due to noise in inputs and outputs). $Bias\left[\widehat{f}(x)\right] = E\left[\widehat{f}(x) - f(x)\right]$ is the method's tendency to consistently produce solutions $\widehat{f}(x)$ that deviate from the truth $f(x)$. Systematic bias can be introduced, for example, by using an inappropriate model, e.g., using a linear model when the true function is nonlinear, or using optimization algorithms that tend to converge at a local optimum (e.g., greedy search). $Variance\left[\widehat{f}(x)\right] = E\left[\widehat{f}(x)^2\right] - E\left[\widehat{f}(x)\right]^2$ is the method's tendency to produce different solutions (move around its mean) as a result of changes in the training set (even though different training sets are generated by the same underlying process) or randomness that is part of the learning algorithm (e.g., Monte Carlo methods).

There is a trade-off between bias and variance: typically bias decreases as the model complexity increases, while variance increases with model complexity. An increasingly complex model will reach a point where its prediction error on the training set is very small but it overfits the training data and leads to an increase in the error on the test data. This is illustrated in Fig. 6.1 where the training set error, depicted by the light gray line, decreases steadily as the size of the model (a tree-based model in this example) increases, whereas increase in complexity leads to no further gains in the test set error after a certain point (tree size of 5) as depicted by the black solid line. This is why, perhaps counterintuitively at a first thought, a more complex learner (model) is not necessarily better than a more parsimonious one, and there is typically some intermediate model complexity that provides the best performance on the test (and future) data. In Fig. 6.1, the dotted line represents one standard deviation above the best test error, which may be a good target to select model complexity. This leads us to the next topic—model selection.

6.2.2   Model Selection

For reasons discussed above, model selection is thus an integral part of the machine learning process with the ultimate goal of choosing the model that provides the best generalization performance on new data. One aspect in terms of choosing the right model is related to the choice of model class, for example, using a linear vs. nonlinear model. Another aspect relates to choosing which predictor variables to include in the model as this also directly determines model complexity. The squared bias component of the prediction error discussed above can itself be decomposed into two parts: average model (specification) bias and average

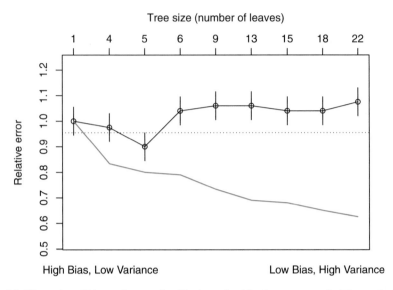

Fig. 6.1 Illustration of bias-variance trade-off using a classification tree example. The x-axis shows the tree size (model complexity); the y-axis shows the relative classification error. The black line is the generalization error (here estimated via tenfold cross-validation), and the gray line is the error estimated from the training set. The error bars are estimates of standard error associated with the cross-validation estimates. The graph suggests that the tree model starts picking up noise when the number of leaves (terminal nodes) exceeds 5

estimation bias. Model bias represents the error between the best-fitting approximation within the chosen class (e.g., a linear model based on a set of chosen predictors) and the true function. The estimation bias is the error between the average estimate of the model parameters and the best-fitting approximation in the class.

For example, for linear models $\widehat{f}(X) = X^T\beta$ using a vector of predictor variables X and parameter vector β, the best-fitting approximation corresponds to the parameter settings $\beta_* = arg\ min_\beta E[(f(X) - X^T\beta)^2]$. The average squared bias of a specific approximation $\widehat{f}_d(x)$ is then decomposed as follows:

$$\left(E_x\left[E\left[\widehat{f}_d(x)\right] - f(x)\right]\right)^2 = \left(E_x\left[x^T\beta_* - f(x)\right]\right)^2 + \left(E_x\left[x^T\beta_* - E\left[x^T\widehat{\beta}_d\right]\right]\right)^2,$$

where the first term on the right-hand side is the model bias and the second term is the estimation bias.

The expectation over the estimated linear predictor $E\left[x^T\widehat{\beta}_d\right]$ is equal to that from the ideal best-fitting linear predictor $x^T\beta_*$ for linear models estimated using the ordinary least squares method, and in this case the estimation bias is zero. For other estimation methods, for example, penalized or ridge regression, the average estimation bias is positive, but then the models obtained with this approach typically reduce the variance component and thus can be used to achieve a desired bias-variance trade-off.

Model selection in terms of choosing the most relevant subset of predictors can be done in many ways. One traditional approach often described in statistics textbooks is based on stepwise variable selection (e.g., forward, backward, or hybrid stepwise selection), where statistical significance of effects associated with each variable are tested in some sequential way and variables are dropped or added to the model one at a time depending on their significance. This approach uses a locally greedy strategy and suffers from several other important drawbacks (e.g., multiple statistical hypothesis testing performed without proper Type I error control, unstable performance, and low prediction accuracy).

In general, data analysis involving a model selection step can be broken down into the following tasks:

1. Choosing a general form of the model (e.g., logistic or linear regression).
2. Specifying the model space (e.g., as defined by original variables X, expanding them into main effects and interactions, expanding them using spline basis functions, etc.).
3. Specifying a model search strategy, i.e., a strategy for obtaining a path or multiple paths through the model space that are likely to capture "promising" models (e.g., stepwise model selection produces a sequence of the best models for the number of predictors $k = 1, 2, 3, \ldots$; coefficient paths obtained by varying the amount of penalty in lasso/elastic net; stochastic model search).
4. Specifying model selection criteria in order to identify the final best model(s).
5. Estimating parameters of the final model(s) while taking into account the uncertainty associated with the model selection step (estimation *after* model selection).
6. Predicting outcomes for new data using the selected model(s).

Typically, the general form of the model (task 1) is chosen by the researcher given domain knowledge. Some common approaches to model selection that take into account model selection uncertainly are highlighted below:

- Strategies that build a sequence of possibly overfitted models (e.g., using stepwise selection algorithms or other heuristic methods) and select from that sequence the best model using goodness-of-fit measures (based on penalized likelihood such as AIC (Akaike information criterion), BIC (Bayesian information criterion), cross-validation, or multiple testing procedures).
- An important special case is strategies based on penalized estimation procedures (e.g., lasso, elastic net) produce sparse coefficient paths corresponding to increasing model dimensionality by varying values of the tuning parameter(s) that control the amount of penalty placed on model complexity; the final model is selected by choosing the optimal tuning settings, e.g., by cross-validation (described further below in this section).
- Bayesian and frequentist model averaging where the "final model" is a weighted average over many models that fit data reasonably well (see review papers,

Hoeting et al. 1999; Wang et al. 2009); and other methods of *ensemble* learning such as random forest and boosting (see further in this section).

Although many analytical tools are packaged as "all-in-one" with specific choices for tasks 2 to 6 outlined above, it is useful to evaluate them on individual components. Sometimes a procedure may be reasonable for one aspect but very unsatisfactory for others, and an improved one can be constructed by borrowing approaches from different procedures and recombining their elements.

6.2.3 Variable Importance

A concept closely related to the problem of model selection is that of variable importance (VI)—an integral measure of the relative importance or contribution of a variable in predicting the response. Variable importance is used in many machine learning approaches where a single variable may contribute multiple times in different parts of the model, hence the need to obtain a single score presenting its overall importance. It can be defined in different ways that suit or reflect the construction of specific types of learners. For example, in classification and regression trees (CART, Breiman et al. 1984), variable importance can reflect improvements in the classification error achieved by using this variable to define splitting criteria across all the tree nodes where it is used as a splitter. Another way of determining variable importance (as was first introduced in random forests by Breiman 2001a, b) is to evaluate the reduction in predictive accuracy after a random permutation of the values of a given variable across all training samples. If the variable is strongly associated with response, then after randomly permuting its values, substantial decreases in prediction accuracy can be expected. Other versions of the permutation-based variable importance have been suggested in the literature, e.g., Sandri and Zuccolotto (2008); Strobl (2008); Altmann et al. (2010); and Lipkovich et al. (2017). A recently developed alternative approach to variable importance is based on SHAP values inspired by the Shapley interaction index from game theory (Lundberg and Lee 2017; 2018). The importance of each feature is defined at the level of individual observations by posing an *additive feature attribution model* that decomposes the fitted value into a sum of contributions from each feature (when present in the model). The importance score for a feature reflects its contribution into conditional expectation of the outcome averaged over all possible subsets of other features conditioned upon. Therefore, this approach is different from others in that it summarizes the contributions of a feature into a fitted model (a "black box") irrespective of how good or poor the fit may be. We will discuss several approaches to variable importance in more detail in the context of subgroup identification in Sect. 6.3.3 and in an application of random forest for computing inverse probability of censoring weights in Sect. 6.5.3.

6.2.4   Multiple Testing

The problem of multiple hypothesis testing is well recognized in statistics and relates to the probability of rejecting a null hypothesis when it is in fact true (referred to as Type I error). In machine learning and data mining applications where analysis tends to be more exploratory, it is not uncommon that tens or hundreds of hypothesis tests are performed by the learning algorithm, and thus care must be taken in this context as well. Some methods, both from classical statistics and machine learning, may have some sort of multiple hypothesis testing performed as part of the internal workings of their algorithm. This is true, for example, of model selection methods that rely on significance findings to select predictor variables. But multiple testing can occur in many other contexts as well, e.g., in medical applications in analyses of genomics data to discover genes, among thousands considered, exhibiting significant expression patterns of interest, or in evaluation of clinical safety data based on a multitude of safety tests and types of adverse events. Today there are many approaches for multiplicity control, some being more conservative or powerful than others while being well disciplined, and so some methods may be more appropriate than others in the context of machine learning.

It has been argued that especially in machine learning, where the number of tests can be very large, it is useful to distinguish between the false positive rate and false discovery rate (Glickman et al. 2014). The false positive rate is the probability of rejecting a null hypothesis given that it is true. The false discovery rate (FDR, introduced by Benjamini and Hochberg 1995) is the probability that a null hypothesis is true given that the null hypothesis has been rejected by a test.

A classical Bonferroni procedure that safeguards against *any* false positive findings is very conservative and has a consequence that the power to reject truly false null hypotheses is greatly reduced as the number of hypotheses tested increases. In the context of exploratory analysis where a large number of hypotheses are tested with an intent to generate promising hypotheses for further investigation and confirmation, it may be more relevant to accept a possibility that some discoveries will be false as long as their proportion among all significant findings is acceptably low. This point of view is taken by approaches that control the FDR. Multiplicity control involves establishing an appropriate adjusted significance level against which the P-values should be compared or conversely adjusting the raw P-values directly. This can also be achieved by resampling/permutation approaches (e.g., Westfall and Young 1993; Westfall and Troendle 2008; Vsevolozhskaya et al. 2015) which can provide empirical distribution of P-values. Resampling/permutation-based methods are particularly useful for multiple testing with high-dimensional data as they do not require specific distributional assumptions and utilize the data-based correlation structure among variables which can provide important power advantages. Efron (2010) provided an extensive discussion of issues in large-scale inference, including a novel interpretation of Benjamini and Hochberg's procedure from the empirical Bayes perspective, and introduced the *local FDR* which is defined as posterior probability of false discovery for a single hypothesis given test statistics for tested hypotheses. Another recent advance is developing a very general class of variable selection procedures that control FDR via so-called knockoff variables—a special type of irrelevant or "dummy" variables that mimic the correlation structure in the original variables (Barber and Candès 2015).

6.2.5 Cross-Validation

Cross-validation (Allen 1974; Stone 1974; Geisser 1975) is a method widely used in machine learning for estimation of the true error rate a.k.a. *generalization error* (model assessment) as well as for variable selection and for estimating tuning parameters that control the complexity of the model and machine learning algorithms. In a nutshell, the motivation and general idea behind the cross-validation is as follows. If we had a sufficiently large data set, we could partition it into a training data set, to which a model can be fit, and a validation set, on which performance of the model could be assessed. However, if the size of the available data set is not large, a more efficient use of data, which also would lead to more stable estimates of the model performance, can be achieved using K-fold cross-validation. In this case, the original data set is split into K nonoverlapping data sets (folds) of equal size, typically in a random fashion. For each fold $k = 1, \ldots, K$, a model is fit to a training data set comprised of all data except the kth fold. We will denote such models as $\widehat{f}^{-k}(x), k = 1, \ldots, K$. For each observation $i = 1, \ldots, N$ in the original full data set, let's denote by $k(i)$ the fold index to which the ith observation was assigned. The cross-validation estimate of the prediction error can be obtained as follows, based on some measure of error or loss $L\left(y, \widehat{f}(x)\right)$ defined for any given pair of predictors x and response y:

$$\widehat{Error}^{CV} = \frac{1}{N} \sum_{i=1}^{N} L\left(y_i, \widehat{f}^{-k(i)}(x_i)\right).$$

The choice of the number of folds K influences a potential bias of the error estimate (smaller K can result in a larger bias due to smaller sizes of the training data sets) and its variance (larger K leading to higher variance as the training data sets will tend to be more similar, i.e., having more observations in common). A special case when $K = N$ is referred to as leave-one-out (LOO) cross-validation, in which case N different models are fit, each to all data excluding only the ith observation. This estimator is approximately unbiased but can have a high variance. In general, the bias will depend on the size of the original data set and a slope of the error curve versus the size of the training data set. Frequently used choices of the number of folds K are 5 or 10 which attain a good balance between bias and variance in practice (Breiman and Spector 1992; Kohavi 1995).

Cross-validation can be used not only to obtain an estimate of the generalization error of a chosen type of model but also to tune parameters of the fitting method, e.g., the size of the model or the amount of penalty placed on the magnitude of the regression coefficients.

If modeling is carried out using several model selection steps, e.g., variable selection and parameter tuning, cross-validation must be applied across the entire sequence of steps: dividing data into k folds at the very beginning, carrying out all modeling steps on all k-1 training sets (leaving the kth fold out), and estimating model performance on the kth test fold. Otherwise, steps performed outside of the cross-validation procedure (e.g., variable selection) may have an unfair "advantage" in terms of basing their criteria on all available data, including those that would later be used as new, test examples (see, e.g., Ambroise and McLachlan 2002). While model selection and model assessment tasks both require cross-validation, it may be done using different cross-validation approaches applied in a nested manner (Varma and Simon 2006). One exception to the rule of subjecting the whole learning procedure to cross-validation is that the steps based on unsupervised learning (not involving outcomes) may be performed based on all available data, before creating the folds.

Recent research (Krstajic et al. 2014) also investigated some variants on the basic idea of K-fold cross-validation, e.g., with repeated random splits of the data and/or stratification on the outcome variable.

6.2.6 Bootstrap

The bootstrap method was introduced by Efron (1979) and has been used extensively ever since both in statistics and machine learning. In the course of any analysis, some kinds of summaries (statistics) are typically generated to describe the data set, the patterns, characteristics, and relationships underlying its variables. It is useful to characterize the variability and distribution of the estimated statistic induced by the sampling variability, but to do it through gathering many data sets from the population is rarely feasible, and we have to content with having only one data set for analysis. The basic idea of bootstrap is to use the data set at hand as a "surrogate population" and to generate multiple data sets, called bootstrap samples, by resampling with replacement from the original data for the purpose of approximating the distribution of the estimated statistic, which is referred to as the empirical distribution. In the most generic application of bootstrap, one needs to estimate the statistic of interest from each of these bootstrap samples, and these multiple estimates serve as samples from the statistic's distribution. Using these values, one can estimate different characteristics of the underlying sampling distribution, for example, bias, standard error and associated confidence interval, and P-values for testing statistical hypotheses, which were the primary goals of bootstrap when it was invented. However, later bootstrap found other "unintended" uses within the realm of machine learning, most notably a bootstrap-based point estimate also known as bagging estimator that plays a key role in algorithms of bagging and random forest. The motivation for bootstrap averaging was that it reduces variability at the expense of small amount of bias for unstable estimation processes where small perturbations in the data may incur substantial differences in estimated models. We will further discuss the application of bootstrap by "bagging" methods in Sect. 6.3.1. Many machine learning procedures belong to this class owing to their inherent instability.

One type of instability is caused by model (variable) selection where bootstrap can be very useful to evaluate model selection uncertainty, as we can fit a model of the same type, such as stepwise selection or lasso, to multiple bootstrap training data sets and obtain different characteristics such as the proportion of times a given variable was selected across all samples which can be plotted against some tuning parameters that control the selection process.

Another use of bootstrap is that it can also help to address the challenge with estimation of the generalization error. Recall the earlier discussion that when constructing a regression or classification model, we are mostly interested in model's predictive accuracy on test data not included in the training data set. Remarkably, bootstrap can be used as a source for generating "test samples," as when we create bootstrap training data sets by resampling with replacement from the original data set, naturally every bootstrap sample will include some observations multiple times, whereas some will not be selected. In fact, it is easy to verify that the probability of an observation to be included in any given bootstrap data set is $1 - \left(1 - \frac{1}{N}\right)^N$, approximately 0.632. In order to estimate the generalization error on samples that were not included in the training data, we can use the leave-one-out bootstrap approach, similar to the LOO cross-validation approach discussed above. To estimate the LOO generalization error on test data using some error or loss function $L\left(y, \widehat{f}(x)\right)$, for each of the N observations (x_i, y_i) in the original full data set, we only look at the predictions from the models that were built with bootstrap training samples where the ith observation was not included, indicated as a subset of indices $J^{(-i)} \subset \{1, .., B\}$, and thus can be designated as a new, test example for this model:

$$\widehat{Error}^{\,LOOB} = \frac{1}{N} \sum_{i=1}^{N} \frac{1}{|J^{(-i)}|} \sum_{b \in J^{(-i)}} L\left(y_i, \widehat{f}^{b}(x_i)\right).$$

Observations that appear in all B bootstrap samples can be omitted from the error calculation.

One drawback of the LOO bootstrap estimator of the generalization error is that the average number of distinct observations in each bootstrap sample is about 0.632 of the original full data set size N and the quality of the model can decline with the reduction of the training set size. In this case, the LOO bootstrap estimate will tend to overestimate the true generalization error. The so-called .632 estimator addresses this issue by estimating the generalization error as a weighted average:

$$\widehat{Error}^{.632} = 0.632 \times \widehat{Error}^{LOOB} + 0.368 \times \widehat{Error}^{train},$$

where the $\widehat{Error}^{train}$ is the training error calculated as the average prediction error over all original training examples when the model is fitted to the full original data set.

The ".632 estimator" corrects bias due to the reduction of the bootstrap training set size, but the second bias-correcting term may be inappropriate if the amount of overfitting is very large and the training error is close to zero, in which case the bias of LOO estimator may be considerable. The ".632+ estimator" (Efron and Tibshirani 1997) improves on this estimator by adjusting the 0.632 and 0.368 weights to reflect the amount of overfitting through the "no-information error rate" estimated as the error rate of the model fit to a data set with no true association between the predictors and outcome. This estimator was shown to outperform the LOO bootstrap and five- and tenfold cross-validation in Efron and Tibshirani (1997), providing low variance and moderate bias.

6.2.7 Ensemble Learning

Several approaches for supervised learning that emerged over the years share a similar basic idea and can be considered as ensemble learning. The general principle of ensemble learning is to build multiple, relatively simple prediction models (referred to as base models or learners, often weak learners, i.e., capable of prediction accuracy at least slightly above random guessing) and combine them into one overall model, which can combine their strengths. As such, ensemble learning consists of two tasks: estimation of a population of base learners from the training data and combining them to produce overall predictions, e.g., by (weighted) voting or averaging. One of the influential works in this area which propelled further research and applications of these methods was done by Hansen and Salamon (1990), who showed that predictions made by a combination of classifiers can be more accurate than predictions from a single classifier as long as each base learner is accurate and the classifiers are diverse. In this context, a classifier is considered accurate if it is better than random guessing. Diversity means that different classifiers make different errors on new data, so that if their errors are uncorrelated, the majority vote or averaging will likely lead to a correct overall classification. We further discuss these ideas in the context of bagging, random forests, and boosting approaches in Sect. 6.3.1.

It should be mentioned that Bayesian model averaging approaches can also be regarded in the framework of ensemble learning, for example, as a large number of models are averaged according to their "credibility"—the posterior distribution of their parameters (see, e.g., Madigan and Raftery 1994; Neal and Zhang 2006). At the same time as pointed out, for example, by Domingos (2000) and Minka (2002), ensemble methods and Bayesian model averaging differ fundamentally in that ensembles change the hypothesis space (e.g., from single decision trees to linear combinations of them), while Bayesian methods weight hypotheses in the original space according to a fixed formula. Bayesian model averaging is implicitly geared towards model selection rather than model combination, so that weights attributed to individual models can get extremely skewed due to overfitting, as too much weight is placed on the maximum likelihood model, to the point where the single highest-weight model usually dominates. In this case, performance of the Bayesian strategies can be worse than that of bagging or boosting. However, if Bayesian method is modified to integrate over combinations of models rather than over individual learners, it can achieve much better results (Monteith et al. 2011; Kim and Ghahramani 2012). These findings also lend support to the view that the power of ensembles lies primarily in the changes in representational and preferential bias inherent in the process of combining several different models.

6.3 Overview of Selected Methods

6.3.1 Supervised Learning

In Sect. 6.1, we discussed supervised machine learning as a counterpart of statistical modeling for regression and classification, where the goal is to approximate a relationship between the dependent variable (outcome) and one or more independent variables (predictors). Regression analysis typically aims at estimating a regression function—the conditional expectation of the outcome Y given the predictors X, $E(Y|X)$. For classification problems, where the outcome variable represents class labels $k = 1, \ldots, K$, the objective may be to estimate a model of the posterior probabilities $P(Y = k|X)$ or define a rule that would assign to each case a class label. Linear regression and logistic regression as well as modeling of other types of outcomes and underlying distributions via generalized linear models and models of time to event are examples of classical approaches widely used in statistics.

6.3.1.1 Penalized Regression

Penalized regression methods have been developed to provide a better prediction accuracy while being computationally efficient and feasible to use even with a large number of predictors. They had been independently proposed by different researches for solving somewhat different tasks: (1) incorporating in the same model a large number of potentially relevant but jointly redundant ("overlapping") predictors (sometimes exceeding the number of observations) without incurring instability in estimated coefficients (multicollinearity) and (2) dealing with a large number of irrelevant (noise) covariates among candidate predictors whose impact on estimation should be minimized (sparsity). These methods estimate model parameters by minimizing the residual sum of squares (more generally, some appropriate loss function, e.g., likelihood-based), but add a constraint (penalty) on the magnitude of the parameters. While this penalty causes the parameter estimates to be biased, it also decreases their variance that may achieve better performance via variance-bias trade-off. Penalized methods work by shrinking estimated model coefficients to zero. Some methods can shrink a coefficient exactly to zero (effectively eliminating the variable from the model), whereas others shrink all coefficients to some non-zero values. These methods are also referred to as shrinkage or regularization methods. In penalized regression, chosen parameters satisfy the following constrained minimization condition, based on a set of N training samples:

$$\widetilde{\beta} = arg\min_{\beta}\left(\sum_{i=1}^{N}\left(y_i - \boldsymbol{x}_i^T\boldsymbol{\beta}\right)^2\right),$$

subject to $Penalty(\beta) < k$.

Various penalized regression methods differ in terms of the penalty $Penalty(\beta)$ that they impose. The most popular methods are the ridge regression (Hoerl and Kennard 1970), lasso (Tibshirani 1996), adaptive lasso (Zou 2006), and elastic net (Zou and Hastie 2005).

These methods rely on one or more tuning parameters that determine the amount of shrinkage. Thus, a penalized regression method can produce a set of models, each associated with a specific setting of its tuning parameter(s). For the final model selection, the analyst must employ a tuning method to choose the optimal setting of these parameters. Among widely used approaches are model fit criteria, such as the Mallow's C_p statistic (Gilmour 1996) or Akaike information criterion (AIC) (Akaike 1974), Bayesian information criterion (BIC) (Schwarz 1978), average squared error on the validation data, and cross-validation.

Penalized regression is implemented in commercial statistical packages, including SAS®, as well as in R packages such as **lasso2** (L_1 constrained regression), **lars** (Least Angle Regression [LARS], lasso, and forward stepwise selection), **grplasso** (Group lasso), **glmpath** (L_1 Regularization Path for Generalized Linear Models and Cox Proportional Hazards Model), **stepPlr** (L_2 penalized logistic regression with a stepwise variable selection), **elasticnet** (elastic net regularization), **glmnet** (lasso and elastic net regularized generalized linear models), and **penalized** (lasso and ridge penalized estimation in generalized linear models and Cox regression model).

6.3.1.2 Classification and Regression Trees

Tree-based models became very popular in data mining solutions since the mid-1980s of the last century and later made their way as building blocks in many modern procedures (e.g., ensemble learning). Therefore, we describe them with more details than others in this review.

Tree-based models can be used both for regression and classification. These models are easily visualized as decision graphs resembling upside-down trees (see

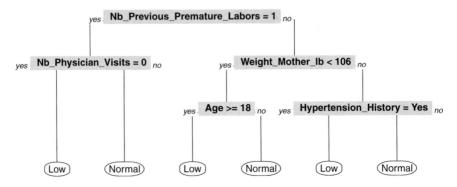

Fig. 6.2 Example of a classification tree for prediction of low/normal birth weight based on mother's characteristics (produced using R package **rpart.plot**)

example in Fig. 6.2): with a single node at the top, called a root node, and where each node can branch out into several (typically, two) child nodes. The nodes at the end of each branch, i.e., nodes that do not have any children, are referred to as terminal or leaf nodes. Each internal (non-leaf) node represents a split of the input space along the axis of one predictor, e.g., Age $\geq$ 18 vs. Age $<$ 18. Each branch culminating at a leaf node—a sequence of internal nodes—specifies a set of conditions with respect to input variables involved in the splits along the branch which define a region in the p-dimentional input space. Therefore, at the end of each branch, a leaf node represents a corresponding region and is assigned a predicted outcome associated with that region—either a numeric constant in the case of regression or a class label in the case of classification. Hence tree-based models are often called piecewise constant.

More specifically, a prediction model represented by a tree with M leaf nodes where each region is denoted as R_m, $m = 1, \ldots, M$ can be described as follows:

$$\widehat{f}(x) = \sum_{m=1}^{M} \widehat{c}_m I\{x \in R_m\},$$

where $I\{x \in R_m\}$ is an indicator function for whether the values of input vector x belong to the region R_m or not and c_m are numerical constants or class labels associated with the regions. For regression, one choice of c_m is the average of outcome values corresponding to training input samples that fall into the corresponding region:

$$\widehat{c}_m = average\{y_i | x_i \in R_m\}.$$

For classification, a class representing majority of y_i values can be chosen as the one determining the prediction in the leaf node:

$$\widehat{c}_m = \arg\max_k \frac{1}{N_m} \sum_{x_i \in R_m} I\{y_i = k\},$$

where N_m is the number of training samples that fall into region R_m.

Fitting a tree-based model typically involves a recursive procedure which, starting with the root note, looks for a beneficial split to associate with that node, where a split creates two child nodes (here we focus on binary trees, although procedures with multi-way splits have also been developed, see, e.g., Kim and Loh 2001 and references therein), and so forth until some stopping criterion is satisfied. This construction process includes a number of steps or tasks, and a multitude of procedures have been developed that differ in how they go about them:

- How to choose splits at each node.
- How to decide whether splitting should stop.
- How to choose the optimal size of the tree (model complexity).
- How to assign a prediction value at each leaf (e.g., by averaging/voting as described above).

Each split corresponding to a node in the tree is typically defined based on a single predictor variable (although procedures that form splits based on low-dimensional functions of data have also been proposed). If the variable is quantitative (ordinal), the split condition is of the form "$X_j \leq s$" where s can be any number and is typically chosen among the values of X_j that actually occur in the training data. If the variable is categorical, the split condition is of the form "$X_j \in A$" where A is any subset of classes that can be assumed by X_j. If the condition is satisfied, the branch from that node leads to the left child, otherwise to the right child. The same variable can be used for a split in multiple nodes of the tree.

During the recursive tree-fitting procedure, at each node, the algorithm has to choose the best split across all input variables and their values. This decision is made based on some measure of goodness of split, which is a measure of reduction in node "impurity" due to the split. The most common measures (for classification trees) are the Gini index and entropy (or information gain), while the misclassification error is less frequently used although available in software implementations. Gini impurity index measures how often a randomly chosen element from the set would be incorrectly labeled if it were randomly labeled according to the distribution of labels in the tree node, being the sum of $p_k(1 - p_k)$ across all categorical outcomes (labels) $k = 1, \ldots, K$, where p_k is the probability of kth outcome, estimated by the proportion of values $\{y_i = k\}$ in a given node. Statistically, each component is the variance of a Bernoulli random variate associated with the kth outcome category.

Information gain is defined as the reduction in entropy (an information theory measure of uncertainty) due to the split. The entropy associated with each node is a measure of "expected surprise" of the node's outcome and is defined as the sum of $-p_k \log_2(p_k)$ across $k = 1, \ldots, K$, which from the statistical perspective is simply related to the negative multinomial log-likelihood. Gini and entropy measures, unlike the classification error measure, are sensitive to class proportions in a node and can lead to more "pure" splits where one class is largely predominant. Thus, for the node splitting decisions during the tree construction, the former two measures are preferred. Nevertheless, all three measures can be useful for another aspect of the tree optimization—pruning—which we briefly discuss further below.

For regression trees, a popular measure of impurity is variance, and the best split is selected as the one that maximizes the reduction of the total corrected sum of squares due to the split. It is equivalent to choosing the split that maximized the between-group sum of squares in analysis of variance with the candidate split as an independent variable.

Other splitting criteria based on statistical tests have also been developed. For example, the CHAID algorithm (Kass 1980) for classification trees is based on a chi-square statistic that tests for a chance difference of the observed distribution of the categorical outcome across child regions. Similarly, the CHAID method for regression trees uses the F-test from ANOVA models to test the null hypothesis of equality of means between the child regions.

It should be noted that the splitting procedure outlined above tends to suffer from a variable selection bias in that the input variables with more distinct values are favored: the more choices are available for a given variable, the more likely it is to find a good split using that variable for a training set at hand. This may amplify a problem with noise variables if they have more unique values than strong predictors. Several approaches have been developed to alleviate this problem, e.g., FACT (Loh and Vanichsetakul 1988), QUEST (Loh and Shih 1997), CRUISE (Kim and Loh 2001), GUIDE (Loh 2002), and linear discriminant-based approach (Kim and Loh 2003). Another tree-based approach that selects variables in an unbiased way is designed in a conditional inference framework—conditional trees (CTree) by Hothorn et al. (2006). The latter approaches are also based on recursive procedures, but when a split is being selected at a tree node, a splitting variable is selected first, independently of the splitting value (and without an exhaustive search over all splits for all candidate variables).

When values of some predictor variables are missing for some training observations, a question arises how to handle this in the splitting process. In the case of categorical predictors, one can treat missing values as a separate category, which may be beneficial if missingness itself is predictive of outcome. Another approach is based on the use of surrogate variables. This strategy provides trees with a built-in mechanism to deal with missing predictor values in a way that exploits correlations between predictors.

When the best split is identified at the current node, two child nodes are created, and the splitting process is repeated from each of these children, as well as all other leaf nodes. There are several ways to decide when the splitting should stop. One can impose a limit on the minimum number of training samples that fall into a region associated with a leaf node, and when that limit is reached, splitting that node should be stopped. Another possibility is to continue splitting until the reduction of node impurity becomes smaller than some threshold. Yet another option is to stop when

Table 6.2 Summary of approaches for tree-based modeling

Step	Classification trees (categorical response)	Regression trees (quantitative response)	Survival trees (time-to-event response)
Variable selection	Exhaustive search based on splitting criteria (CART)	Exhaustive search based on splitting criteria (CART)	Exhaustive search based on splitting criteria (LeBlanc and Crowley 1992)
	Pre-selection by F-test or χ^2-test (FACT, CHAID, QUEST, GUIDE), association measures (CTree)	Pre-selection by F-test (CHAID) or χ^2 test for sign of residuals vs. predictors (GUIDE), association measures (CTree)	Pre-selection by association measures (CTree)
Splitting criteria	Reduction in Gini index (CART), information gain (CART, C.4.5), change in log-likelihood due to split (test statistic or adjusted P-value, JMP), χ^2 test of independence (CHAID)	Reduction in total sum of squares (CART, JMP), adjusted P-value from F-test (CHAID, JMP)	Reduction in deviance residual (LeBlanc and Crowley 1993)
Stopping criteria/ pruning	Pruning based on cost-complexity (CART, QUEST, GUIDE), pessimistic pruning (C4.5), reduction in test error; stopping rules based on (adjusted) P-values (CHAID, CTree), direct stopping rules (FACT), limits on minimum size of the leaf, number of levels, etc.		

the best split is not statistically significant at a pre-specified level. This approach is referred to as "forward selection" and is implemented in the CHAID algorithm. These approaches will likely result in large trees, susceptible to overfitting, so the initial large tree construction can be followed by pruning—reducing the size of the tree—with the goal of optimizing some cost-complexity criterion involving a penalty parameter interpreted as costs associated with each additional split that determines a trade-off between the goodness of fit to the data and the size of the tree. Tree pruning is considered a "backward elimination" strategy, and one popular approach is known as the weakest link pruning. An appropriate value of the penalty parameter can be found, for example, by cross-validation.

Table 6.2 provides a summary of different approaches available for classification, regression, and survival trees across the three main steps of the tree building procedure.

The key reference for the modern approach to tree-based machine learning is that of Breiman et al. (1984). Books on statistical learning, e.g., by Ripley (1996) and Hastie et al. (2009), and a recent comprehensive review by Loh (2014) can provide further reading.

An early example of applications of tree-based models for clinical data predictive modeling was construction of a diagnostic tool to identify patients with acute myocardial infarction in non-traumatic chest pain patients on admission to the emergency department (Mair et al. 1995). Other notable examples include classification (diagnosis and prognosis) of pulmonary hypertension in mixed connective tissue disease (Kotajima et al. 1997); study of the effects of risk factors on time to hip fracture using tree structures survival analysis (Lu et al. 2003); use of CART as alternatives to logistic regression for the estimation of propensity scores in the context of observational data analysis (Lee et al. 2010); determination of baseline predictors of remission with placebo for patients with major depressive disorder (Nelson et al. 2012); and tools for cancer prognosis and prediction (Konstantina et al. 2015).

The discussion above focused mainly on methods pertaining to the CART (classification and regression tree) methodology. Other tree-based methods developed over the years include ID3, C4.5, and C5.0 (Quinlan 1986, 1993, 2004). The latter, in particular, includes a scheme for deriving rule sets—simplifications of conditions along a tree branch without altering the subset of observations that fall in the branch leaf, which makes them easier to interpret. The multivariate adaptive regression splines (MARS) method (Friedman 1991) can be viewed as a modification of CART designed to improve smoothness of resulting models, the lack of which is inherent in piecewise constant models realized by the trees, as well as to allow fitting additive models, which are difficult to fit with trees. Hierarchical mixture of experts (HME) (Jordan and Jacobs 1994) can also be viewed as a variant of tree-based strategies, where splits are probabilistic functions of a linear combination of multiple inputs. Tree-based models can also be built for survival outcomes (Gordon and Olshen 1985). For example, Therneau et al. (1990) suggested using regression trees with null martingale residuals from a Cox proportional hazards model as the outcome variable. Various splitting criteria for survival trees have been proposed, e.g., a measure of within-node homogeneity based on the negative log-likelihood of the exponential model within a node (Davis and Anderson 1989), deviance residual (LeBlanc and Crowley 1992), weighted impurity based on the observed times and proportions of censored and uncensored subjects in a node (Zhang 1995), and two-sample log-rank statistics for the separation in survival times between child nodes (Segal 1988). Approaches have also been developed to extend the tree-based models to piecewise linear Poisson and logistic regression (e.g., Chaudhuri et al. 1995; Loh 2006) and longitudinal and multi-response variables (e.g., Loh and Zheng 2013) including in a context of identification of subgroup with differential treatment effect (Loh et al. 2016).

One issue with trees is their notorious instability, which is difficult to reduce even with tree pruning strategies. Small changes in the training data set may lead to trees with very different splits. Due to a hierarchical process of tree fitting, any errors in the top layers of the tree propagate all the way down. One way of dealing with this problem is bagging and random forests discussed below. These methods are based on averaging over a collection of trees fitted to different random samples of the data, which substantially reduces variability inherent in individual trees and typically results in improved prediction accuracy.

There are several R packages that implement decision tree methods, for example, the **rpart** (essentially implementing the CART algorithm), **party** (based on conditional tree platform), and **RWeka** packages. Other R packages such as **rattle**, **rpart. plot**, and **RColorBrewer** (a general-purpose color palette package) provide additional functions for visualizing the trees. Other examples of CART commercial implementations include SAS® Enterprise Miner, IBM® SPSS® Decision Trees, and a package by the Salford Systems. The non-R-based package GUIDE implements a number of methods developed by W-Y Loh and colleagues over the last 20 years with a common thread of unbiased variable selection (signified by the "U" letter in the acronym).

6.3.1.3 Bagging

We have mentioned earlier the general idea of ensemble learning as a way to reduce inherent variability in predictive models. Tree-based models, for example, can benefit greatly from this approach as they are flexible enough to represent complex functions (low bias), yet suffer from the high variance. One type of ensemble learning is bagging (Breiman 1996)—a term that is a contraction of *bootstrap aggr*egation. As the component terms suggest, the idea is to form B bootstrap data sets from the original data and fit a separate prediction model $\widehat{f}^b(x), b = 1, \ldots, B$ to each of them. Then an aggregated (bagged) prediction is obtained as

$$\widehat{f}_{bag}(x) = \frac{1}{B} \sum_{b=1}^{B} \widehat{f}^b(x).$$

Bagging reduces the variance component of the generalization error, especially when used with highly unstable models, such as regression trees. Because averaging leaves the bias component unchanged, it improves the predictive accuracy in general. Typically, to ensure the low bias, averaging is applied to full-sized (unpruned) trees.

Analyses using bagging can be carried out using R packages **ipred** and **adabag**.

6.3.1.4 Random Forests

Random forest (Breiman 2001a, b) is another ensemble learning approach that adds to bagging yet another stochastic element: for each candidate split in the learning process, only a random subset of variables is considered ($r \leq p$ of input variables). This is done to reduce the correlation in the base trees leading to enhancing variance-lowering advantages of bagging. When a collection of B trees is obtained on bootstrap samples as in bagging, the trees can exhibit high correlation if there are variables that are strong predictors of outcome, as these same predictors are very likely to be selected as primary splitters in many trees. For bagging to be effective, the base learners should be less dependent (ensuring larger diversity). This is because the average of B identically distributed random variables has the variance of

$$\rho\sigma^2 + \frac{1-\rho}{B}\sigma^2,$$

where ρ is a pairwise correlation and σ^2 is a variance of each variable. The trees estimated from bootstrap samples are identically distributed, and so the second term diminishes with increasing number of bootstrap samples B, but the first term becomes a bottleneck for variance decrease if the correlation ρ is high.

Selecting the best split from a random subset of variables increases the diversity of the ensemble and prevents few "winners" to dominate all the trees. A discussion of how bagging and random subspace projection together improve accuracy can be found in Ho (2002). The smaller the number of variables used to select each split is, the more reduction in correlation could be achieved (thus reduction in variance). At the same time, as the total number of variables grows, and the fraction of relevant variables decreases, the performance of random forests will degrade with a small number of variables sampled for each split because the bias of each tree will increase. A general recommendation is to use $\sqrt{p}$ variables to choose each split in classification problems and $p/3$ (with a minimum of 5) variables in regression problems. This number can also be treated as one of the tuning parameters of the algorithm. The number of trees in the random forest, B, is another tuning parameter, and both can be optimized, for example, using cross-validation. In principle, the depth of the individual trees could also be a tuning parameter, but Segal (2004) demonstrated that only small gains in performance could be achieved by optimizing this aspect, and so full-grown trees are typically used.

After B full-sized (unpruned) trees are constructed using the random forest algorithm, the overall predictor is determined in the same way as in bagging, e.g., as the average of all trees' predictions for regression, and a majority vote across predictions from all trees for classification.

The performance of random forests is often very similar to boosting—another powerful approach that we summarize below—and it often requires relatively little tuning (offer a more "automated" approach compared to boosting).

One of the bonus features of the random forest algorithm is that it provides an estimate of the generalization accuracy based on the out-of-bag (OOB) samples. As previously discussed (Sect. 6.2), test samples not included in the training data play a key role in estimating the generalization error. In the context of random forests, it can be achieved by constructing the overall prediction for each observation x_i in the original full training set by using predictions only from those trees that were estimated from the bootstrap samples where the observation (x_i, y_i) was not included. Although the OOB error estimates are very similar to those produced by cross-validation, with random forests, generalization error estimation can utilize the same bootstrap replicates that were used for model fitting and thus does not create a computational overhead. Wager et al. (2014) extended an earlier work on estimation of the variance for bagged predictors and proposed an efficient approach to variance estimation based on jackknife and infinitesimal jackknife estimators. In this work, Wager et al. addressed potential upward bias in bagged variance estimates due to the Monte Carlo noise resulting from a finite number of bootstrap replicates. They developed bias-corrected versions of the jackknife and infinitesimal jackknife estimators.

The random forest method also provides variable importance scores to rank predictive strengths of all input variables. Variable importance is naturally defined in the context of tree-based models. Any input variable X_j, $j = 1, \ldots, p$ can be involved in multiple splits across the tree and thus contribute to the reduction of node impurity. One way of defining the relative importance of variable X_j in a tree T is as follows:

$$I(j, T) \propto \sqrt{\sum_{\tau \in T} a(s_j, \tau) \Delta Q(\tau)},$$

where the sum is over nodes τ in the tree T, function $a(s_j, \tau)$ reflects whether variable X_j is involved in a main or surrogate splitting rule s_j in node τ, and $\Delta Q(\tau)$ is a reduction in node impurity due to a split of this node. Variable importance scores estimated within each individual tree are then accumulated over all trees for each variable. Additionally, permutation-based variable importance is also computed by random forests utilizing the OOB samples. This is done by first estimating prediction accuracy on the OOB samples for each tree separately. Then, to estimate the variable importance of variable X_j, values of this variable are randomly permuted across OOB samples, and prediction accuracy is again estimated in those permuted observations for each tree (i.e., without refitting the trees). The decrease in prediction accuracy as a result of permutation is then calculated and averaged across all trees. Although the ranking of variables according to their variable importance scores tends to agree for these two methods, there are some differences in the distribution of the scores.

Other useful features of random forests include computation of proximities between observations that can be used for clustering and locating outliers. Marginal effects of the individual variables on the outcome can also be estimated, which we will illustrate in a case study in Sect. 6.5.3.

The elements of the random forest method as discussed here were introduced by Breiman (2001a, b) following his development of bagging (1996); of note, the term "random forest" was introduced earlier by Ho (1995) in the context of a method based on a consensus of trees estimated in random subspaces of input features. Research and improvement of the random forest methodology continue, e.g., by Xu (2013). Random forests have had many uses in large applications in genomics and proteomics as well as in the analysis of clinical data. The following are just some examples of the latter applications: predicting disease risk from medical diagnosis history using Healthcare Cost and Utilization Project data set (Khalilia et al. 2011), detection and prediction of Alzheimer's disease (Lebedev et al. 2014), multidimensional clinical phenotyping of an adult cystic fibrosis patient population (Conrad and Bailey 2015), and clustering of patients based on tissue marker data (Shi et al. 2005).

Several variants, extensions, and methods related to the random forest methodology have been introduced over the years. A relationship between random forests and the adaptive nearest neighbor algorithm was pointed out by Lin and Jeon (2006)—both approaches can be viewed as so-called weighted neighborhoods schemes. Friedman and Hall (2007) suggested that subsampling without replacement can be used as an alternative to bagging and demonstrated that fitting trees on samples of size $N/2$ achieves approximately the same performance as bagging, and using smaller fractions of N can reduce the variance even further. The "extremely randomized forest" is an extension of the random forest method where both a subset of input variables and their possible split values are selected randomly when considering candidates for each split (Geurts et al. 2006).

Instead of fitting decision trees as base learners in the random forest, other alternatives have been proposed, e.g., multinomial logistic regression and naive Bayes classifiers (Prinzie and Van den Poel 2008) and naïve Bayes models (Aridas et al. 2016). Other variants of random forests include multivariate random forests (Segal and Xiao 2011), enriched random forests (Amaratunga et al. 2008), quantile regression forests (Meinshausen 2006), and random survival forests (Ishwaran et al. 2008).

Random forest software maintained by a collaborator of Leo Breiman, Adele Cutler, is publicly available online (http://www.math.usu.edu/~adele/forests/). There are also several R packages, such as **randomForest**, **randomSurvivalForest**, **extraTrees** (extreme random forest), and **varSelRF** (variable selection using random forest) implementing this methodology.

6.3.1.5   Boosting

Boosting represents another family of ensemble learning algorithms. It was originally introduced for classification as a way to combine many weak learners to produce a powerful "committee." One of the most popular boosting algorithms introduced by Freund and Schapire (1997), called AdaBoost, relies on a set of weak classifiers whose error rate is only slightly better than random guessing. The weak classification algorithm is applied M times to modified—weighted—training data sets. At the first iteration, weights of all data samples are equal $w_i = 1/N$, and a classifier $\widehat{f}_1(x)$ is estimated based on a data set with such weights. At subsequent iterations, $m = 2, 3, \ldots, M$, weights are increased for those observations that were misclassified by the classifier from the previous iteration, $\widehat{f}_{m-1}(x)$, and decreased for observations that were classified correctly. As the algorithm progresses, successive classifiers are compelled to focus on "difficult" cases missed by previous classifiers. The overall classification at the end is obtained as

$$\widehat{f}_{AdaBoost}(x) = sign\left[\sum_{m=1}^{M} \alpha_m \widehat{f}_m(x)\right],$$

where α_m are the weights determining the contribution of each learner based on its weighted training error. Boosting can dramatically increase the accuracy of very weak single classifiers (those that are just slightly better than random guessing) and outperform large single classification trees. Breiman called AdaBoost as the "best off-the-shelf classifier in the world," and the ideas have since been extended to regression as well.

As it was shown later (Friedman et al. 2000), the AdaBoost is a special case of a general class of forward stagewise additive modeling, where the overall predictor consists of an additive model in some basis functions (base learners) $h(x, \beta)$, with each function fitted and added sequentially without changing parameters of the previously fitted functions so that the overall prediction can be improved. After fitting an initial model, at each subsequent stage, $m = 2, 3, \ldots, M$, the overall additive model from the previous stage is expanded as $\widehat{f}_m(x) = \widehat{f}_{m-1}(x) + h_m\left(x, \widehat{\beta}\right)$, so that the additional component $h_m\left(x, \widehat{\beta}\right)$ improves the performance of the previous model. Least Angle Regression is a computationally efficient version of the stagewise approach. Its details and connections to the lasso regression can be found in Efron et al. (2004).

The base learner $h(x, \beta)$ can be selected from a variety of choices: a linear model (e.g., ordinary linear regression with few best selected predictors), a smooth model (e.g., spline), or a shallow tree (perhaps the most common choice). The complexity of the base learner (e.g., the number of terminal nodes of the tree) is controlled by the user.

Gradient boosting (Friedman 2001; Mason et al. 2000) is a generalization of the stagewise modeling approach that allows the optimization of any differentiable loss function and applies to both regression and classification. Stochastic gradient boosting proposed by Friedman (1999) also incorporated some "elements" of bagging, where each successive base learner is fitted on a subset of the training data set drawn at random without replacement. Friedman reported significant improvements with the stochastic gradient boosting when the size of the subsample is between 50% and 80% of the original data set size. The subsampling strategy also allows for estimation of the generalization error using "out-of-sample" observations, similar to as it was described for bootstrap.

Another element that may help prevent overfitting and improve the accuracy of boosting is introduction of regularization (shrinkage) parameter $0 < \nu \leq 1$, so that instead of adding the "full fit" for each successive learner, only a portion of the fit $\nu h_m\left(x, \widehat{\beta}\right)$ is added. The meta-parameter ν is also called "learning rate" parameter because it controls how much is learned from the training data at each step. To summarize, gradient boosting implements several elements of "slow learning" that prevents adapting to the random features of the training data and ensures its ability to generalize well to the "new" data (prediction performance):

- Forward stagewise strategy (not updating previously fitted components of the ensemble when adding new fit)
- Subsampling (fitting a subsequent learner to a random fraction of the training data)
- Shrinkage (adding only a portion of the new fit)

The two most important complexity parameters that control gradient boosting are the number of iterations (fitted models, M) and learning rate (ν), and they are selected by cross-validation. Typically, the smaller the learning rate, the larger is the number of iterations required to achieve a good fit (i.e., until the model starts overfitting training data).

Both random forest and gradient boosting are ensemble methods and have shown comparable performance on a variety of benchmark data sets. However, as boosting is connected with forward stagewise modeling, its theoretical properties are more amenable to analyses compared to random forest that appears more as a "black box" and a highly heuristic method. In particular, the fact that model complexity of the base learner is controlled by the analyst and kept at relatively low level makes boosting a useful tool for understanding the underlying structure of the data. By fitting different boosting models with a tree as the base learner and having varying depths (the number of terminal nodes, K), one can assess the presence of k-order interaction effects in the data. For example, if $K = 2$, only main effects can be captured by a boosting model, as each fitted tree is a "stump" (split on a single variable) capturing only the main effect of that variable; if $K = 3$, two-way interactions can be captured, etc. Friedman and Popescu (1999) developed a procedure based on parametric bootstrap for conducting formal significance testing for the presence of interaction effects.

An excellent discussion of boosting from a statistical perspective for estimating complex parametric and nonparametric models, including generalized linear, additive, and survival analysis models, as well as its application to variable selection, can be found in Bühlmann and Horthorn (2007).

Analyses using boosting approaches can be carried out using various R packages: **adabag** (AdaBoost and bagging), **ada** (AdaBoost with some Friedman's modifications), **gbm** (tree-based gradient boosting), **GAMBoost** (boosting with penalized B-splines), **mboost** (boosting with high-dimensional (generalized) linear or smooth additive models and a possibility to supply own implementation of any negative gradient for general surrogate loss functions), and **xgboost** (Extreme Gradient Boosting, which can automatically do parallel computation on a single machine and includes many common objective functions with the flexibility of allowing for customized objective functions). Two recent additions worth noting are **bujar** (implementing boosting for survival data) and **bst** (implementing a method called twin boosting; Bühlmann and Hothorn 2010).

6.3.1.6 Support Vector Machines

A support vector machine (SVM) is a supervised learning method which was originally developed for classification and later extended to regression. In the context of classification, it is based on a concept of decision boundary or a hyperplane that separates a set of objects in the space of their attributes belonging to different classes. The algorithm tries to learn a parameterized hyperplane that maximizes the margin between the hyperplane and the closest training examples in each class. For example, in a p-dimensional input space and a binary classification problem, a linear SVM classifier is the one that can separate two response classes using a $(p-1)$-dimensional hyperplane. If data cannot be perfectly separated and classes overlap in the input space, one can define a hinge loss function that allows some samples to fall on the wrong side of the margin (giving zero penalty to samples inside the margin and linearly increasing penalty for those on the wrong side), thus introducing a cost of each misclassification. This leads to a constrained optimization problem, and a classifier of this type can be estimated using a quadratic programming solution with Lagrange multipliers. An extension of this idea is that if a satisfactory linear classifier cannot be obtained, then the input space can be mapped/transformed to a higher-dimensional feature space and then a linear classifier can be built in that feature space. This is reminiscent of other linear methods that expand the model complexity by using, for example, basis expansions such as polynomials or splines. In the case of SVMs, the feature space is allowed to have a very high dimensionality, but the learning algorithm deals with this efficiently by using a hinge loss function and a form of regularization. Indeed, it can be shown (Hastie et al. 2009) that the solution to the constrained optimization posed by SVM is equivalent to estimating a classification model with the hinge loss function and quadratic (ridge) penalty on the coefficients.

The elements that form the foundation of SVMs have been introduced by Vapnik (1996). Other references for introductory reading include a tutorial by Burges (1998) and Evgeniou et al. (2000). Examples of SVM use for clinical data analysis include applications in diabetes research (Kavakiotis et al. 2017), classification of major depressive disorder (Sacchet et al. 2015), breast cancer diagnosis (Zheng et al. 2014), predicting Alzheimer's disease using linguistic deficits and biomarkers (Orimaye et al. 2017), etc.

SVMs are a member of a more general class of kernel methods (Shawe-Taylor and Cristianini 2004) based on the use of kernel functions that operate in a high-dimensional feature space by computing inner products between mappings of data pairs in the feature space. This approach is sometimes referred to as a "kernel trick" because the operations involving inner products in the feature space are computationally cheaper than the ones in the original space. Kernel-based algorithms include Gaussian processes, principal components analysis (PCA), canonical correlation analysis, ridge regression, spectral clustering, and others.

SVM implementations are available in R in the **SVM** and **svmpath** packages, SAS® Enterprise Miner®, a C-based **SVM**[light] package from Cornell University (available at http://svmlight.joachims.org/), and many other packages publicly available online.

6.3.1.7 Artificial Neural Networks

The roots of neural networks can be traced back both to statistics and machine learning. The basic principle is to create features as linear combinations of inputs and then to fit a predictive function as a nonlinear function of these derived features. In statistics, this idea was used, for example, in the projection pursuit regression, which is based on an additive model of a collection of nonlinear nonparametric functions of the linear combination of the original predictors. The richness of such models in terms of their capacity to represent arbitrary complex functions increases as the number of these feature functions grows, but this also comes at the cost of low interpretability—resulting in a so-called "black box" method.

The term artificial neural network emerged in the fields of artificial intelligence and machine learning, where parallels between the underlying computational model and brain functioning were drawn. A basic artificial neural network model is often represented in the form of a directed graph consisting of several layers of units, the first layer representing the original predictor variables and the last layer the outcome for regression or classification. Values (signals) from one layer are fed into units of the subsequent layer, where units are thought of as representing neurons. Signals pass through the connections representing synapses, which can "weight" the input signals upon entry to the neuron. Each unit then represents a weighted linear combination of its inputs and produces an output signal when the weighted combination exceeds some threshold (i.e., the neuron fires). The outputs from the units in one layer can then be fed as inputs to the units of the subsequent layer. The function regulating "firing" of each neuron can be a step function or a smoother alternative such as the sigmoid function. Fitting such models can be done using a gradient descent approach, referred to in the neural network literature as back-propagation, as it relies on the chain rule for differentiation. Neural networks can be prone to overfitting, and approaches similar to regularization have been developed to deal with the issue. Performance can be sensitive to the initial values of the synaptic weights and to the scale of the input values. The number of units and inner layers typically also needs to be tuned, for example, using cross-validation. The gradient descent-based learning is prone to converge to local optima and benefits from introducing randomness into the starting values of synaptic weights as well as from the use of bagging. Some researches consider artificial neural networks to be a foundation for advances in large-scale machine learning due to their ability to produce highly accurate predictive models in a wide range of applications, including image and sound recognition, text processing, time series analysis, etc. Recently neural networks experienced a revival under the name of "deep learning," to a large extent due to the availability of increased computational power allowing building networks with a larger number of layers than before and some additional improvements in the network architecture (Efron and Hastie 2016). The black box nature of neural networks and the fact that they can be difficult to tune represent some of their disadvantages, which may be particularly important in the context of clinical data mining where the focus is often on generating new, interpretable insights about the data patterns.

Projection pursuit method is due to Friedman and Tukey (1974) and Friedman and Stuetzle (1981). Modern approaches to neural networks are developed by Werbos (1975) and Rumelhart et al. (1986). The book by Ripley (1996) provides an excellent further reading. Applications of neural networks in the clinical data analysis are numerous. Recent examples include a cardiac health prognostic system

(Sunkaria et al. 2014), cancer prognosis and prediction (Konstantina et al. 2015), applications in prostate cancer (Cosma et al. 2017), prediction of pregnancy outcomes in women with systemic lupus erythematous (Paydar et al. 2017), etc.

The original neural networks algorithm has been extended in many ways over the years, giving rise to feed-forward, recurrent, probabilistic, modular, and neuro-fuzzy neural networks and many other variations.

Several R packages offer neural networks learning, such as **nnet**, **neuralnet**, **H2O**, **DARCH**, **deepnet**, and **mxnet**; SAS® Enterprise Miner® provides neural networks functionality, and there are many publicly and commercially available software packages online.

6.3.2   Unsupervised Learning

6.3.2.1   Clustering

Clustering is one of the major applications of unsupervised machine learning. The goal of clustering is to find a grouping (a set of clusters) of a collection of objects, described by their input attributes so that the objects assigned to the same cluster are more similar to each other than to objects in other clusters. Sometimes clusters may need to be arranged in a hierarchy to reflect some natural structures in the data. Once clusters are learned from the data, some descriptive summary attributes may be of interest to describe specific properties of objects within each cluster.

A key concept in clustering is a definition of similarity measure, or conversely dissimilarity measure, based on which the relationship between objects can be evaluated. There are several frequently used measures, but an appropriate choice is often dictated by domain knowledge. In general, the choice of the dissimilarity measure is very important and can have a crucial effect on the resulting clustering (some say that even more so than the choice of the clustering algorithm).

The classical K-means algorithm can be used, for example, when all input variables are quantitative, and the dissimilarity measure is based on the average squared distance—the Euclidean distance. When the Euclidian distance is used as a measure of dissimilarity, the algorithm may be sensitive to outliers, as the observations with the largest distance will have a significant influence on the loss function. For this reason as well as to allow non-quantitative input attributes, the algorithm can be generalized to use other appropriate dissimilarity measures. This more general approach is often referred to as K-medoids method.

The term K-means clustering was first used in MacQueen (1967) although the underlying ideas were introduced by Lloyd (1957) and basically the same algorithm was published by Forgy (1965). The more general K-medoid procedure was described in Kaufman and Rousseeuw (1990). Description of this algorithm can be found in many machine learning textbooks, e.g., Hastie et al. (2009). Some recent examples of applications of K-means clustering in the analysis of clinical data include identifying subgroups of fibromyalgia patients with different forms of disease and outcomes (Docampo et al. 2013; Lipkovich et al. 2014), identifying clinical phenotypes in chronic obstructive pulmonary disease patients with multiple comorbidities (Burgel et al. 2014), phenotyping of severe asthma patients (Wu et al. 2014) and bipolar disorder patients (Wu et al. 2017).

K-means clustering is closely related to the Expectation-Maximization (EM) algorithm. Parallels between the two can be drawn in that the K-means clustering approach, for example, in the case of continuous variables, models each cluster by a spherical Gaussian distribution, but assigns each data sample to a single cluster and uses equal weights to mix cluster distributions. Both algorithms are special cases of modeling with Gaussian mixtures. Another approach that can be viewed as a generalization of the K-means clustering is the K-SVD algorithm (Aharon et al. 2006). It uses a set of K so-called dictionary functions (e.g., wavelets, curvelets, etc.) to create sparse representations of high-dimensional data as linear combinations of dictionary functions. The algorithm then iterates by alternating between sparse coding of the data samples based on the current dictionary and updating the dictionary to fit the data better. Self-organizing maps (Kohonen 1989) is a related method that can be viewed as a constrained variant of K-means clustering where cluster centers are placed on one- or two-dimensional manifolds in a feature space constructed from original variables.

K-means clustering is readily available in R **stats** package through the **kmeans** function. The R package **cluster** implements the algorithm for partitioning around medoids. This package also implements a CLARA algorithm specifically designed to work with large data sets. The R package **clustMixType** implements an extension of K-means to mixed data types and package **kml** to longitudinal data. SAS® offers multiple procedures for clustering, including FASTCLUS implementing the K-means algorithm.

Hierarchical clustering is another approach which produces a hierarchical representation of data groupings, often graphically depicted by a tree-like structure known as dendrogram: individual observations are associated with the lowest level of the hierarchy (leaves), and the entire data set is represented by the highest level—single cluster (root). There are two approaches for hierarchical clustering: agglomerative and divisive based on either recursive merging or partitioning of the data from the previous level of the hierarchy. Hierarchical algorithms work with a measure of dissimilarity between disjoint groups of observations represented by nodes in the hierarchy, which in turn is based on a measure of dissimilarity between individual observations. In agglomerative strategies, the dissimilarity between clusters that are merged from one level to the next is monotone increasing, and the dendrogram is typically drawn such that the height of each node is proportional to the dissimilarity between its two child nodes. Dendrograms provide a graphical summary of the data, but not an obvious description of the clusters, and represent the structure imposed by the algorithm as applied to a particular training sample, which may not necessarily reflect any natural hierarchy in the domain.

Early approaches to agglomerative hierarchical clustering are due to Ward (1963), Macnaughton Smith et al. (1965), Sibson (1973), and Defays (1977). The books by Kaufman and Rousseeuw (1990) and Hastie et al. (2009) provide a good discussion of various clustering algorithms, including hierarchical approaches. Some recent applications of hierarchical clustering in clinical data analysis include finding groups of fibromyalgia patients with similar efficacy outcomes across multiple symptom scales (Abtroun et al. 2016), identification of biomarkers for tuberculosis susceptibility (Luo et al. 2014), identifying distinct hemostatic responses to trauma and key components of the hemostatic system that vary between responses (White et al. 2015), etc.

In the R **stats** package, hierarchical clustering can be carried out using the **hclust** function. Other R packages implementing hierarchical approaches include **cluster**, **fastcluster**, **fastClust**, **genie**, and **pvclust**. SAS® procedure CLUSTER provides an implementation of hierarchical clustering. Open-source Cluster 3.0 software is available for most operating systems. Most commercial statistical software packages provide hierarchical clustering functionality.

6.3.2.2 Principal Components and Related Methods

Principal component analysis is a dimensionality reduction method where the goal is to find a low-dimensional representation of the data that captures most of the information (variability) of interest in the data. The classical approach relies on the orthogonal linear transformation of the data to a new coordinate system where the principal components are linear manifolds approximating a set of N p-dimensional data points. Some nonlinear generalizations of PCA have also been developed where the principal components are curved manifold approximations. In the linear case, each component is a linear combination of the p original variables. Principal components are constructed as a sequence of components that are mutually uncorrelated and ordered by variance, so that the first principal component accounts for the largest amount of variability in the data, and each subsequent component has the highest variance subject to a constraint that it is orthogonal to the preceding components.

Principal components are typically constructed by eigenvalue decomposition of a data covariance or correlation matrix or a singular value decomposition of a data matrix usually after applying appropriate standardization of variables (e.g., to have 0 mean and standard deviation of 1, corresponding to PCA on the correlation matrix). The decision of whether PCA should be applied to raw or transformed data and the selection of appropriate transformation depends on various subject-matter considerations. For example, PCA on data covariance allows one to capture nontrivial differences in variances among variables, whereas applying PCA to correlations effectively standardizes the data to have the same (unit) variances. The former makes sense when variables are commensurate: for example, reflecting similar rating scales or the same outcomes measured at different time points. However, if the variables are incommensurate, the differences in variance are not meaningful and may reflect trivial differences in measurement scales. As an "extreme case," consider difference in the variance of two variables representing the same variable "body weight" measured first in pounds and then in kilograms. In such cases, of course, data should be standardized before applying PCA. However, one may consider standardizing to unit variances too radical, as it completely washes away any differences in variability among variables, and prefer other standardization procedures, such as transforming data to vary within a unit range. It is also a common practice to remove outliers from the data before applying the PCA if they can be identified, as the results may be quite sensitive to them. Some variants, such as weighted PCA, have been proposed to improve robustness in this respect.

It is a common practice to visualize multivariate data sets by low-dimensional scatter plots using the first 2–3 principal components. This is a special case of a broad class of *multidimensional scaling* procedures (MDS, Kruskal and Wish 1978). A related visualization technique is the *biplot* display, based on singular value decomposition of (appropriately transformed) data matrix (Gower and Hand 1996; Lipkovich and Smith 2002). In biplots, both data columns and rows are represented graphically: as rays and dots, respectively. The cosines of angles between rays roughly reflect the correlations between variables, and the projections of data points onto the rays reflect the data coordinates (values) in the underlying multidimensional space.

The founding ideas behind the PCA date back to 1901 due to Pearson and 1933 due to Hotelling. PCA is covered in many textbooks, e.g., Jolliffe (2002) is devoted entirely to this method, its applications, and many of its variants. PCA was used to identify distinct patterns of coagulopathy after trauma in Kutcher et al. (2013), to uncover important differences in how patients and informants perceive and report Alzheimer's disease symptoms using the Clinical Meaningfulness in Alzheimer Disease Treatment scale (Jacova et al. 2013), and to explore the association between anemia (hepcidin and hemoglobin levels) and clinical disease activity and acute phase response in patients with rheumatoid arthritis (Padjen et al. 2016).

A counterpart of PCA for analysis of nominal categorical data is a multiple correspondence analysis (MCA) (Greenacre 1984). PCA forms principal components as linear combinations of all input variables which may be problematic in sparse domains where $p > N$. Sparse PCA (Zou et al. 2006) addresses this challenge by looking for linear combinations that involve a subset of just a few input variables. PCA is related to the factor analysis (FA, Cattell 1952) and the independent component analysis (Hyvärinen and Oja 2000) that aim to explain joint variations in input variables by unobserved latent variables. Probabilistic PCA (Tipping and Bishop 1999) is a closely related method where principal axes are determined through maximum likelihood estimations of parameters in a latent variable model. Kernel PCA (Schölkopf et al. 1997) uses a "kernel trick" that forms the basis of support vector machines, where data is first nonlinearly mapped into a high-dimensional feature space, and then the PCA is performed in that space, thus generalizing the PCA to a nonlinear setting.

PCA is implemented in many publicly and commercially available packages. In the R's **stats** package, the functions **princomp** and **prcomp** provide the PCA functionality, as well as such packages as **FactoMineR** and **ade4**. In SAS®, procedures PRINCOMP and FACTOR implement the PCA.

6.3.3 Semi-supervised Learning

6.3.3.1 Methods for Biomarker and Subgroup Identification from Clinical Trial Data

Various methods for subgroup and biomarker identification have been proposed during the last decade in statistical literature as a response to the need for precision/personalized medicine: to provide the best treatment for a patient with specific characteristics at a particular time. A comprehensive review can be found in Lipkovich et al. (2017). See also recent review papers focusing on special types of modeling by Lamont et al. (2016), Henderson et al. (2016), Ondra et al. (2016), and Janes et al. (2013).

Broadly, these methods fall within the class of semi-supervised learning, as the goal is predicting treatment contrast for a patient given his or her biomarker profile. Here a biomarker is understood as any patient-specific measure (covariate) taken prior to assigning a treatment. Unlike patient's outcomes, treatment contrasts are not fully observed in the training sample when patients are exposed to only one of the set of possible treatment options (which is typically the case unless a crossover design is entertained). In the literature on the analysis of medical data, biomarkers that are predictive of treatment contrast are called *predictive*, and biomarkers that are predictive of patient's outcomes if left untreated are called *prognostic*. This is somewhat confusing and inconsistent with the general statistical and machine learning terminology where prediction and predictive covariates/variables (predictors) are understood in a broader sense. Nevertheless, we will adopt the above distinction between predictive and prognostic biomarkers that has been accepted by researchers in the area of subgroup analysis. A biomarker can be predictive and prognostic, only prognostic, and only predictive. The latter case corresponds to rare occasions when a biomarker is not predictive of outcomes for the untreated (more broadly, "control") population but is predictive of outcomes in patients who underwent experimental treatment. The distinction depends on the definition of the estimand for measuring treatment contrast: for example, a biomarker may be predictive when measuring the treatment effect in a binary outcome as the difference in proportions but not predictive when using odds ratios and vice versa. Figure 6.3 depicts several situations: when a biomarker is (a) prognostic but not predictive, (b) both prognostic and predictive, (c) predictive but not prognostic, and (d) neither predictive nor prognostic.

A plethora of methods for identifying predictive biomarkers and subgroups (defined in terms of underlying predictive biomarkers) emerged in the recent literature from diverse research areas: machine learning, causal inference, multiple testing, and design and analysis of clinical trials (see Lipkovich et al. 2017). To facilitate our review, we will introduce some minimal notation that will help us in describing common features and differences across subgroup identification methods.

Define a vector of p measurements for candidate biomarkers $X_1, \ldots, X_p$ on the ith subject as $\boldsymbol{x}_i = (x_{i1}, \ldots, x_{ip})$ and (for the sake of simplicity) two treatment arms

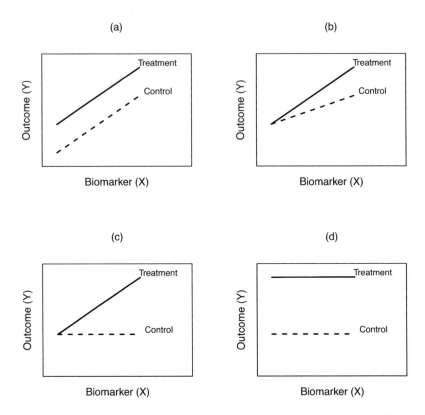

Fig. 6.3 Schematics of predictive and prognostic markers: (**a**) prognostic but not predictive, (**b**) both prognostic and predictive, (**c**) predictive but not prognostic, and (**d**) neither predictive nor prognostic

(control and experimental treatment) indexed by variable $T = \{0, 1\}$ and the outcome variable Y (for simplicity, assume Y is continuous or binary).

Assume the true response function has the following simple representation: $f(x, t) = h(x) + (t - p) \times z(x)$, where $f(x, t) \equiv E(Y|X = x, T = t)$; therefore, $z(x) = f(x, 1) - f(x, 0)$ is the "personalized" treatment contrast, and $h(x)$ is an unspecified "baseline" function. The constant p is often conveniently used to represent the probability of treatment, $p = \Pr(T = 1)$.

Adopting potential outcomes framework (see a review paper by Little and Rubin (2000) and references therein), for each subject we define two potential (hypothetical) outcomes $Y(1)$ and $Y(0)$ with only one being observed. These outcomes are connected with the observed data via the consistency assumption as $Y = Y(1)T + Y(0)(1 - T)$ and with the above quantities as $f(x, t) = E(Y(t)|X = x)$, $t = 0, 1$ and $z(x) = E(Y(1) - Y(0)|X = x)$.

Treatment regime is a function, $g(x)$, that maps x to treatment 1 or 0. Optimal treatment regime is defined as $g_{opt}(x) = I(f(x, 1) > f(x, 0))$, where $I(a)$ is an indicator function that assumes values 1 or 0 when its argument a is true or false, respectively. In terms of potential outcomes, it is the regime that maximizes the expected potential outcomes assuming everyone follows the regime.

Subgroup $S(X)$ is defined by a rule that assigns a subject to the subgroup based on a biomarker vector x. For example, $S(X) = \{x : X_1 \leq a, X_2 > b\}$. The subgroup definition is also referred to as subgroup signature. Then treatment effect in the subgroup $S(X)$ is defined as $E(z(X)|X \in S(X))$, where the expectation is computed with respect to the distribution of X. A measure of how interesting a subgroup may be is the excess of treatment effect in the subgroup over that in the overall population: $E(z(X)|X \in S(X)) - E(z(X))$.

The distinction between predictive and prognostic biomarkers can be formalized as follows: prognostic biomarkers are those that contribute only to $h(x)$ (the "main effects"), whereas predictive biomarkers are those that also contribute to $z(x)$ (and perhaps to $h(x)$ as well).

Based on the above definitions, we can classify different methods that have been proposed recently for selection of predictive biomarkers (and choosing biomarker cutoffs to define subgroups of patients) in terms of what *estimands* (functions or components of these functions) they aim to estimate.

- *Global outcome modeling*: estimating the underlying outcome function $f(x, t)$
- *Global treatment effect modeling*: directly estimating the underlying treatment effect $z(x)$
- *Global modeling of treatment regimes:* identifying an optimal treatment assignment rule that produces positive treatment contrast given patients' covariates $g_{opt}(x) = I(z(x) > 0)$
- *Local modeling*: direct search for subgroups with a beneficial treatment effect, i.e., identifying subgroups $S(X)$ in the covariate space with large values of treatment effect, such that $z(x) > \delta$, for all $x \in S(X)$

As a by-product or an intermediate step of many of these approaches, predictive biomarkers can be identified and ranked; also, optimal cut points associated with biomarkers are often evaluated.

This typology is meant to facilitate the discussion of different methods for subgroup modeling and search and show connections between them. Clearly, these classes are not mutually exclusive as the quantities that different methods estimate are interconnected.

In what follows, we provide a brief description of existing approaches within each class.

Global outcome modeling. Many approaches within this class estimate a single response model that incorporates both main effects (prognostic effects) and treatment by covariate interactions (predictive effects). Alternatively, separate regression models for estimating outcomes within each treatment arm can be entertained. Constructing subgroups typically requires multistage procedures: for example, at the first stage of the Virtual Twins method of Foster et al. (2011), $f(x, t)$, $t = 0, 1$ is estimated using a *black box* model (random forests) fitted to the observed data, which is used to compute hypothetical individual treatment differences $\widehat{z}(\boldsymbol{x}) = \widehat{f}(\boldsymbol{x}, 1) - \widehat{f}(\boldsymbol{x}, 0)$ for each subject with an observed covariate vector $\boldsymbol{x}$. These differences are modeled at the second stage as outcomes via CART procedure. Some researchers advocate for more traditional parametric regression approaches. Since fitting parametric models with a large number of interaction terms poses a lot of problems, methods of penalized regression and their extensions have been proposed to mitigate some of these issues. One challenge in modeling outcomes via penalized regression is that it may fail to detect important treatment-by-bio-marker interactions that may be obscured by much stronger main effects (i.e., the effects of prognostic biomarkers), which may require using different penalties for the main and interaction terms (as in FindIt, approach by Imai and Ratkovic 2013). Some methods use a combination of parametric and nonparametric modeling. For instance, Cai et al. (2011) use a combination of a proportional hazards Cox regression at the first stage and nonparametric smoothing at the second; and Dusseldorp et al. (2010) fit simultaneously an additive model (STIMA) for prognostic effects and a tree-based regression model for predictive effects. Bayesian hierarchical modeling of the response function with prognostic and predictive effects includes an early proposal by Dixon and Simon (1991), Smoothing ANOVA by Hodges et al. (2007), and methods based on Bayesian lasso (Gu et al. 2013). Recently, Henderson et al. (2017) have proposed a fully nonparametric Bayesian approach to subgroup evaluation in the context of accelerated failure time models (AFTM) for survival outcomes where the regression function is modeled using Bayesian additive regression trees (BART) and the error function—via a flexible location mixture of normal densities.

Global treatment effect modeling. Approaches in this class obviate the need to model prognostic or "main effects" which "cancel out" in the course of modeling. As a result, procedures in this class may be more robust compared to the global outcome modeling, as they would not be so prone to model misspecification inevitable in global outcome models. For example, in trees, pricewise constant estimates of $z(\boldsymbol{x})$ are obtained simply as treatment effect statistics computed within each terminal node of a tree. The key contributions are Interaction Trees (IT) of Su et al. (2008, 2009) and several new tree-based procedures proposed in Loh et al. (2015, 2016) within the GUIDE recursive partitioning platform. Similarly, Seibold et al. (2015) illustrated how the model-based recursive partitioning (MOB) platform could be adopted for the purpose of subgroup identification by incorporating treatment effect in the models considered within each leaf of the tree. Dusseldorp and Van Mechelen (2014) introduced a tree-based algorithm (QUINT) for subgroup identification that specifically aims at recovering qualitative interactions.

Individualized treatment regimes modeling. Note that the optimal regime can be determined based on the estimated treatment contrast (as in the previous approaches): $g_{opt}(\boldsymbol{x}) = I(z(\boldsymbol{x}) > 0))$. This approach, however, obviates the need of estimating $z(\boldsymbol{x})$ and directly targets the sign of $z(\boldsymbol{x})$ as a binary outcome; it aims at identifying *qualitative* interaction effects. If $z(\boldsymbol{x}) > 0$ for all $\boldsymbol{x}$ (i.e., the drug has beneficial effect for all patients), the potential outcome $Y(1)$ can often be redefined by taking into account a fixed "treatment burden" or "cost." $\delta > 0$. For example, defining $\widetilde{Y}(1) = Y(1) - \delta$ results in shifting the treatment contrast downward: $\widetilde{z}(x) = z(x) - \delta$, so that values become negative for some x and nontrivial optimal regimes can be identified.

Broadly, this class includes any approach that matches patients to one set of candidate treatments, based on available patient-level data. For example, Qian and Murphy (2011) formulated the problem of finding an optimal individual treatment regime (ITR) using traditional outcome modeling ("global outcome modeling," using our terms). They proposed a two-step procedure that first estimates the conditional mean response using penalized regression (with lasso penalty) allowing the inclusion of a large number of candidate biomarkers and associated treatment interactions and at the second stage derives the optimal treatment assignment rule by inverting the model for the conditional mean.

It became apparent, however, that determining optimal treatment regimes does not require estimating the entire mean response function (which is driven by both prognostic and predictive biomarker effects) but critically depends on identifying only predictive biomarkers associated with *qualitative* (as opposed to *quantitative*) treatment-by-covariate interactions. Gunter et al. (2011) proposed some methods for identifying only biomarkers contributing to qualitative interactions with treatment (and therefore to personalized rules) using resampling procedures that ensure family-wise error rate control. Zhang et al. (2012) and Zhao et al. (2012) showed that estimating optimal individualized treatment policies could be cast as a classification problem. For example, in the weighted outcome learning (OWL) methodology of Zhao et al. (2012), the optimal treatment regime $g_{opt}(x)$ is found as the one that minimizes the *weighted* misclassification loss: $E\{I(T \neq g(X))w(Y,X)\}$, where the expectation is taken with respect to the triple of random variables $\{Y, X, T\}$, and the subject weights $w(Y, X)$ are proportional to the outcome Y (here assuming larger values are desirable) and inversely proportional to the probability of patients following the regime prescribed by the rule $g(X)$. Then the optimal rule can be found by standard methods of predictive learning aiming at minimizing misclassification loss via appropriate smooth "surrogate" loss functions (e.g., hinge loss resulting in the SVM classifier, well-known in the machine learning community, or negative binomial log-likelihood, familiar to statisticians, resulting in the penalized logistic regression). Intuitively, minimizing the above weighted loss would tend to recover the optimal rule $g_{opt}(x)$ that would recommend the actually received treatment for those patients who achieved good outcomes while suggesting switching the treatment for those who failed the treatment they were assigned to in the trial. This method applies to observational trials as well as randomized clinical trials. In the latter case, the inverse weighting by the probability of treatment assignment is trivial and determined by the randomization ratios; in the former case, estimating propensity of the treatment as a function of baseline covariates X needs to be done as a separate modeling step. Other key references include tree-based approaches by Zhang et al. (2015) and Fu et al. (2016) and penalized regression methods by Huang and Fong (2014) and Xu et al. (2015).

We note that from the perspective of optimal treatment regimes, identified subgroups are the two subpopulations based on the sign of the estimated individual treatment difference, $sign(z(x))$. Some researchers would argue that it may be not sufficient to adequately describe the optimal treatment strategy by considering only two subpopulations of patients ("treat" vs. "non-treat"). For example, Dusseldorp and Van Mechelen (2014) consider three groups: patients who benefit from treatment A vs. B, patients who benefit from B vs. A, and the rest allocated to "indifference" zone comprised of patients for whom either treatment may work equally well or not work. On the other hand, the perspective of subgroups defined by the optimal treatment regime may be different from the idea of identifying "natural subgroups," say, as rectangular regions or "bumps," which brings us to the last category in our classification of subgroup methods.

Local modeling. The last class of subgroup search methods focuses on the direct search for treatment-by-covariate interactions and selecting subgroups with desirable characteristics, for example, subgroups with enhanced treatment effect. This approach obviates the need to estimate the response function over the entire covariate space and focuses on identifying specific regions with large differential treatment effect. Some of the approaches under this heading (Kehl and Ulm 2006; Chen et al. 2015) were inspired by bump hunting (also known as PRIM, Patient Rule Induction Methods) by Friedman and Fisher (1999) which is a method of predictive modeling that aims at estimating only regions where a target function (here, the treatment contrast, $z(x)$) is large. They argued that it may be better to search directly for such "interesting" regions in the covariate space rather than estimating $z(x)$ first in the entire space and then discarding the regions that are "uninteresting." The main goal of bump hunting methods such as PRIM is to define sets of multivariate rectangular regions based on the candidate covariates $X_1, X_2, \ldots, X_p$. The limits of the region are determined in a data-driven manner using a *peeling* technique. Specifically, extreme values of continuous/ordinal covariates or individual levels of nominal covariates are removed. The peeling algorithm is sequentially applied to single covariates, one at a time, and the order of the covariates is determined by the value of an appropriate objective function.

Another strategy for direct subgroup search was first implemented via a recursive partitioning process in the SIDES method (Subgroup Identification based on Differential Effect Search, Lipkovich et al. 2011) and later extended to the SIDEScreen method (Lipkovich and Dmitrienko 2014). In Sect. 6.5.1 of this chapter, we will apply these methods to a case study and provide additional technical details.

Another member of this group of algorithms is Activity Region Finder (ARF), by Amaratunga and Cabrera (2004), that combines algorithms of CART and the bump hunting to search for high or low response (activity) subgroups. Bayesian methods for local modeling were inspired by the idea to treat each subgroup as a model and apply model averaging to a collection of generated subgroups (Berger et al. 2014; Bornkamp et al. 2016). Schnell et al. (2016) implemented a procedure for identifying subgroups as *credible sets* which comprise points in the covariate space with the sufficiently high posterior probability of associated treatment effect $z(x)$ exceeding a pre-specified threshold.

Any method within the four groups can be further characterized with respect to the following features, forming a checklist that a user of any subgroup identification method should bear in mind when evaluating whether the method may be appropriate for the problem at hand (Lipkovich et al. 2017).

- Modeling type: frequentist/Bayesian and within either subtype, parametric, semi-parametric, or nonparametric
- Dimensionality of the covariate space that the method can handle: low (1–5), medium (6–15), or high (>15)
- Results produced by the method: selected biomarkers or biomarker ranking that can be used for tailoring, predictive scores for individual treatment effects, optimal treatment assignment, or identified subgroup(s) as biomarker signatures
- Application of complexity control to prevent data overfitting and selection bias when evaluating candidate subgroups
- Evaluation of the Type I error rates/false discovery rates for the *entire* subgroup search strategy
- Availability of "honest" (bias-corrected) estimates of treatment effects in the identified subgroups

The dimensionality of covariate space that can be handled by a proposed method may vary dramatically. Some methods were originally developed for evaluating treatment by covariate interaction in the context of a *single* continuous covariate and later extended to a small number of pre-selected biomarkers (e.g., the method of fractional polynomials by Royston and Sauerbrei (2004, 2013); the STEPP method by Bonetti and Gelber (2000, 2004); Jones et al. (2011)). These can be contrasted with methods developed with the idea of handling high-dimensional covariate vectors and incorporated variable selection as part of the model building strategy (e.g., Virtual Twins by Foster et al. (2011) and many others referenced below). The middle grounds are occupied by methods assuming that a medium-sized set of candidate biomarkers has been specified, e.g., in the statistical analysis plan (SIDES by Lipkovich et al. 2011; Gi method by Loh et al. 2015). Mayer et al. (2015) describe some findings from a survey with respect to the dimensionality of covariate space and other features of subgroup analysis tasks routinely dealt with by Pharma statisticians.

Depending on the method, different results may be produced. For example, some methods are searching for "biomarker signatures." These are often defined as rectangles in covariate space (requiring predictive biomarkers and associated cutoff points), which is motivated by the desire to base clinical decisions on simple and easily interpretable rules, e.g., Foster et al. (2015). Other approaches look for arbitrary biomarker signatures (e.g., additive scoring functions) that would allow ranking all patients by a score reflecting predicted individual treatment effect; and some methods provide selection or scoring for predictive biomarkers (such as variable importance scores) that can be used for tailoring in subsequent clinical development programs.

All subgroup selection methods considered here have data-driven elements. However, the scope of search may vary dramatically from selecting a subgroup based on estimated patient's predictive score as a linear combination of, say, 3 pre-specified continuous biomarkers to identifying a subgroup as a "region" formed by selecting 2 out of 1000 candidate biomarkers with an optimal cut point determined within each of these in a data-driven fashion. Depending on the scope of search in the "covariate space" induced by a specific method, different types of complexity control may be needed. The idea is to ensure that the finally selected biomarker signatures defining subgroups are not unnecessarily "complex" (e.g., by including irrelevant or noise covariates), resulting in spurious findings with little chance to be replicated in the future trials. Such situations occur when the set of candidate subgroups/biomarker signatures includes the elements of different "complexity." For example, of two candidate subgroups, one defined by a single biomarker as {Age $\leq$ 20} and the other defined by two biomarkers, {Age $<$ 20} and {Gender = "Female"}, the latter is more "complex." When using a greedy search over possible signatures, it may appear to fit the observed data better and therefore will look more promising than the former simpler subgroup. As in other applications of machine learning, the chance of spurious findings ("overfitting") increases with model complexity, and to offset that, some forms of complexity penalty are required.

Different approaches of complexity control to prevent data overfitting have been proposed in the context of subgroup/biomarker search including:

- Frequentist penalized regression (e.g., Imai and Ratkovic 2013) and Bayesian shrinkage (e.g., Jones et al. 2011)
- Frequentist ensemble learning methods (e.g., Foster et al. 2011) and Bayesian model averaging (Berger et al. 2014; Bornkamp et al. 2016) that aggregate results over a large number of "learners" (here, subgroups or signatures) to shrink the contribution of noise covariates to zero
- Using "indirect" or less direct criteria for variable/subgroup selection that avoid the exhaustive search for subgroups with desired features (Loh et al. 2015, 2016)

Another example of data overfitting (often called biomarker selection bias) arises when making a choice between subgroups based on biomarkers with widely different sets of candidate cutoff points. For example, a subgroup based on patient's age as a continuous variable with a data-driven cutoff, e.g., {Age $\leq$ 20}, has a higher potential for overfitting than a subgroup of seemingly equal complexity based on gender, e.g., {Gender = "Female"}. This is because variable Age has a much larger number of candidate splitting points (basically, all values of Age realized in the database except the extreme ones leading to subgroups not passing the minimal sample size requirement), whereas only two subgroups can be selected based on patient's gender. Therefore, if both biomarkers Age and Gender are irrelevant (noise variables), we would have a higher chance of selecting Age as a promising marker if our selection is based on exhaustive evaluation of all possible subgroups based on Age and Gender. Several approaches were proposed in the literature to deal with variable selection bias (Loh et al. 2015; Seibold et al. 2015).

One may think that "complexity control" would be unnecessary if at the end of the subgroup search, we can correctly evaluate the Type I error or false positive rate associated with the selected subgroups. This would be the case if all candidate subgroups in the covariate space were of the same complexity; then it is straightforward to select the one having the largest apparent treatment effect while controlling for multiplicity (selection bias, winner's curse, etc.) by computing an adjusted *P*-value and a bias-corrected treatment effect. However, as was discussed, the fact that different subgroups may have very different "complexity" requires imposing a penalty for complexity *during* the process of selection, thus preventing us from "chasing noise." Adjusting the finally selected subgroups which may be purely driven by noise *after* selection would be too late, as it would merely suggest that our selected subgroup (after appropriate adjustment) has a very large associated *P*-value and therefore would have little reproducibility in future trials. Indeed, the goal is to avoid making such an unfortunate selection by putting a "constraint jacket" on the selection process.

Of course, even with complexity control, we need to account for multiplicity inherent in subgroup identification by computing adjusted *P*-values associated with treatment effects in the selected subgroups. However, procedures that are less "greedy" would require less adjustment of *P*-values than the "greedier" procedures. This is because a less greedy procedure induces a smaller search space by restricting search to models satisfying complexity constraint, hence less multiplicity burden. For example, the multiplicity adjustment for *P*-values in subgroups selected using a very greedy stepwise selection method (in the context of a linear regression with the main effects and treatment by covariate interactions) would be much harsher than the adjustment of *P*-values when the selection is made using much less greedy methods of penalized regression (e.g., lasso). The analytical expressions for multiplicity-adjusted *P*-values in subgroup search methods are typically not available, and researchers have to resort to approximate *P*-values based on various resampling methods (permutations or bootstrap under null scenarios).

Finally, once the subgroup(s) have been identified, the sponsor would need to make a decision based on anticipated treatment effects in these subgroups (e.g., by computing probabilities of success for different designs involving enriched populations versus the overall population). It is important to understand that even if the identified subgroup may be very close to the true one, the apparent treatment effect computed using the same data that was used for subgroup search (a naive method of data "resubstitution") is likely to overestimate the true treatment effect contained in that subgroup. Like with multiplicity-adjusted *P*-values, the size of the treatment effect can be estimated using resampling methods such as bootstrap or cross-validation (see Foster et al. 2011; Faye et al. 2011; Simon et al. 2011; Loh et al. 2016; Rosenkranz 2016); Bayesian methods implementing shrinkage such as an empirical Bayes correction (Ferguson et al. 2013) or model averaging (Bornkamp et al. 2016) can also be used (see Thomas and Bornkamp 2017 for comparison of several methods for estimating treatment effect in data-driven subgroups). The amount of over-optimism in the naïve estimates of treatment effect computed by resubstitution depends on the richness of the search space and the "greediness" of the search algorithm.

Many applications of subgroup identification to real data sets can be found in the original papers introducing the discussed methods. Here, we provide additional references for applications of existing methods to clinical or observational data. Hardin et al. (2013) applied SIDES to conduct an exploratory analysis of a large multinational, randomized, open-label trial in patients with type 2 diabetes to identify subgroups where the effect of an insulin lispro mix versus insulin glargine was substantially different from that in the overall population. Dmitrienko et al. (2015) applied SIDES methods to the ATTAIN program based on two Phase III multinational trials to evaluate the safety and efficacy of telavancin (test antibiotic) compared to vancomycin (active control antibiotic) for treatment of adults with nosocomial pneumonia. Hou et al. (2015) compared the results of several tree-based subgroup identification methods including Interaction Trees and Virtual Twins to the data from an alcohol dependence pharmacogenetic trial of ondansetron. Patel et al. (2016) analyzed patients with low back pain using data pooled from 19 randomized clinical trials applying Interaction Trees, SIDES, and Indirect Network Meta-analysis to identify subgroups defined by multiple parameters. Doubleday (2016) adopted recursive partitioning methods to evaluate individualized treatment assignment rules from both randomized and observational data and applied it to diabetes data from electronic medical records (see also Fu et al. 2016). Seibold et al. (2016) adopted methods of model-based recursive partitioning to construct individual treatment effect predictions for patients with amyotrophic lateral sclerosis pooled from several randomized clinical trials.

Links to several packages that implemented popular subgroup identification methods could be found at the site maintained by the QSPI (Quantitative Sciences in the Pharmaceutical Industry) Subgroup Analysis Working Group: http://biopharmnet.com/subgroup-analysis-software/. These methods include both R packages available in CRAN (**aVirtualTwins, SIDES, quint, FindIt, partykit, model4you, personalized**) and implementations with R and other software provided by the developers for public dissemination: an R package RSIDES implementing SIDES and SIDEScreen methods (Lipkovich and Dmitrienko 2014), R code for ROWSi (Regularized Outcome Weighted Subgroup identification) by Xu et al. (2015), the GUIDE package implementing methods by Loh et al. (2015), and BLASSO by Gu et al. (2013).

The above packages focus on the problem of biomarker/subgroup identification. For situations when one or two markers are pre-selected, Janes et al. (2014) propose a statistical framework for evaluating a candidate treatment selection marker and comparing two continuous markers; an R package developed by the authors implementing these methods is available at http://labs.fhcrc.org/janes/index.html.

6.3.3.2   Q-Learning for Dynamic Treatment Regimes

Q-learning is an approximate dynamic programming algorithm for estimation of optimal dynamic treatment regimes (DTRs). DTRs are the sequences of decision rules, one per decision/intervention stage, that map up-to-date patient information to a recommended treatment. The key is that a patient's treatment at each stage is not known at the start of the treatment sequence, as it depends on time-varying variables that may be influenced by earlier treatment choices. In many health disorders, especially chronic conditions, the sequential decision-making is necessary to adapt treatment over time in response to the evolving health status of the patient. This is especially important if there is a high degree of heterogeneity in an individual response to treatment and when treatment may need to be adjusted as a result of emerging side effects. In such cases, the treatment that appears optimal in the short term may not be best in the long term. Thus, the goal is to optimize a long-term outcome of interest which may be measured at the end of the last treatment stage or may encompass intermediate outcomes, e.g., represent a (weighted) average of clinical outcomes across all intervention stages.

Q-learning can be viewed as an extension of regression to multistage decision problems based on backward induction. It starts with an estimation of the optimal treatment rule at the last stage of treatment based on patient-level data up to the last treatment decision, which may include baseline characteristics, treatment decisions, and intermediate outcomes up to that point. This information is used as "independent variables" for a regression model of the long-term outcome measured after the last treatment decision. Based on this regression model, the last stage optimal treatment is estimated for each patient so that it optimizes the expected long-term outcome. Subsequently, Q-learning performs a similar regression and optimization step for a preceding decision stage to find a treatment that would result in optimal long-term outcome assuming that subsequent, last stage treatment will be determined by the optimal rule constructed in step 1 of the procedure. This backward re-estimation and optimization are performed iteratively until the first decision point, allowing the method to account for future decisions when making treatment choices at earlier stages.

Ideally, DTRs should be estimated from trials with a Sequential Multiple Assignment Randomized Trial (SMART) design (Collins et al. 2007; Almirall et al. 2014), where subjects are randomized multiple times during the course of the trial. At each randomization stage, the set of available treatments may depend on subject-specific characteristics and evolving health status. SMART would be a "gold standard" for determining optimal DTRs as they remove any confounding of treatment assignment with subject characteristics, just like randomized controlled trials are a gold standard for confirmatory clinical trials. For ethical and logistical reasons, SMART are rare in the pharmaceutical industry practice. DTRs can also be constructed using observational data from trials with flexible dosing or evolving treatment assignment, e.g., long-term open-label trials in chronic pain or dynamic second, third, etc. line of treatment selection in cancer. Such studies are more common in practice; however, care must be taken to account for potential confounding.

Maintaining a balance between treatment efficacy and limiting undesirable side effects is an important aspect of successful dynamic treatment regimes, but is a relatively open area of research. Composite scores that integrate measures of treatment efficacy and safety could be used. For example, in Wang et al. (2012), a composite score was constructed by eliciting from the Principal Investigator of the trial subjective numerical values to quantify the clinical desirability of efficacy, toxicity, and progressive disease response to a prostate cancer treatment. In many circumstances, it may be difficult to obtain a single composite measure that encompasses patient and physician preferences across several competing and potentially time-varying outcomes. Laber et al. (2014a) proposed an approach to deal with such challenges by using set-valued functions and recommending a set of possible treatments which are non-inferior across outcomes at each decision point and which can then be considered by individual patients and physicians. Another approach, which avoids using subjective composite measures and works directly with the original efficacy and safety outcomes, is to optimize treatment efficacy using Q-learning under constraints of the risk of adverse events so that DTRs can be designed to achieve specific levels of efficacy tailored to patient's adverse event tolerance limit.

Original ideas behind Q-learning can be found in Watkin (1989) and Watkin and Dayan (1992). These ideas have been further developed and adapted to the context of estimation of dynamic multistage treatment strategies, e.g., by Murphy (2005), Schulte et al. (2014), and Laber et al. (2014b). They have also been extended to survival outcomes by Goldberg and Kosorok (2012) and to discrete utilities (long-term outcomes) and to nonlinear relationships between covariates and outcomes by Moodie et al. (2014). A general overview of SMART design considerations can be found, for example, in Almirall et al. (2014).

Examples of clinical applications of Q-learning for estimation of optimal treatment regimes can be found in a number of recent publications. For example, Wu et al. (2015) applied DTR for treatment of acute bipolar depression; Chakraborty et al. (2013) and Chakraborty and Moodie (2013) for chronic illnesses including major depressive disorder; Laber et al. (2014b) and Nahum-Shani et al. (2012) for attention deficit hyperactivity disorder; Laber et al. (2014a) and Shortreed et al. (2011) for schizophrenia; Moodie et al. (2007) and Sterne et al. (2009) for HIV/AIDS; Strecher et al. (2006) for cigarette addiction; and Lei et al. (2012) for prevention of alcoholism relapse.

The term Q-learning refers to the estimation of a Q-function, which stands for the "quality" associated with a specific treatment choice at each stage given the patient's history up to that point and following the optimal regime thereafter. Having an estimate of the "quality" of each possible treatment decision, we can select the best one at each stage. The challenge, in this case, is to obtain a good unbiased estimate of the Q-function over the entire space of histories and possible treatment choices, which may be difficult to achieve, especially over high-dimensional spaces and with relatively sparse data. A-learning (Blatt et al. 2004) is an alternative method, which estimates an "advantage" for each treatment, i.e., the difference between the quality of a given treatment choice and the optimal treatment at each stage. This approach may be less sensitive to bias introduced by the mismodeling of the Q-function. However, A-learning may have a disadvantage of high variability and require variance reduction techniques, such as bagging or random forests, for successful implementations, and its complexity increases with the number of possible treatment choices.

Both Q-learning and A-learning use regression to estimate some function representing the value of the treatment choice and then obtain the optimal decisions by inverting that function. On the other hand, outcome-weighted learning (OWL) uses a different paradigm by attempting to estimate the optimal DTR directly, casting it as a weighted classification problem. Treatments actually received by patients with good observed outcomes are considered to be "correctly classified," i.e., corresponding to the optimal treatment assignment, whereas treatments actually received by patients with poor outcomes are considered to be "misclassified." The method tries to minimize a weighted misclassification error where the weights are proportional to the observed outcome and inversely proportional to the probability of receiving a given treatment given patient history. Powerful classification methods from machine learning, e.g., support vector machines, can be applied in this context. Two variants of this approach, backward outcome weighted learning (BOWL) and simultaneous outcome weighted learning (SOWL), applicable to multistage treatment regimes were proposed by Zhao et al. (2015).

Publicly available tools for Q-learning applicable to DTRs are limited. The **iqLearn** package in R (Linn et al. 2015) can be used for estimating optimal DTRs from data obtained from a two-stage trial with two treatments at each stage. The **DTRlearn** package in R implements both single- and multiple-stage Q-learning OWL approaches. Proc QLEARN developed for SAS v9.1 or higher for Windows by Ertefaie et al. (2012) at the University of Michigan and the Pennsylvania State University (https://methodology.psu.edu/downloads/procqlearn) can be used with data from a sequential, multiple assignments, randomized trial (SMART) but is limited to situations where the outcome is continuous; there are two decision stages and up to two treatment options at each decision.

6.4   Principles of Data Mining with Clinical Data

Here, we focus on data mining in randomized clinical trials (RCTs). As RCTs are conducted in a highly regulated environment, the interpretation of data mining activities with such data may be considered particularly controversial and therefore calls for clearly defined principles to ensure their validity. It is often argued that data mining with clinical data has limited validity since by its nature it cannot be pre-specified and therefore occupies the lowest rank in the Statistical Analysis Plan.

The relative ranking of the importance of analyses undertaken in a Phase 3 trial can be loosely described as follows: the primary analysis of primary outcome, the primary analysis of secondary outcomes, the secondary analyses of primary outcome, the secondary analyses of secondary outcomes, supportive analyses and sensitivity analyses, and exploratory analyses. We note the striking contrast between the wealth of (often underutilized) data collected in the course of clinical trials and the "minimalistic" focus on the primary analysis as the basis for major study conclusions.

On the other hand, in exploratory Phase 2 studies, it is often felt by the sponsor that any data exploration is allowed as long as it is used only for "internal decision-making." However, when the drug development program is driven by unprincipled and unconstrained data exploration in Phase 2, it often results in a failed Phase 3 study, further contributing to a lack of respect for data mining.

As a result of the described mind-set, the exploratory analysis is felt as belonging to the lowest category of analysis on the above scale and is typically described in the section "Exploratory analysis" which is often a polite word for a "garbage collector" to store various poorly conceived data analysis strategies. This practice blurs the subtler distinction of and the relationship between exploratory and confirmatory data analyses (as originally proposed by J. Tukey in his famous "exploratory data analysis") where the former paves the road to the latter. The exploratory analysis in this framework is a well-thought activity that forms a continuous process of learning from the data that requires flexible methods of model selection and model fitting (robust to model misspecification) combined with various ways of looking at the data and graphical display. Findings from exploratory analyses may be confirmed in the future trials.

The key idea is that data mining should be understood as a flexible data analytic strategy with various data-driven elements. While "data-driven" means that some elements are not specified in advance, the strategy itself can be pre-specified. This is similar to adaptive clinical trial designs, where the exact trial parameters (e.g., the final sample size or doses that remain under investigation) are not fixed at the design stage, but the adaptation strategy is nevertheless fully pre-specified. Here we list some principles for conducting data mining activities in the context of clinical data mining.

6.4.1 Documenting Business Need and Scientific Rationale for Data Mining

This document may include the following components:

- Statement of hypothesis(es) of interest based on the current understanding of the phenomena (based on relevant literature).
- Scientific assumptions and current relevant scientific theories.
- Relationships of interest and type of research: association/causation/prediction/search for patterns.
- Anticipated findings based on current knowledge (e.g., of biological mechanisms) and a priori considerations of how "unanticipated" findings, if happen, could be further explored. It is not uncommon that when findings are not in line with the current understanding of biologically plausible mechanisms, the researchers come up all too quickly with ad hoc "explanations" of the results. If variables with no a priori-known relationships to the outcome are included in analysis, there should be some plan as to how any potential findings on these predictors can be further explored/investigated/confirmed.
- Definition of "success" and "failure" for the data mining application. Here "success" does not necessarily mean obtaining findings "favorable" to

experimental treatment but rather a success in modeling the data that leads to new insights (e.g., identifying biomarkers predictive of treatment effect). It is important, however, that "failed" analyses are also reported. For example, data mining of an integrated database in depression indicating a lack of reliable predictors of placebo response in itself constitutes an important (negative) finding.

- "Stopping rules" for data mining activity should be specified here (or in the analytics plan section), which helps avoid endless search for "a significant effect."

6.4.2 Developing a Data Mining Analytic Plan

As model selection is an integral component of DM, it is impossible within a DM process to "pre-specify" exactly what statistical models will be used. However, it is important that the analytic strategy is outlined in sufficient detail prior to the beginning of the data analysis.

The scope of data used should be clearly identified; specifically, the following should be defined:

- The target population of interest
- Studies/data sources to be included
- Clinically defined outcomes: e.g., response/relapse/remission criteria
- Outcome variable(s)
- Covariates that potentially may affect the outcome of interest

It is a good practice to list all "data-driven" components and "tuning parameters" of the analytic strategy upfront and explain how they will be identified in the course of the study.

The possibility of replicating findings with additional data sets that were not used in model fitting and selection (test data) should be addressed. If this is not possible due to limited data, other approaches should be used, e.g., bootstrap and cross-validation.

If hypothesis testing is the primary objective, all adjustments for multiplicity and control of Type I error rates should be explained.

If the model selection is a part of the DM strategy (which is almost always the case), the DM Analytic Plan should explain how potential data overfitting would be handled (e.g., via cross-validation, using separate validation data sets).

If inference about causal parameters is the primary objective, all non-randomized covariates that may potentially cause selection bias should be listed and methodology that will be used to overcome it outlined.

If the analytic strategy involves a multistage data analysis (i.e., when selection of an analytic procedure at a later stage may depend on the results at previous stages), the DM plan should contain a discussion on how uncertainty in the multistage process could be accounted for (e.g., via bootstrapping the *entire* multistage analysis sequence, or model averaging). It is often the case that only uncertainty associated with the final stages of such complex analytic strategies is taken into account, while the steps leading to final analyses are left undocumented and obliterated from the "collective memory" of the research team. Also in many exploratory analyses, some stages of analysis involve "human intervention" where decisions are made subjectively which makes it challenging to automate the entire analytic strategy by implementing it in a programming code and prevents the use of resampling methods for evaluating such strategies. When implementing multistage procedures and applying them to resampled data, it is important to account for the fact that on some samples the result may be negative or null, for example, when an empty set is returned for a subgroup search or when no predictive bookmakers are found. In such situation it is important that the analysis strategy should be well-defined in the sense that it is applicable for any data, not only for the specifically observed data set on which it was used.

The DM analysis plan should include "sensitivity analyses" to validate the robustness of the findings to various departures from (often untestable) assumptions. This may relate to assumptions about missing data mechanisms, unmeasured confounders, or possible "structural" changes (e.g., in the relationship between outcomes and predictors) in the future populations that may affect the generalizability of findings. As part of sensitivity analyses, sensitivity to methodology (e.g., frequentist vs. Bayesian) could be explored as well. Visualization tools should be used at all stages of analyses, primarily to investigate potential issues such as outliers, influential observations, etc.

Many data mining techniques are simulation based (e.g., cross-validation, bootstrap); therefore, retaining seed values is recommended to ensure the *reproducibility* of findings.

Finally, we emphasize the importance of proper quality control and validation of analyses, just like in the standard stat analysis of clinical trial data.

6.4.3   Ensuring Data Integrity

Integrating and aggregating information from multiple studies may pose challenges such as:

- Using different clinical outcomes (e.g., rating scales) and different definitions for the same outcomes across multiple data sources.
- The extent of and approach to data cleaning may not be the same across multiple studies. DM often utilizes various patient characteristics and time-dependent covariates that may not be fully cleaned and validated even in locked databases, as they might not have been a focus for analyses intended for clinical study report (e.g., the time of occurrence of certain events or concomitant treatments).
- Many challenges of data aggregation (e.g., using combined regional, ethnic, etc. groups; grouping adverse events, concomitant medications; alignment across common time points) require careful consideration and close collaboration between the statistician and medical team and may require a substantial amount of time in the absence of integrated databases.

When integrated databases are available, it is tempting and often seems reasonable to form initial analysis plan around variables available in the integrated database; however, the absence of important potential predictors in the integrated database cannot serve as a justification for not considering them as potential predictors in the DM analysis plan.

Further, study populations may be somewhat different and/or recruited at significantly different times, and this heterogeneity may need to be accounted for in the model/analysis. This should be done keeping in mind the target population the findings need to be generalized for, possibly leading to re-weighing current data so as to better match the target population.

6.5 Case Studies

In this section, we present three case studies that illustrate several data mining/machine learning methods as applied to clinical trial data. While some of them are taken to a greater level of detail, others are presented in a briefer manner.

6.5.1 Evaluation of Subpopulations Using SIDES Methodology

In this subsection, we illustrate some of the methods introduced in Sect. 6.3.3, specifically variants of the SIDES methodology by applying them to a data set simulated to mimic a realistic data from a Phase 3 study.

6.5.1.1 SIDES Methodology

Here, we provide a brief outline of SIDES method. An interested reader may refer to Lipkovich et al. (2011) and Lipkovich and Dmitrienko (2014) for further details. In our example, SIDES is applied to a binary outcome, and the description is tailored to this type of outcome, although the approach is not limited to it. Also for simplicity, we assume that all covariates are continuous as is the case for our data set, but this is not a requirement.

First, we apply to the data set the SIDES subgroup generation procedure that starts with evaluating a differential splitting criterion at every allowable split of every candidate covariate, which is defined as follows:

$$D = 2\left(1 - \Phi\left(\frac{|Z_{left} - Z_{right}|}{\sqrt{2}}\right)\right).$$

Here $\Phi(\cdot)$ is the normal CDF; the statistics Z_{left} and Z_{right} are scaled by the pooled standard error of treatment differences between proportions evaluated for the experimental treatment and control in two child groups resulting from splitting a continuous variable X into the *left* $\{X \leq x_0\}$ and the *right* child groups $\{X > x_0\}$, based on a provisional cutoff x_0. Note that the criterion is on the probability scale with smaller values indicating larger differentials.

For each candidate covariate, the best cutoff associated with the smallest value of D is determined. Based on this value, the covariates are ordered from best to worst, and the first M covariates (the *width* parameter) are selected. For any covariate, we have two child groups resulting from splitting at the optimal cutoff, and the child with the largest treatment effect is retained as "promising." Therefore, from M top covariates, M promising subgroups are retained. These are called *promising* subgroups of level 1. Depending on the maximal number of levels L (the *depth* parameter), the process continues recursively by applying the same splitting process to each of the promising groups. The resulting *terminal* groups are considered as final promising subgroups. For example, if $L = 1$, the process stops with the M level 1 groups which will be the terminal groups, whereas if $L = 3$, the process is recursively applied two more times resulting in up to M^3 terminal subgroups. The size of the candidate subgroups is controlled by the user-specified minimal required subgroup size, n_{min}. Only subgroups of size at least n_{min} are considered as allowable splits, and the recursion might stop even before achieving the specified *depth* once no subgroups of required size can be formed.

The above process, which we refer to as base SIDES, results in generating a potentially large pool of subgroups. A greedy approach to subgroup selection would be to simply choose the subgroup from the pool with the largest observed treatment effect (or few subgroups with largest effects). Of course, the observed effect(s) and the associated P-value(s) would be highly overoptimistic. These can be adjusted by using resampling methods. For example, the multiplicity adjusted P-value can be obtained by randomly permuting treatment labels, reapplying the same subgroup search procedure to each null (permuted) set, and computing the smallest P-value over all promising subgroups for each null data set. Based on a large number of null sets, the adjusted P-value can be computed as the proportion of such sets where the minimum P-value is as small as or smaller than the one found in the best subgroup of the actual data set.

However, this greedy process is likely to generate the top subgroups that will be subsequently penalized very severely in terms of having very large adjusted P-values (suggesting that the findings are driven by chance and are not likely to generalize to the future data).

To develop more sensible subgroup search procedures, several methods of restraining the greediness of the search have been proposed. One approach is to introduce a complexity parameter that constrains the search by placing a requirement on how much better the treatment effect in a child group should be compared to that in the parent group at each split. The split is made only if the candidate child group exceeds that threshold.

The second approach, called "SIDEScreen" (pursued in this example), uses a variant of model averaging. From the harvesting process, a variable importance index is evaluated for each covariate that reflects its overall predictive worth. This is defined as the average contribution of a covariate across all generated promising subgroups (counting only terminal subgroups of the harvesting process). Specifically

$$VI(X) = K^{-1} \sum_{i=1}^{K} \nu_i,$$

where $\nu_i = -\log d_i(X)$, if the ith subgroup contains biomarker X, and $\nu_i = 0$ otherwise; K is the number of promising subgroups; and $d_i(X)$ is the splitting criterion evaluated for biomarker X for the selected split.

Thus, computed variable importance scores are screened by applying a screening rule

$$VI(X) > \widehat{E}_0 + k\sqrt{\widehat{V}_0},$$

where $\widehat{E}_0$ and $\widehat{V}_0$ are the mean and variance of the maximal (over all biomarkers), VI score under the null distribution obtained by permuting the treatment labels. These mean and variance are estimated from a large number of such samples. The multiplier k is a free parameter that can be calibrated as $k = \Phi^{-1}(1 - \kappa)$, where κ is interpreted as the probability of selecting at least one noise biomarker in the absence of predictive biomarkers in the data set.

At the second stage, the basic SIDES is applied only to biomarkers selected at the first stage. The final adjusted p-values are computed by replicating the entire two-stage procedure on a large number of additional null sets. Note that the same multiplier k is applied to each null set; therefore, regardless of the value of multiplier at the first stage, the overall Type I error rate of the final subgroup(s) can be controlled at any desired level.

6.5.1.2   Analysis Data

Our example data set *sepsis_ex.csv* is available at QSPI working group site along with the **RSIDES** package: http://biopharmnet.com/subgroup-analysis-software/. The data set is based on a Phase 3 trial conducted to examine the efficacy and safety profiles of a novel treatment for severe sepsis. There are 470 patients (317 patients in the experimental treatment arm and 153 patients in the control arm) with a binary outcome variable *mortality* (the primary endpoint) that represents the survival status of patients after 28 days of treatment: the value of 1 for subjects who died within 28 days and 0 for those who survived. There are eight candidate covariates, including demographic and clinical characteristics listed in Table 6.3, all of which are numerical variables. Note that the results for baseline serum concentration (*il6*)

Table 6.3 Candidate covariates in the severe sepsis data example

Candidate covariates	Description	Median (range)
Time	Time from first sepsis-organ failure to start of treatment (hours)	30.67 (10, 3775.9)
Age	Patient age (years)	59.871 (33.2, 93.3)
Platelets	Baseline local platelets ($1000/mm^3$)	153 (45, 650)
Sofa	Sum of baseline SOFA scores (cardiovascular, hematologic, hepatic, renal, neurological, and respiratory scores)	8 (3, 17)
Creatinine	Baseline creatinine (mg/dL)	1.5 (1, 20)
Apache	Pre-infusion APACHE-II score	23 (19, 48)
IL6	Baseline serum IL-6 concentration (pg/mL)	406.6 (37.1, 296,550)
Bilirubin	Baseline bilirubin (mg/dL)	1 (0.4, 20.4)

exhibit some extreme values which are not uncommon for this lab measure. We comment that with parametric regression methods, this would be a problem requiring special treatment (e.g., variable transformation), but the tree-based methods are immune to that as they essentially treat a numerical covariate as ordinal and are invariant to any monotone transformation of a covariate.

6.5.1.3 Results

Table 6.4 shows the results of applying base SIDES with parameters

- Width $= 3$
- Depth $= 2$
- $n_{min} = 30$

To illustrate the subgroup generation process, the three intermediate subgroups of the first level (based on variables *time*, *age*, and *il6* with optimal cutoffs 30.67, 59.871, and 519.4) are highlighted in bold. The associated splitting criterion (on the $-\log$ scale, with larger values being better) is shown in the third column. The terminal subgroups are obtained after splitting the above three level 1 groups by the best three variables selected from the candidate list excluding the one selected at the first level. There are eight rather than nine groups because one group based on *time* and *age* occurred twice with the same cutoffs for both variables and was removed as a duplicate. The penultimate column contains the *P*-value for the overall treatment effect (one-tailed) and unadjusted *P*-values for promising subgroups. Note that the overall treatment effect is negative while some subgroups show apparently large treatment effect with subgroup *time* ≤ 30.67 and age > 59.871 appearing best with an unadjusted *P*-value of 0.00196. However, the adjusted *P*-values based on 10,000 sets of randomly permuted treatment labels are hopelessly large. In particular, the adjusted *P*-value for the above subgroup is 0.5.

Table 6.4 Subgroups generated using base SIDES for sepsis data (*width* = 3, *depth* = 2, n_{min} = 30)

Subgroup	Size	Splitting criterion (−log scale)	P-value (unadjusted)	P-value (adjusted)
Overall population	470		0.8301	
Time ≤ 30.67	253	5.29	0.0588	0.99
Time ≤ 30.67 and age > 59.871	123	3.37	0.00196	0.50
Time ≤ 30.67 and IL6 > 162.65	171	1.09	0.0136	0.88
Time ≤ 30.67 and bilirubin ≤ 2.5	199	0.74	0.0496	0.99
Age > 59.871	217	4.25	0.0718	0.99
Age > 59.871 and IL6 > 92.8	169	2.29	0.0362	0.97
Age > 59.871 and sofa > 5	183	1.98	0.0172	0.91
IL6 > 519.4	180	2.55	0.1800	1.00
IL6 > 519.4 and age > 56.098	99	4.68	0.0076	0.78
IL6 > 519.4 and creatinine > 1.4	104	1.85	0.0168	0.91
IL6 > 519.4 and time ≤ 30.67	117	1.60	0.0328	0.97

Next, we evaluate subgroups using a less greedy and more powerful Adaptive SIDEScreen approach. First, we apply base SIDES with even less restrictive parameters on generated subgroups than for the first run, specifically setting *width* = 5 and *depth* = 3 resulting in up to 5^3 = 125 subgroups based on three covariates. While the resulting subgroups may be picking up a lot of noise and would likely not generalize to the future data, we are not using these subgroups as candidates for the final selection but rather use them as an intermediate step for computing variable importance scores used for covariate screening. Averaging over a broader set of subgroups (models) in general helps to obtain more reliable variable importance scores.

Figure 6.4 contains variable importance and an associated benchmark from 1000 null sets. The threshold rule is $VI(X) > \widehat{E}_0 + \sqrt{\widehat{V}_0}$ with the multiplier $k = 1$. As we can see, two variables, *time* and *age*, stand out having larger scores. Also, they both exceed the threshold based on 1 standard deviation from the null mean.

Table 6.5 shows the results of the second-stage analysis where base SIDES is applied only to variables that passed the screening stage. Predictably, the subgroup is the same as the best one that was found by a greedy base SIDES. However, the adjusted P-value is very different from the one computed for the base SIDES.

To understand this seemingly contradictory result, first recall that the adjusted P-values are computed for the SIDEScreen procedure by applying to each null set the two-stage procedure, including computing anew the variable importance scores based on subgroups generated from each null set and comparing them with the same null threshold as was applied to the observed data. Of the null sets where some covariates pass the threshold, we identify those having subgroups with P-values such as or smaller than the one found in the observed data. Naturally, many null sets would not have any covariates that pass the screening threshold (about 84%, assuming the normal distribution for VI scores under the null and the threshold with $k = 1$). Even if each of the remaining ≈16% of the null sets produced a

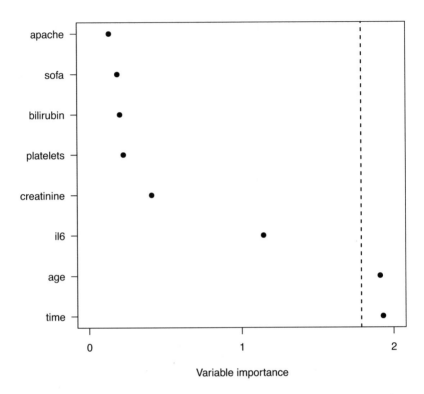

Fig. 6.4 Variable importance scores (shown as filled circles) and the threshold based on null distribution (shown as the dashed line)

Table 6.5 Subgroups generated using Adaptive SIDEScreen for sepsis data

Subgroup	Size	Splitting criterion (–log scale)	P-value (unadjusted)	P-value (adjusted)
Overall population	470		0.8301	
Time ≤ 30.67	253	5.29	0.0588	0.112
Time ≤ 30.67 and age > 59.871	123	3.37	0.00196	0.036
Age > 59.871	217	4.25	0.0718	0.116

subgroup better than the one found on the observed data, the adjusted *P*-value would be no larger than about 0.16. One might consider the application of this "shrinkage factor" to compute adjusted *P*-values as a kind of cheating. However, note that the selection rules are the same whether we apply them to the observed or null data. Only in the case when at least one covariate will pass the threshold on the observed data would we have the opportunity to adjust an associated *P*-value, which under the true null will amount to the same 0.16. As a result, data with no real predictive marker would likely not proceed to the second stage, thus reducing the probability of spurious findings.

6.5.2 Evaluating Optimal Dynamic Treatment Regimes via Q-Learning

This case study is a brief summary of recently reported analyses of a STEP-BD trial by Wu et al. (2015).

6.5.2.1 The STEP-BD Trial, Analysis Objectives, and Available Data

STEP-BD (Systematic Treatment Enhancement Program for Bipolar Disorder) is a long-term study of bipolar disorder funded by the National Institute of Mental Health (NIMH), the results of which were reported in Sachs et al. (2003). The study enrolled more than 4000 patients from the United States and lasted about 7 years including options for several treatment pathways: an observational trial (standard care pathway, SCP) and several randomized trials (randomized care pathway, RCP). First, all patients entered SCP and then some were eligible to follow one of the RCPs. Within the latter, there were several options (pathways) depending on the depression features. The Wu et al. (2015) analysis is focusing on one of them: acute depression randomized pathway (RAD).

The purpose of RAD was to explore the effectiveness of two antidepressant treatments (bupropion or paroxetine) versus placebo, in addition to a number of mood stabilizers (lithium, valproate, and others) that were used in combination with the two drugs or placebo. Initially, patients were randomly assigned to one antidepressant (150 mg of a sustained release formulation of bupropion or 10 mg of paroxetine) or placebo. After 6 weeks, patients with non-response on the placebo were randomized to either paroxetine or bupropion; patients with non-response on the antidepressant would have the dose of their current antidepressant increased. The schematic of the RAD sub-trial is presented in Fig. 6.5. The reader should bear in mind that patients under active treatments or placebo received mood stabilizers at physician's discretion, which is not reflected in the labels of the figures.

The objective of the analyses in Wu et al. (2015) was estimating optimal DTRs for both stages 1 and 2 to minimize the expected depression score at week 12 (SUMD), based on all available data at the decision time. Note that our ability to search for optimal treatment options is naturally limited by the available (or *feasible*) treatment options restricted by design. Specifically, as we see from Fig. 6.5, the second-stage randomization was only applied to patients who failed on placebo during stage 1. Therefore, the Q-learning algorithm would not be able to "learn" from the data a regime that recommends, for example, to treat with bupropion (at stage 2) those patients who had previously failed on paroxetine (at stage 1).

Patient covariates and intermediate outcomes available for analysis are listed in Table 6.6.

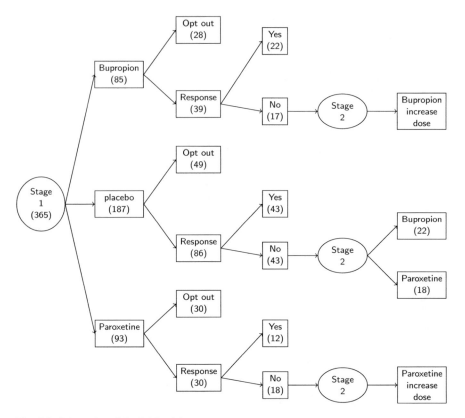

Fig. 6.5 Schematics of the RAD trial

6.5.2.2 Q-Learning Methodology for the RAD Trial

Here we briefly outline the Q-learning method adapted for estimating optimal regimes in the RAD trial of the STEP-BD design. Although the Q-learning applies for a more general m-sage learning, our exposition is tailored to the two-stage decision setting and a terminal continuous outcome (here, depression score at week 12).

As described in Sect. 6.3.3, Q-learning is an approximate dynamic programing algorithm that can be viewed as an extension of regression to multistage decision problems. In our case, this amounts to sequentially fitting regressions for the outcome, with pretreatment covariates, earlier treatments, and outcomes fitted as predictors. Starting from the last (i.e., the second stage) decision, Q-learning first finds an optimal decision rule at the second stage as the one maximizing expected outcome after stage 2, given earlier patient outcomes and covariates available prior to treatment decision for stage 2 as well as the treatment choice that has been made at decision stage 1. Then going backward, it regresses the (expected) outcome (that would have resulted if optimal treatment rules at stage 2 were applied) on treatment assigned at stage 1 and covariates available at the decision stage 1. The optimal regime for stage 1 is found as the one maximizing the response of this second regression. The key element is that covariate-by-treatment interactions have to be included in the regressions; otherwise, the estimated optimal regime will be assigning the same treatment to all patients regardless of their covariate values.

The backward induction allows Q-learning to factor in future decisions when making treatment decisions at earlier stages. This can be contrasted with a "myopic" strategy that only looks at intermediate (proximal) outcomes of a current treatment assignment. For example, treatments at stage 1 may lead to temporary alleviation of symptoms and therefore appear beneficial; however, the long-term benefits may become questionable after a later (e.g., second)-stage decisions are factored in.

Several challenges are encountered when applying the Q-learning algorithm to this data, including the need to make model selection given a large number of candidate covariates (Table 6.6) and handling a substantial number of missing data on the outcomes and covariates. These problems, typical of data mining/machine learning applications to clinical data, need to be integrated within estimating the optimal DTR.

Another challenge that appears unique for DTRs (although, more broadly, is present in any "estimation after model selection") is obtaining confidence intervals for outcomes under an estimated DTR. Because the DTR estimator is irregular (non-smooth), the standard bootstrap theory may not apply and other methods (such as *m-out-of-n* bootstrap (Chakraborty et al. 2013)) need to be used.

Finally, even relatively simple rules based on linear regressions with a few selected covariates may appear rather unwieldy for decision-makers (such as prescribing physicians); therefore, more visual and easy-to-use presentation of the rules is desired. This can be accomplished by approximating the estimated DTR with classification trees, in an additional step.

Following Wu et al. (2015), we first describe how the Q-learning would proceed for this case, assuming the correct (e.g., linear) models for Q-functions have been pre-specified, and no data are missing; then we explain how missing data imputation and model selection were integrated within the Q-learning strategy.

First, we define stage 1 and stage 2 Q-functions in terms of available treatment choices, patent-level covariates, and outcomes. Specifically, the ith patient in a hypothetical complete data set can be characterized with a trajectory $(X_{1i}, T_{1i}, X_{2i}, T_{2i}, Y_i)$, $i = 1, \ldots, n$, where X_1 denotes a vector of baseline covariates available at decision stage 1, X_2 comprises post-baseline outcomes collected during stage 1 and potentially informing treatment choice at stage 2, and T_1 and T_2 indicate randomized treatment choices at stages 1 and 2, respectively. That is $T_1 = \{Bupropion, Paraxetime, placebo\}$ and $T_2 = \{Bupropion, Paraxetime\}$; Y is the SUMD score at the end of stage 2, with lower values indicating clinically desirable outcome (low depression score).

The Q-functions are essentially the response functions that map patients with particular treatment choices and covariate profiles to expected outcomes, similar to our response functions $f(x, t)$ introduced in Sect. 6.3.3 (in the context of subgroup

Table 6.6 Candidate predictors for regression models in Q-learning (based on Table 5 of Wu et al. 2015)

Variable (label)	Description	Type	Values (range or levels)	Mean (SD) or frequency
AGE	Age at entry (years)	Numerical	18–77	40.59 (11.74)
RACE	Race	Binary	White or Caucasian, non-White	90.4%, 9.6%
GENDER	Gender	Trinary	Male, female, transgender	43%, 56%, 1%
MARSTAT	Marital status	Trinary	Never married, married, separated	35.6%, 33.8%, 30.6%
HINCOME	Annual household income (×$1000)	Binary	<40, ≥40	58.5%, 41.5%
EMPLOY	Employment status	Binary	Employed, unemployed	46.9%, 53.1%
EDUCATE	Education level	Binary	College or below, technical school or above	53%, 47%
MEDINS	Indicator of medical insurance	Binary	Yes, no	72.8%, 27.2%
BITYPE	Bipolar type at entry	Binary	Type I, type II	70.4%, 29.6%
PRONSET	Clinical episode immediately preceding current depressive episode	Trinary	Remission, hypo(manic), mixed	45.9%, 33.2%, 20.9%
SUMD0	Scaled depression at entry	Numerical	0.75–18	7.47 (2.30)
SUMD1[a]	Scaled depression at the end of stage 1	Numerical	0–14	4.49 (3.07)
SUMM0	Scaled mood elevation at entry	Numerical	0–7	1.19 (1.09)
SUMM1[a]	Scaled mood elevation at the end of stage 1	Numerical	0–6.75	0.95 (1.30)
Trt1[a]	Treatment received at stage 1	Trinary	Bupropion, paroxetine, placebo	23.3%, 25.5%, 51.2%
SIDE1	Tremor	Binary	Yes, no	26.9%, 73.1%
SIDE2	Dry mouth	Binary	Yes, no	21.1%, 78.9%
SIDE3	Sedation	Binary	Yes, no	17.1%, 82.9%
SIDE4	Constipation	Binary	Yes, no	5.7%, 94.3%
SIDE5	Diarrhea	Binary	Yes, no	12%, 88%
SIDE6	Headache	Binary	Yes, no	13.7%, 86.3%
SIDE7	Poor memory	Binary	Yes, no	14.3%, 85.7%

[a]Covariates that were available only for the second-stage regression model

identification). The stage-specific Q-functions are defined recursively, starting with the last stage function. In our case

- $Q_2(x_1, t_1, x_2, t_2) = E(Y|X_1 = x_1, T_1 = t_1, X_2 = x_2, T_2 = t_2)$,
- $Q_1(x_1, t_1) = E(\min_{t_2} Q_2(X_1, T_1, X_2, t_2)|X_1 = x_1, T_1 = t_1)$.

The Q_2 is a usual regression, here estimating the "quality" of treatment assignment t_2 for a patient presented with his or her "history" up to that point. Similarly, the function Q_1 measures the quality of assigning treatment t_1 for a patient presented with his/her pretreatment covariates and *assuming optimal decision at subsequent stage 2*, defined by minimizing Q_2 (SUMD score) over t_2.

We assume that $Q_1(\cdot, \theta_1)$ and $Q_2(\cdot, \theta_2)$ are parametrized as linear functions of patient covariate history and prior treatments with vector θ_1 containing regression coefficients associated with X_1, T_1, and X_1 by T_1 interactions and θ_2 containing coefficients for X_1, X_2, T_1, T_2, and (X_1, X_2) by T_2 interactions. The parameters of Q-functions are estimated in three steps:

1. Estimate parameters in θ_2 using only data on *placebo non-responders* who were randomized at the second stage to bupropion or paroxetine, by regressing Y on X_1, X_2, T_1, T_2.
2. Compute new "response" vector $\widetilde{Y}$ to be used for estimating the first stage Q-function, defined as

$$\widetilde{Y} = \begin{cases} \widehat{Q}_2(t_2^{opt}), & \text{for placebo nonresponders} \\ Y, & \text{for the rest of patients} \end{cases},$$

where $\widehat{Q}_2(t_2^{opt})$ is the predicted response from the regression model at the previous step with treatment T_2 set for each patient at the *optimal* value t_2^{opt} corresponding to the minimum of estimated $\widehat{Q}_2$.
3. Estimate parameters in θ_1 using all patients by regressing $\widetilde{Y}$ on X_1, T_1, and compute the optimal first-stage treatment t_1^{opt} by minimizing the estimated $\widehat{Q}_1$.

The variables for modeling Q_1 and Q_2 are selected from 24 potential predictors listed in Table 6.6 using stepwise forward variable selection with the entry and stopping conditions determined by the Bayes information criterion (BIC). This was combined with multiple imputation procedures for missing values. The imputation was done using Fully Conditional Specification (chained equations) procedure available in the R package **mice** (van Buuren 2018). This method imputes missing values using sampling from posterior distributions and does not require explicit specification of joint likelihood. Instead, conditional models are defined for each variable given all the rest. This is especially convenient for data sets of mixed type, combining numerical and categorical variables, where joint distributions are hard to specify. In our case, for continuous variables, Predictive Mean Matching was used, and logistic regression models were used for binary variables.

The stepwise forward selection was conducted in such a way that each candidate variable to be added was evaluated using the BIC averaged across m generated complete data sets. The final model was then selected based on the best average BIC across all models in the list formed by the stepwise selection. First, the optimal model for estimating θ_2 in step 1 of the outlined three-step Q-learning procedure was selected in this fashion. Then the optimal model for Q_1 was selected by applying the same stepwise selection (based on average BIC) to estimating θ_1 (step 3) given $\widehat{\theta}_2$ estimated with the model selected for Q_2. For details of the procedure, see Wu et al. (2015).

Once models for Q_1 and Q_2 have been selected, they were applied to each of the m completed data sets, the resulting m estimates of Q-functions averaged, and optimal treatment regimes found as the minimizers of the averaged Q-functions.

Finally, the optimal treatment assignments t_1^{opt} and t_2^{opt} for each patient were approximated with classification trees using R package *rpart* to provide more easily interpretable rules. To achieve that, classification tree algorithm was applied separately to new variables capturing estimated t_1^{opt} and t_2^{opt} as categorical response variables with covariates, selected for modeling Q_1 and Q_2, as candidate splitting variables. The resulting trees are presented in the left and right panel of Fig. 6.2.

6.5.2.3   Results of Q-Learning

Details of estimated Q-functions and associated regression coefficients can be found in Wu et al. (2015). Here we will briefly discuss the tree representation of the optimal DTR shown in Fig. 6.6. The tree on the left shows assignment rules at the first stage. Interestingly, patients who experienced a (hypo) manic episode immediately preceding the current major depressive episode are not recommended any of the two available antidepressant treatments but rather using only mood stabilizers (note that "placebo" actually refers to treating with mood stabilizers only). For the rest of the patients, bupropion is recommended to younger patients, and paroxetine is

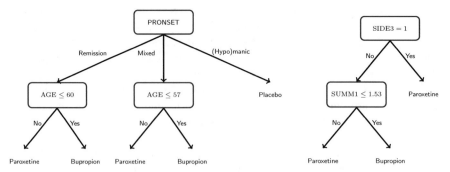

Fig. 6.6 Estimated optimal regimes at stages 1 (left) and 2 (right). Note that the optimal regime at the second stage is evaluated only for those patients who are assigned to placebo at the first stage and fail to show response

Table 6.7 Point estimates and confidence intervals for the expected depression score SUMD at week 12 under estimated DTR and some static regimes (labeled by a pre-specified combination of a first-stage and a second-stage treatment)

Regime	Estimated SUMD	Estimated 90% confidence interval
Estimated optimal DTR	2.13	(1.34, 2.86)
(Bupropion, high-dose bupropion)	6.91	(6.27, 7.71)
(Paroxetine, high-dose paroxetine)	8.25	(7.39, 9.07)
(Placebo, bupropion)	3.71	(3.38, 4.04)
(Placebo, paroxetine)	4.51	(4.10, 4.90)

The lower scores indicate clinically preferred outcome (based on Table 4 from Wu et al. 2015)

recommended to older patients. The tree on the right illustrates the assignment of the second-stage treatment for patients who had failed on placebo during the first stage: variables SUMM1 (mood severity after stage 1) and SIDE3 (presence of sedation side effect) dictate treatment selection; subjects with no sedation side effects and low mood severity are recommended to bupropion, and all others are recommended to paroxetine.

It is also instructive to compare the expected outcomes assuming patients undergo the optimal treatment to outcomes expected under some pre-specified fixed (static) regimes. To estimate expected outcomes under static regimes, an inverse probability weighted estimator was used (Zhang et al. 2013; see also our last case study in Sect. 6.5.3), and confidence intervals were computed using nonparametric bootstrap. The confidence intervals for the optimal DTR estimator were computed using the m-out-of-n bootstrap. Table 6.7 summarizes the results, suggesting some advantages of the estimated dynamic regime.

6.5.3 Estimating Treatment Effect in an Oncology Trial Using Inverse Probability of Censoring Weights

6.5.3.1 Introduction

Demonstrating statistically significant and clinically meaningful gains in overall survival (OS) remains the gold standard to provide evidence of the benefits of new anticancer drugs (Johnson et al. 2015). In clinical trials, in patients with advanced or metastatic cancer, however, it is very common for participants to switch from the treatment to which they were initially randomized to other therapies (Latimer and Abrams 2014), typically after disease progresses on the initially randomized treatment. For both ethical and practical reasons, this option may be built into oncology trial protocols. Switching may also be allowed from the study control treatment to experimental treatment, which is not part of the standard treatment pathway, if no other non-palliative treatments are available.

When patients switch to and benefit from active post-progression therapies, a standard ITT analysis may inaccurately estimate the "true" OS benefit associated with the investigational product the patients were initially randomized to and will affect the cost-effectiveness analyses in the context of economic evaluations that make use of the OS evidence. In general, switching to active post-progression therapies that do not form part of the standard treatment pathway should be adjusted for (Latimer and Abrams 2014).

Several switching adjustment methods that seek to estimate the true treatment effect are available, ranging from simple to complex techniques. Simple or naïve methods such as simple censoring (when data from patients who switched are censored at the point of switching) or exclusion techniques (patients who switched are excluded entirely from the analysis) are highly prone to selection bias and should be avoided (Latimer and Abrams 2014). More complex statistical techniques are classified as *randomization based* (e.g., the rank-preserving structural failure time model or iterative parameter estimation algorithm) or *observational based* (e.g., the two-stage accelerated failure time model [two-stage method] or inverse probability of censoring weights [IPCW]) (Latimer and Abrams 2014). Different switching adjustment methods may be appropriate under certain scenarios, and none is optimal in all circumstances. All of them involve untestable assumptions, as is always the case with causal inference from observational data. Here, for illustration, we will focus on IPCW.

In the IPCW approach, patients are artificially censored at the time of switching, and the weight/influence of uncensored patients with similar prognostic character- istics is increased based on covariate values and a model of the probability of being censored. The key assumption made by the IPCW method is the "no unmeasured confounders" assumption; that is, data must be available for all baseline and time- dependent prognostic factors for mortality that independently predict informative censoring (switching) (Latimer et al. 2014; Robins and Finkelstein 2000). This assumption cannot be tested using the observed data (Robins and Finkelstein 2000). In practice, this is unlikely to be perfectly true, but the method is likely to work adequately if the "no unmeasured confounders" assumption is approximately true; that is, there are no important independent predictors missing (Latimer et al. 2014). Additionally, the method assumes that the model for computing weights is correctly specified and that the probabilities of treatment switching conditional on given covariates are bounded away from zero. The latter would not be the case if physicians were switching patients based on deterministic rules (e.g., all female patients are switched to treatment A and male patients switched to treatment B). As correct model specification plays an important role in implementing the IPCW analysis strategy, modern methods of statistical learning that are free of parametric model assumptions can be very useful because they allow automating the strategy, making it less prone to misspecification error.

6.5.3.2   Example Data Set in Prostate Cancer

The data set used to illustrate the IPCW in this section represents a randomized, double-blind trial with 800 subjects with prostate cancer in each of the two arms—

experimental and placebo. The endpoint of interest for this analysis is overall survival. All subjects were followed up for OS after discontinuing study treatment.

Treatment switching is defined as the switch from the control treatment to the experimental treatment for those subjects randomized to the control arm or from either treatment group to other post-study treatments that are not part of the standard treatment pathway. Treatment switching often occurs upon disease progression or when conclusive evidence accrues about the benefit of the experimental treatment and therefore the study is stopped and unblinded. We assume this typical scenario for our case study.

In our example data set, all subjects in the control group and 27.5% (220/800) of subjects in the experimental arm discontinued the treatment they were randomized to by the data cutoff. In this case study, we are concerned with one type of switch only—when the subject switches from the randomized treatment to another therapy that was not part of the standard treatment pathway, e.g., as per the NICE clinical guideline for prostate cancer (NICE 2014), and we are not concerned with possible multiple switches thereafter. The data set contains a total of 376 switchers, with a larger proportion of switchers in the placebo arm: 18.0% (144/800) and 29.0% (232/800) of subjects in the experimental and placebo groups, respectively.

6.5.3.3 IPCW Methodology

We illustrate herein the IPCW approach for adjusting estimates of a treatment effect in the presence of informative censoring. Censoring is informative when a subject with specific characteristics is more likely to be censored than another (e.g., a subject who has poor prognosis discontinues treatment and is censored because of this). In this case study, we consider treatment switching as the only informative censoring mechanism. All other censoring reasons are modeled as non-informative (as part of the proportional hazard partial likelihood of the Cox regression).

The IPCW method represents a type of Marginal Structural Model (MSM), which was originally developed for use with observational data (Hernán et al. 2001). The IPCW method involves censoring subjects at the time of treatment switch and then controlling for this potentially informative censoring by weighting. Specifically, the follow-up information for subjects who remain at risk for the event is weighted, so that they account not only for themselves but also for subjects with similar characteristics (both baseline and time-dependent) whose follow-up was censored by informative censoring (Robins and Finkelstein 2000).

The IPCW method entails the following general steps. First, for all subjects, follow-up time from randomization until failure (e.g., death) or censoring (informative or otherwise) is partitioned into intervals. At the beginning of each interval, time-dependent variables that may be predictive of informative censoring (switching) or failure are calculated and updated. For each subject and interval, so-called stabilized weights (SW) are then calculated as described by Hernán et al. (2001). The numerator of each weight is the cumulative probability of remaining uncensored by informative censoring from the beginning of follow-up to the end of the interval given only baseline covariates. The denominator of the weight is the cumulative probability of remaining uncensored by informative censoring to the end of the interval given both baseline and time-dependent covariates. In the original formulation of Hernán et al. (2001), an individual's treatment history up until the end of the previous interval is included in both the numerator and denominator. Given that in our case study the cause of informative censoring is the *first* switch from the randomized treatment to another antineoplastic therapy, "past treatment history" is reduced to the initial randomized treatment that is conditioned upon simply by performing computations of weights separately by treatment arms.

Specifically, patient-specific estimates of the stabilized weights at the jth interval, $SW_i(j)$, are obtained as follows (here we drop the patient index from all terms to simplify notation):

$$SW(j) \equiv \frac{\prod_{k=0}^{j} P[C(k) = 0 | C(k-1) = 0, X(0)]}{\prod_{k=0}^{j} P[C(k) = 0 | C(k-1) = 0, X(0), Y(k)]},$$

where

- $C(k)$ is an indicator function representing censoring/treatment switch status at the end of interval k (1, censored due to switching, 0, uncensored).
- $X(0)$ is a vector of subject characteristics measured at baseline (see Table 6.8).
- $Y(k)$ is a vector of time-dependent subject characteristics measured at or prior to the beginning of interval k (see Table 6.8).
- $P[C(k) = 0 | C(k-1) = 0, X(0)]$ is the probability of remaining uncensored (not switched) at the end of interval k given uncensored at the end of interval $k-1$ and conditioned on baseline characteristics $X(0)$.
- $P[C(k) = 0 | C(k-1) = 0, X(0), Y(k)]$ is the probability of remaining uncensored (not switched) at the end of interval k given uncensored at the end of interval $k-1$ and conditioned on baseline characteristics $X(0)$ and time-dependent patient characteristics $Y(k)$.

Probabilities of remaining uncensored by informative censoring are unknown and therefore need to be estimated. Here, we use two approaches to illustrate the difference between traditional parametric modeling and methods of machine learning: logistic regression and random forest models (see Sect. 6.3.1). In each case, we fit one model for the denominator and one model for the numerator, with informative censoring (switching) as the dependent variable. Details on how these methods were applied in this case study are provided further below. Both the logistic regression and the random forest models are estimated within each treatment arm separately, to account for potential differences in the reasons that led to switching treatment in each arm. Covariates included in these models represent measurements typically collected in the studies of prostate cancer and are presented in Table 6.8.

A hazard ratio (HR) for the outcome of interest is then estimated using a weighted Cox proportional hazards regression model that includes only baseline variables and the treatment arm indicator (i.e., the indicator of the initial randomized treatment) as

Table 6.8 Covariates for modeling weights in IPCW estimators

Covariates
Baseline covariates:
Age (years, continuous)
Time since diagnosis (categorical; <5 years vs. ≥ 5 years)
Number of bone metastases at screening (categorical; ≤ 5 vs. >5)
Presence of visceral disease at baseline (categorical; yes vs. no)
Type of disease progression at study entry (categorical; PSA progression only vs. radiographic progression with or without PSA vs. no disease progression at study entry)
Baseline EQ-5D utility index (continuous)
Baseline FACT-P total score (continuous)
Time-dependent covariates:
ECOG Performance Status (categorical; 0 vs. >0)
History of grade 3/4/5 adverse events (categorical; yes vs. no)
Occurrence of grade 3/4/5 adverse events since last visit (categorical; yes vs. no)
Corticosteroid use (categorical; yes vs. no)
PSA level (continuous)
Laboratory tests: LDH level (categorical; ≤ 240 IU/mL vs. >240 IU/mL)
EQ-5D utility index (continuous)
FACT-P total score (continuous)
Time since treatment discontinuation (continuous)
Time to treatment discontinuation (continuous)[a]
Disease progression (categorical; yes vs. no)[a]

ECOG Eastern Cooperative Oncology Group, *FACT-P* Functional Assessment of Cancer Therapy-Prostate, *LDH* lactate dehydrogenase, *PSA* prostate-specific antigen
[a]Although disease progression and time to treatment discontinuation do not vary with time, they could be important covariates to be accounted for in the estimation of the weights

covariates. The weights are the subject- and interval-specific stabilized weights as described above.

Because the standard errors for the HRs obtained from the Cox regression analysis do not account for the variability associated with the estimation of the stabilized weights, 95% confidence intervals for HR estimates are obtained by bootstrapping (Hernán et al. 2001; see also Sect. 6.2). This method involves resampling with replacement from the experimental and placebo arms to obtain B (here $B = 100$ for illustration, but we would recommend 2000) bootstrap samples of the original data and repeating all the steps above for each of these samples to calculate B bootstrap estimates of the HR. A 95% CI for the HR is estimated based on the 2.5 and 97.5 percentiles of B bootstrap replicates.

6.5.3.4   Estimating Stabilized Weights with Logistic Regression

To estimate the numerator of the stabilized weights, a logistic regression (model 1) was fitted to the "stacked data" (i.e., with multiple records per patient) from all patient intervals from randomization until treatment switch or failure or censoring, defined as death, withdrawal of consent, or end of study, whichever occurred first. The probability of remaining uncensored was modeled conditional on patient baseline factors listed in Table 6.8 and a time-dependent intercept. The time-dependent intercept was estimated by including a variable indicating the number of days elapsed since randomization at the start of the interval and its quadratic term. The dependent variable in the logistic model was a binary variable (1/0) indicating whether the patient had switched treatment or not during the interval.

To estimate the denominator of the stabilized weights, a similar logistic regression (model 2) was fitted in which the probability of remaining uncensored was modeled conditional on the same baseline factors as above plus patient time-dependent covariates measured at the start of each interval, as listed in Table 6.8. Upon randomized study drug discontinuation, patients are typically followed mainly in terms of their survival status and initiation of new therapies, while other regular study assessments, e.g., ECOG, LDH, SPA, etc., are no longer performed. Therefore, only data as observed at the time of study treatment discontinuation (fixed) and time since treatment discontinuation (time-varying) are used as predictors of treatment switching in our models for the denominator of the weights. In a typical study, the probability of treatment switching prior to study treatment discontinuation is zero by trial design (alternatively, the probability of remaining uncensored is 1). Therefore, the probability of being uncensored was set to 1 for patient intervals prior to study treatment discontinuation, and these observations were not used in the estimation of this logistic model.

For all patient intervals prior to the date at which patients were assumed to be at risk of informative censoring (treatment switching, i.e., the date of study treatment discontinuation), stabilized weights were calculated. The numerator of $SW(j)$ was obtained using the estimates of the first model as described above, and the denominator of $SW(j)$ was set to 1.0 (i.e., the time-dependent probability of switch set equal to zero). Thus, these weights are always less than 1.0. For subsequent intervals, the numerator of $SW(j)$ was calculated using model 1, and the denominator was calculated using model 2. These weights may be greater than 1.0.

6.5.3.5   Estimating Stabilized Weights Using Random Forests

Stabilized weights were also estimated using random forests, in a manner similar as described above for the logistic regression, i.e., fitting separate models within each treatment arm as well as for the numerator and denominator of the weights, using the same baseline and time-dependent covariates, and data from the same patient intervals. This analysis was carried out using the R package **randomForest**. The model can be fit using the following function:

$$model = randomForest(predictors, as.factor(outcome), ntree = 1000),$$

where

- "predictors" contains a matrix with the values of patient covariates included in the model with rows corresponding to patient intervals used to fit the model.
- "outcome" is a vector of binary values representing the switching indicator for each patient interval as previously described.
- "ntree" is a parameter of the random forest algorithm specifying the number of classification trees that are fit as part of the random forest.

A default setting is used for the number of covariates that are randomly chosen as candidates for the splits (the "mtry" parameter) when building the classification trees so that the square root of the number of all available predictors is used. Once the model is estimated, predicted probabilities of not switching (remaining uncensored due to the non-ignorable reason) can be obtained using the function "predict" from the **randomForest** package:

$$pred = as.data.frame\left(predict\left(model, newdata = predictors, type = \text{``prob''}\right)\right)$$

where

- "model" is a "randomForest" object estimated above.
- "newdata = predictors" specifies that predictions should be provided for the same data set of patient intervals and covariate values.
- type = "prob" argument requests predictions in the form of probabilities as opposed to binary outcomes. These predicted probabilities are used for the calculation of the numerator or denominator of the stabilized weights.

6.5.3.6 Results

When applying the IPCW method, it is important to explore the distributions of the weights estimated in the first part of the method. A necessary condition for the correct model specification is that the stabilized weights have a mean of 1 (Hernán and Robins 2006).

Summary statistics on the stabilized weights for the IPCW analysis are presented in Table 6.9. Irrespective of the method used to estimate the probability of not being informatively censored (logistic regression or random forest), for both treatment

Table 6.9 Descriptive statistics for stabilized weights in IPCW models

Treatment arm	N	Mean	STD	Min	Max	Q1	Median	Q3
Logistic regression								
Placebo	10,692	1.01	0.25	0.87	12.10	0.98	0.99	1.00
Experimental	11,039	1.00	0.07	0.92	2.78	0.98	1.00	1.00
Random forest								
Placebo	10,692	1.02	0.24	0.27	9.60	1.00	1.00	1.00
Experimental	11,039	1.01	0.11	0.28	3.67	1.00	1.00	1.00

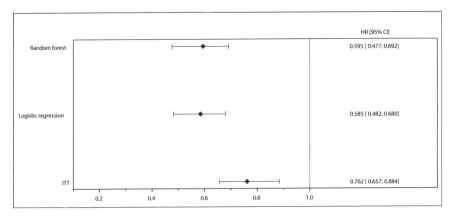

Fig. 6.7 Results of the unadjusted analysis and the IPCW method. The 95% CI are obtained from bootstrapping

arms, the mean of the stabilized weights is very close to 1, as expected. The median of the weights is also close to 1.

The results of the unadjusted analysis and the IPCW method using stabilized weights obtained from both logistic regression and random forest method are provided in Fig. 6.7. The unadjusted results were obtained with the analysis where all ITT subjects were included in the analysis set and no censoring was applied at the point of treatment switching.

Adjusting for the treatment switching, as well as for other baseline characteristics, indicates that the experimental treatment was associated with reduction in the risk of mortality of approximately 41% irrespective of the method used to obtain the stabilized weights (HR = 0.59; 95% CI [0.48; 0.68] using logistic regression and HR = 0.60; 95% CI [0.48; 0.69] using random forest). The unadjusted HR was 0.76, 95% CI [0.66; 0.88]. A smaller HR from the adjusted analysis is expected because there are more switchers in the placebo arm than in the experimental arm which is appropriately accounted for in the adjusted analysis.

As discussed in Sect. 6.3.1, random forests can also provide an insight into which covariates are most predictive of the outcome using the estimated variable importance scores. They can be obtained using the function "importance":

$$VI = importance(model, type = 1)$$

where the argument "type=1" requests the VI scores estimated based on the mean decrease in accuracy from permuting out-of-bag data (see Sect. 6.3.1). For example, from the treatment-specific models used for the denominators of the weights including baseline and time-dependent covariates, the VI scores are as illustrated in Fig. 6.8. We can see that in both treatment arms, the top four predictors are the time to treatment discontinuation, PSA level, time from randomization, and age.

Variable Importance

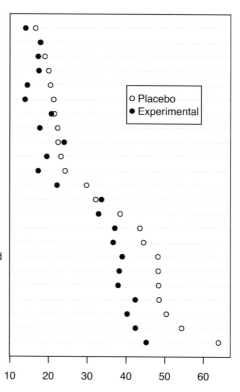

Fig. 6.8 Variable importance scores from random forest models of treatment switching based on baseline and time-dependent covariates (models for denominators of stabilized weights)

To gain further insight into the relationship between the top predictors and the probability of treatment switching, we can obtain partial dependence plots (using the function "partialPlot") that provide a graphical display of the marginal effects of the variables of interest on class probability. Figure 6.9 illustrates such partial dependence plots for the three top predictors in the treatment-specific models of weight denominators.

6.5.3.7   Discussion

The objective of these analyses was to estimate the effect of experimental treatment vs. placebo, adjusting for the potentially confounding effects of receipt of nonstandard anticancer therapy in both treatment groups. This is of particular interest for economic evaluations considering a lifetime horizon where standard ITT analyses are likely to be inappropriate in the presence of treatment switching failing

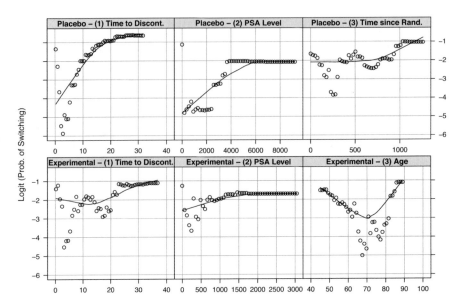

Fig. 6.9 Partial dependence plots for three top predictors from random forest models of treatment switching based on baseline and time-dependent covariates (models for denominators of stabilized weights)

to inform the decision problem (selecting the most effective therapy for a given patient population) from the causal inference perspective.

The IPCW method to adjust for the treatment switching was chosen in this example because a large number of potentially prognostic covariates (that can influence the investigator's decision to switch treatment for a prostate cancer patient) were available for the analysis. Also, as suggested by the theory and existing evidence, IPCW is best suited for studies where the switching proportions are not very high (Latimer and Abrams 2014), which is the case in our example data set. The IPCW method is reliant on the assumption of "no unmeasured confounders" which is not testable from observed data. One strategy is to include in the analysis a comprehensive set of potentially important confounders identified using expert knowledge (which may include redundant covariates) and rely on powerful machine learning methods to extract useful information in the process of model building. Whether the results could substantially change after including covariates entirely missing in the observed data can be evaluated using sensitivity analyses framework (see Brumback et al. 2004; Klungsøyr et al. 2009).

We have applied the IPCW method where weights were estimated using two approaches: a traditional logistic regression and a modern method of statistical learning, the random forest. In our example, the results using the logistic regression and random forest models of treatment switching provided similar results. The random forest model is of particular interest as it is free of parametric model assumptions, can effectively deal with a large number of predictors without overfitting, is known for its good predictive accuracy, and provides useful insights into the predictive strength of considered covariates and their relationship to the outcome.

6.6   Discussion and Conclusions

DMML methods are becoming now an integral part of data analysis at all stages of clinical drug development, which can be contrasted with its primary use in preclinical stage of "drug discovery" in the past. The need in DMML arises whenever a model selection is entertained, which may occur in different tasks including traditional estimation of the overall treatment effect in the presence of potential confounding due to post-randomization events and novel tasks of treatment optimization in the realm of personalized/precision medicine.

A wealth of patient data collected during the clinical development program may be better utilized with the principled use of DMML that should inform a decision-making process across the entire drug development cycle. We hope that the references to examples of various clinical applications and case studies provided in this chapter will give the reader an appreciation of the breadth of areas where the power of DMML can be leveraged.

Application of DMML to clinical data has some unique features. Unlike more traditional applications of DMML (such as speech and character recognition), with potentially unlimited amount of data that can be used for model training, DMML in clinical settings is dealing with relatively small number of records due to substantial costs and other constraints associated with each patient that can be enrolled in a clinical study. Therefore, a typical application of DMML in the clinical world is within the medium or small "n" and medium/large "p." Cross-validation and other resampling-based methods, therefore, play a key role.

Modeling of clinical data, whether randomized or based on observational studies, involves methods accounting for different sources of confounding and missing data. This explains the trend of integrating DMML and casual inference methods in some applications.

Another feature of applications of DMML in drug development is the need to control the Type I error or false discovery rate which is a new trend in the area of machine learning that historically considered the concept of statistical significance irrelevant. Typically, the analytical form of the null distribution for many DMML techniques is not available, and one needs to resort to methods of resampling.

It is important to understand that the multiplicity control is interrelated with model complexity control: the latter effectively restricts the model search space and results in a lesser multiplicity burden.

It is a common trend for DMML applications in clinical data that the decision-makers desire interpretable solutions rather than a "black box" which can often be achieved by post-processing the "black box" to produce interpretable graphical displays, such as trees, marginal plots, low dimensional projections, etc.

"Data mining" in the clinical world sometimes was ascribed a negative connotation as "data dredging." However, we argue that using principled DMML strategies and pre-specification of analytic strategies in the data mining plans may help remove the stigma from data mining, making it a valuable set of tools for improved decision-making in the drug development process.

Acknowledgments The authors would like to thank Matthew Rotelli, Qianyi Zhang, and Chakib Battioui for many stimulating discussions on data mining and its role in drug development process, Alex Dmitrienko for long-standing collaboration on developing the SIDES method, Fan Wu, Eric Laber and Emanuel Severus for their generous help with the case study on Q-learning, and Natallia Katenka and Anthony Zagar for reviewing the draft of the chapter and providing many valuable suggestions that led to substantially improved presentation of the material.

References

Abtroun L, Bunouf P, Gendreau RM, Vitton O (2016) Is the efficacy of milnacipran in fibromyalgia predictable? A data-mining analysis of baseline and outcome variables. Clin J Pain 32:435–440

Aharon M, Elad M, Bruckstein A (2006) K-SVD: An algorithm for designing overcomplete dictionaries for sparse representation. IEEE Trans Signal Process 54(11):4311-4322

Akaike H (1974) A new look at the statistical model identification. IEEE T Automat Contr 19 (6):716–723

Allen D (1974) The relationship between variable selection and data augmentation and a method of prediction. Technometrics 16:125–127

Almirall D, Nahum-Shan I, Sherwood NE, Murphy SA (2014) Introduction to SMART designs for the development of adaptive Interventions: with application to weight loss research. Transl Behav Med 4(3):260-274

Altmann A, Toloşi L, Sander O, Lengauer T (2010) Permutation importance: a corrected feature importance measure. Bioinformatics 26(10):1340-1347

Amaratunga D, Cabrera J. (2004) Mining data to find subsets of high activity. J Stat Plan Inference 122:23-41

Amaratunga D, Cabrera J, Lee Y-S (2008) Enriched random forests. Bio-informatics 24(18):2010-2014

Ambroise C, McLachlan G (2002) Selection bias in gene extraction on the basis of microarray gene-expression data. Proc Natl Acad Sci USA 99:6562–6566

Aridas CK, Kotsiantis SB, Vrahatis MN (2016) Increasing diversity in random forests using Naive Bayes. In Iliadis L, Maglogiannis I (eds) Artificial Intelligence Applications and Innovations, 12th IFIP WG 12.5 International Conference and Workshops, pp. 75–86

Ashley EA (2015) The precision medicine initiative. A national effort. J Am Med Assoc 313 (21):2119-2120

Barber RF, Candès EJ (2015). Controlling the false discovery rate via knockoffs. Ann Stat 43 (5):2055-2085

Benjamini Y, Hochberg Y (1995) Controlling the false discovery rate: A practical and powerful approach to multiple testing. J R Statist Soc Series B 57(1):289-300

Bühlmann P, Hothorn T (2010) Twin Boosting: improved feature selection and prediction, Stat Comput 20:119-138

Berger J, Wang X, Shen L (2014) A Bayesian approach to subgroup identification. J Biopharm Stat 24:110–129

Blatt D, Murphy SA, Zhu J (2004) A-learning for approximate planning. Technical Report 04-63, The Methodology Center, Pennsylvania State Univ., State College, PA

Bonetti M, Gelber RD (2000) A graphical method to assess treatment–covariate interactions using the Cox model on subsets of the data. Stat Med 19:2595–2609

Bonetti M, Gelber RD (2004) Patterns of treatment effects in subsets of patients in clinical trials. Biostatistics 5(3):465–481

Bornkamp B, Pinheiro J, Bretz F. (2009) MCPMod: An R package for the design and analysis of dose-finding studies. J Stat Softw 29(7)1:23

Bornkamp B, Ohlssen D, Magnusson B, Schmidli H (2016) Model averaging for treatment effect estimation in subgroups. Pharm Stat. DOI: https://doi.org/10.1002/pst.179

Breiman L (1996) Bagging predictors. Mach Learn 26:123–140

Breiman L (2001a) Random forests. Mach Learn 45(1):5-32

Breiman L (2001b) Statistical modeling: The two cultures. Stat Sc 16:199–231

Breiman L, Spector P (1992) Submodel selection and evaluation in regression: the X-random case. Int Stat Rev 60:291–319

Breiman L, Friedman JH, Olshen RA, Stone CJ (1984) Classification and Regression Trees. Chapman & Hall, London

Bretz F, Pinheiro JC, Branson M (2005) Combining multiple comparisons and modeling techniques in dose-response studies. Biometrics 61:738-748

Brumback BA, Hernán MA, Haneuse SJ, Robins JM (2004) Sensitivity analyses for unmeasured confounding assuming a marginal structural model for repeated measures. Stat Med 23(5):749-767

Bühlmann P, Horthorn T (2007) Boosting algorithms: regularization, prediction and model fitting. Stat Sci 22(4):477-505

Burgel PR, Paillasseur JL, Roche N (2014) Identification of clinical phenotypes using cluster analyses in COPD patients with multiple comorbidities. BioMed Res Int Article ID 420134

Burges C (1998) A tutorial on support vector machines for pattern recognition. Knowl Discov Data Min 2(2):121–167

Cai T, Tian L, Wong P, Wei LJ (2011) Analysis of randomized comparative clinical trial data for personalized treatment selections. Biostatistics 12:270–282

Cattell RB (1952) Factor analysis. New York: Harper

Chakraborty B, Moodie EE (2013) Statistical reinforcement learning. Gail M, Krickeberg K, Samet J, Tsiatis A, Wong W (eds) Statistical Methods for Dynamic Treatment Regimes. Springer, New York

Chakraborty B, Murphy SA (2014) Dynamic treatment regimes. Annu Rev Stat Appl 1:447–464

Chakraborty B, Laber EB, Zhao Y (2013) Inference for optimal dynamic treatment regimes using an adaptive m-out-of-n bootstrap scheme. Biometrics 69(3):614-723

Chaudhuri P, Lo W-D, Loh W-Y, Yang C-C (1995) Generalized regression trees. Stat. Sinica 5:641–666

Chen G, Zhong H, Belousov A, Viswanath D (2015) PRIM approach to predictive-signature development for patient stratification. Stat Med 34:317–342

Clarke B, Fokoué E, Zhang HH (2009) Principles and Theory for Data Mining and Machine Learning. Springer, New York

Collins LM, Murphy SA, Strecher V (2007) The multiphase optimization strategy (MOST) and the sequential multiple assignment randomized trial (SMART): New methods for more potent e-health interventions. Am J Prev Med 32(5 Suppl):S112-S118

Conrad DJ, Bailey BA (2015) Multidimensional clinical phenotyping of an adult cystic fibrosis patient population. PLoS One 10(3):e0122705

Cosma G, Brown D, Archer M, Khan M, Pockley AG (2017) A survey on computational intelligence approaches for predictive modeling in prostate cancer, Expert Syst Appl 70:1-19

Davis RB, Anderson JR (1989) Exponential survival trees. Stat Med 8:947-961

Defays D (1977) An efficient algorithm for a complete-link method. Comput J British Comput Soc 20 (4):364–366

Dixon DO, Simon R (1991) Bayesian subset analysis. Biometrics 47:871–882

Dmitrienko A, Lipkovich I, Hopkins A, Li YP, Wang W (2015) Biomarker evaluation and subgroup identification in a pneumonia development program using SIDES. Applied Statistics in Biomedicine and Clinical Trials Design. Chen Z, Liu A, Qu Y, Tang L, Ting N, Tsong Y. (editors). Springer

Docampo E, Collado A, Escaramís G, Carbonell J, Rivera J, Vidal J, Alegre J, Rabionet R, Estivill X (2013) Cluster analysis of clinical data identifies fibromyalgia subgroups. Baradaran HR (ed) PLoS One 8(9):e74873

Domingos P (2000) Bayesian averaging of classifiers and the overfitting problem. In: Proceedings of the 17th International Conference on Machine Learning, pp. 223–230

Domingos P (2012) A few useful things to know about machine learning. Commun ACM 55 (10):78-87

Doubleday K (2016) Generation of Individualized Treatment Decision Tree Algorithm With Application to Randomized Control Trials and Electronic Medical Record Data. Master Theses, The University of Arizona, available at http://arizona.openrepository.com/arizona/bitstream/10150/613559/1/azu_etd_14716_sip1_m.pdf

Dusseldorp E, Van Mechelen I (2014) Qualitative interaction trees: A tool to identify qualitative treatment-subgroup interactions. Stat Med 33:219–237

Dusseldorp E, Conversano C, Van Os BJ (2010) Combining an additive and tree-based regression model simultaneously: STIMA. J Comp Graph Stat 19:514–530

Efron B (1979) Bootstrap methods: another look at the jackknife, Ann Stat 7:1–26

Efron B (2010) Large-Scale Inference: Empirical Bayes Methods for Estimation, Testing, and Prediction. Cambridge University Press

Efron B, Hastie T (2016) Computer Age Statistical Inference: Algorithms, Evidence, and Data Science. Cambridge University Press: New York

Efron B, Tibshirani R (1997) Improvements on crossvalidation: The 0.632+ bootstrap method. J Am Stat Assoc 92:548–560

Efron B, Hastie T, Johnstone I, Tibshirani R (2004) Least angle regression. Ann Stat 32(2):407-499

Ertefaie A, Almiral D, Huang L, Dziak JJ, Wagner AT, Murphy SA (2012) SAS PROC QLEARN users' guide (Version 1.0.0). University Park: The Methodology Center, Penn State. Available from http://methodology.psu.edu

Evgeniou T, Pontil M, Poggio T (2000) Regularization networks and support vector machines, Adv Comput Math 13(1):1–50

Faye LL, Sun L, Dimitromanolakis A, Bulla SB (2011) A flexible genome-wide bootstrap method that accounts for ranking and threshold-selection bias in GWAS interpretation and replication study design. Stat Med 30(15):1898-912

FDA (U.S. Food and Drug Administration) (2018) "FDA permits marketing of artificial intelligence algorithm for aiding providers in detecting wrist fractures" FDA News Release, May 24, 2018; https://www.fda.gov/newsevents/newsroom/pressannouncements/ucm608833.htm

Ferguson JP, Cho JH, Yang C, Zhao H (2013) Empirical Bayes correction for the Winner's Curse in genetic association studies. Genet Epidemiol 37(1):60–68

Forgy E (1965) Cluster analysis of multivariate data: efficiency vs. interpretability of classifications. Biometrics 21:768–769

Foster JC, Taylor JMC, Ruberg SJ (2011) Subgroup identification from randomized clinical trial data. Stat Med 30:2867–2880

Foster JC, Taylor JMG, Kaciroti N, Nan B (2015) Simple subgroup approximation to optimal treatment regimes from randomized clinical trial data. Biostatistics 16(2):368-82

Freund Y, Schapire RE (1997) A decision-theoretic generalization of on-line learning and an application to boosting. J Comp Syst Sci 55(1):119-139

Friedman J (1991) Multivariate adaptive regression splines (with discussion). Ann Stat 19(1):1–141

Friedman JH (1997) Data mining and statistics: what's the connection? In: Proceedings of Symposium on the Interface Between Computer Science and Statistics

Friedman J (1999) Stochastic gradient boosting, Technical report, Stanford University

Friedman J (2001) Greedy function approximation: A gradient boosting machine. Ann of Stati 29 (5):1189–1232

Friedman JH, Fisher NI (1999) Bump hunting in high-dimensional data. Stat Comput 9:123–143

Friedman J, Hall P (2007) On bagging and nonlinear estimation. J Stat Plan Inference 137:669–683

Friedman JH, Popescu BE (1999) Predictive Learning via Rule Ensembles. Ann of Appl Stat 2:916–954

Friedman J, Stuetzle W (1981) Projection pursuit regression. J Am Statist Assoc 76:817–823

Friedman JH, Tukey JW (1974) A projection pursuit algorithm for exploratory data analysis. IEEE Transactions on Computers, C–23 (9):881–890

Friedman J, Hastie T, Tibshirani R (2000) Additive logistic regression: a statistical view of boosting (with discussion). Annals of Statistics 28:337–407

Fu H, Zhou J, Faries DE (2016) Estimating optimal treatment regimes via subgroup identification in randomized control trials and observational studies. Stat Med 35(19):3285-3302

Geisser S (1975) The predictive sample reuse method with applications. J Am Stat Assoc 70 (350):320–328

Geurts P, Ernst D, Wehenkel L (2006) Extremely randomized trees. Mach Learn 63: 3–42

Gilmour SG (1996) The interpretation of Mallows's Cp-statistic. J R Stat Soc Ser D 45(1):49–56

Glickman ME, Rao SR, Schultz MR (2014) False discovery rate control is a recommended alternative to Bonferroni-type adjustments in health studies. J Clin Epidemiol 67(8):850-857

Goldberg Y, Kosorok, MR (2012) Q-learning with Censored Data. Ann Stat 40(1):529-560

Goodfellow I, Bengio J, Courville A, Bach F (2016) Deep Learning. MIT Press: Cambridge, MA

Gordon L, Olshen RA (1985) Tree-structured survival analysis. Cancer Treat. Rep 69:1065–1069

Gower JC, Hand DJ (1996) Biplots. Chapman and Hall: London

Greenacre MJ (1984) Theory and Applications of Correspondence Analysis. Academic Press: London

Gu X, Yin G, Lee JJ (2013) Bayesian two-step Lasso strategy for biomarker selection in personalized medicine development for time-to-event endpoints. Contemp Clin Trials 36:642–650

Gunter L, Zhu J, Murphy S (2011) Variable selection for qualitative interactions in personalized medicine while controlling the familywise error rate. J Biopharm Stat 21:1063–1078

Hand DJ (1998) Data mining: statistics and more? Am Stat 52(2):112-118

Hand DJ, Mannila H, Smyth P (2001) Principles of Data Mining. The MIT Press: Cambridge.

Hansen LK, Salamon P (1990) Neural network ensembles. IEEE Trans Pattern Ana. Mach Intell 12 (10):993–1001

Hardin DS, Rohwer RD, Curtis BH, Zagar A, Chen L, Boye KS, Jiang HH, Lipkovich IA (2013) Understanding heterogeneity in response to antidiabetes treatment: A post hoc analysis using SIDES, a subgroup identification algorithm. J Diab Sci Technol 7:420–429

Harpaz R, DuMouchel W, Shah NH, Madigan D, Ryan P, Friedman C (2012) Novel data mining methodologies for adverse drug event discovery and analysis. Clin Pharmacol Ther 91(6):1010-1021

Hastie T, Tibshirani R, Friedman J (2009) The Elements of Statistical Learning. Data Mining, Inference, and Prediction, 2nd Edition. Springer-Verlag: New York

Henderson NC, Louis TA, Wang C, Varadhan R (2016) Bayesian analysis of heterogeneous treatment effects for patient-centered outcomes research. Health Serv Outcomes Res Methodol 16(4):213–233

Henderson NC, Louis TA, Rosner G, Varadhan R (2017) Individualized treatment effects with censored data via fully nonparametric Bayesian accelerated failure time models. Available arXiv preprint arXiv: 1706.06611v1

Herland M, Khoshgoftaar TM, Wald R (2014) A review of data mining using big data in health informatics. J Big Data 1:2

Hernán MA, Robins JM (2006) Estimating causal effects from epidemiological data. J Epidemiol Community Health 60:578–586

Hernán MA, Brumback B, Robins JM (2001) Marginal structural models to estimate the joint causal effect of nonrandomized treatments. J Am Stat Assoc 96(454):440-448

Ho, TK (1995) Random decision forests. In: Proceedings of the 3rd International Conference on Document Analysis and Recognition, Montreal, QC, pp. 278–282

Ho TK (2002) A data complexity analysis of comparative advantages of decision forest constructors. Pattern Anal Appl 5(2):102–112

Hoeting JA, Madigan D, Raftery AE, Volinsky CT (1999) Bayesian model averaging: A tutorial. Stat Sci 14(4): 382–417

Hodges JS, Cui Y, Sargent DJ, Carlin BP (2007) Smoothing balanced single-error-term analysis of variance. Technometrics 49:12–25

Hoerl AE, Kennard R (1970) Ridge regression: Biased estimation for nonorthogonal problems. Technometrics 12:55–67

Hotelling H (1933) Analysis of a complex of statistical variables into principal components. J Educ Psychol, 24:417–441

Hothorn T, Hornik K, Zeileis A (2006) Unbiased recursive partitioning: A conditional inference framework. J Comp Graph Stat 15(3):651-674

Hou J, Seneviratne C, Su X, Taylor J, Johnson B, Wang XQ, Zhang H, Kranzler HR, Kang J, Liu L (2015) Subgroup identification in personalized treatment of alcohol dependence. Alcohol Clin Exp Res 39(7):1253-1259

Huang Y, Fong Y (2014) Identifying optimal biomarker combinations for treatment selection via a robust kernel method. Biometrics 70:891–901

Hyvärinen A, Oja E (2000) Independent component analysis: Algorithms and applications. Neural Networks 13:411–430

Imai K, Ratkovic M (2013) Estimating treatment effect heterogeneity in randomized program evaluation. Ann Appl Stat 7:443–470

Ishwaran H, Kogalur U, Blackstone E, Lauer M (2008) Random survival forests. Ann Appl Stat 2 (3):841–860

Jacova C, Slack PJ, Hsiung G-YR, Beattie BL, Lee P (2013) Patients' self-reports on function and cognition in Alzheimer's disease are strongly influenced by their affective states: Principal component analysis of the CLIMAT scale. Alzheimers Dement 9(4):650

Janes H, Brown MD, Pepe M, Huang Y (2013) Statistical methods for evaluating and comparing biomarkers for patient treatment selection. UW Biostatistics Working Paper Series. Working Paper 389. http://biostats.bepress.com/uwbiostat/paper389

Janes H, Brown M, Pepe M, Huang Y (2014) An approach to evaluating and comparing biomarkers for patient treatment selection. Int J Biostat 10(1):99-121

Johnson P, Greiner W, Al-Dakkak I, Wagner S (2015) Which metrics are appropriate to describe the value of new cancer therapies? Biomed Res Int 2015:865101

Jolliffe IT (2002) Principal Component Analysis, Series: Springer Series in Statistics, 2nd ed., Springer: New York

Jones HE, Ohlssen DI, Neuenschwander B, Racine A, Branson M (2011) Bayesian models for subgroup analysis in clinical trials. Clin Trials 8:129–143

Jordan M, Jacobs R (1994) Hierachical mixtures of experts and the EM algorithm. Neural Comput 6:181–214

Kass GV (1980) An exploratory technique for investigating large quantities of categorical data. App Stat 29:119-127

Kaufman L, Rousseeuw P (1990) Finding Groups in Data: An Introduction to Cluster Analysis, Wiley, New York

Kavakiotis I, Tsave O, Salifoglou A, Maglaveras N, Vlahavas I, Chouvarda I (2017) Machine learning and data mining methods in diabetes research. Comput Struct Biotechnol J 15:104-116

Kehl V, Ulm K (2006) Responder identification in clinical trials with censored data. Comput Stat Data Anal 50:1338–1355

Khalilia M, Chakraborty S, Popescu M (2011) Predicting disease risks from highly imbalanced data using random forest. BMC Medical Informatics and Decision Making 11:51

Kim H, Loh WY (2001) Classification trees with unbiased multiway splits. J Am Stat Assoc 96:589-604

Kim H, Loh WY (2003) Classification trees with bivariate linear discriminant node models. J Comput and Graph Statsit 12:512-530

Kim H-C, Ghahramani Z (2012) Bayesian classifier combination. In: Proceedings of the 15th International Conference on Artificial Intelligence and Statistics 22:619–627

Klungsøyr O, Sexton J, Sandanger I, Nygård JF (2009) Sensitivity analysis for unmeasured confounding in a marginal structural Cox proportional hazards model. Lifetime Data Anal 15 (2):278-294

Kohavi R (1995) A study of cross-validation and bootstrap for accuracy estimation and model selection. In: Proceeding IJCAI'95 Proceedings of the 14th international joint conference on Artificial intelligence - Volume 2, pp. 1137–1143

Kohonen T (1989) Self-Organization and Associative Memory (3rd edition), Springer: Berlin

Konstantina K, Themis PE, Konstantinos PE, Michalis VK, Dimitrios IF (2015) Machine learning applications in cancer prognosis and prediction. Comput Struct Biotechnol J 13:8–17

Kotajima L, Aotsuka S, Nishimaki T, Kashiwagi H, Kunieda T, Tojo T, Yokohari R (1997) Classification tree criteria of pulmonary hypertension in mixed connective tissue disease. Jpn J Rheumatol 7(4):293-303

Kruskal J B, Wish M. (1978) Multidimensional Scaling. Beverly Hills, California: Sage.

Krstajic D, Buturovic LJ, Leahy DE, Thomas S (2014) Cross-validation pitfalls when selecting and assessing regression and classification models. J Cheminformatics 6:10

Kutcher ME, Ferguson AR, Cohen MJ (2013) A principal component analysis of coagulation after trauma. J Trauma Acute Care Surg 74(5):1223-1230

Laber EB, Lizotte DJ, Ferguson B (2014a) Set-valued dynamic treatment regimes for competing outcomes. Biometrics 70:53–61

Laber EB, Lizotte DJ, Qian M, Pelham WE, Murphy SA (2014b) Dynamic treatment regimes: technical challenges and applications. Electron J Stat 8(1):1225–1272

Lamont A, Lyons MD, Jaki T, Stuart E, Feaster DJ, Tharmaratnam K, Oberski D, Ishwaran H, Wilson DK, Horn MLW (2016). Identification of predicted individual treatment effects in randomized clinical trials. Stat Methods Med Res Mar 17. pii: 0962280215623981

Latimer NR, Abrams KR (2014) NICE DSU Technical Support Document 16: Adjusting survival time estimates in the presence of treatment switching. Available from http://www.nicedsu. org.uk

Latimer NR, Abrams KR, Lambert PC, Crowther MJ, Wailoo AJ, Morden JP, Akehurst RL, Campbell MJ (2014) Adjusting survival time estimates to account for treatment switching in randomized controlled trials-an economic evaluation context: methods, limitations, and recommendations. Med Decis Making 34(3):387-402

Lebedev AV, Westman E, Van Westen GJP, et al. for the Alzheimer's Disease Neuroimaging Initiative and the AddNeuroMed consortium (2014) Random Forest ensembles for detection and prediction of Alzheimer's disease with a good between-cohort robustness. NeuroImage: Clinical 6:115-125

LeBlanc M, Crowley J (1992) Relative Risk Trees for Censored Survival Data. Biometrics 48:411-425

LeBlanc M, Crowley J (1993) Survival trees by goodness of split. J Am Stat Assoc 88:457–467

Lee BK, Lessler J, Stuart EA (2010) Improving propensity score weighting using machine learning. Stat Med 29:337-346

Lei H, Nahum-Shani I, Lynch K, Oslin D, Murphy S (2012) A "Smart" design for building individualized treatment sequences. Annu Rev Clin Psychol 8:21–48

Lin Y, Jeon Y (2006) Random forests and adaptive nearest neighbors. J Am Stat Assoc 101 (474):578-590

Linn KA, Laber EB, Stefanski LA (2015) iqLearn: Interactive Q-learning in R J Stat Softw 64(1): i01

Lipkovich I, Dmitrienko A (2014) Strategies for identifying predictive biomarkers and subgroups with enhanced treatment effect in clinical trials using SIDES. J Biopharm Stat 24:130–153

Lipkovich I, Dmitrienko A, D'Agostino BR Sr (2017) Tutorial in biostatistics: Data-driven subgroup identification and analysis in clinical trials. Stat Med 36(1):136-196

Lipkovich IA, Houston JP, Ahl J (2008) Identifying patterns in treatment response profiles in acute bipolar mania: a cluster analysis approach. BMC Psychiatry 8:65

Lipkovich I, Dmitrienko A, Denne J, Enas G (2011) Subgroup identification based on differential effect search (SIDES): A recursive partitioning method for establishing response to treatment in subject subpopulations. Stat Med 30:2601–2621

Lipkovich IA, Choy EH, Van Wambeke P, Deberdt W, Sagman D (2014) Typology of patients with fibromyalgia: cluster analysis of duloxetine study patients. BMC Musculoskeletal Disorders 15:450-460

Lipkovich IA, and Smith EP (2002) Biplot and singular value decomposition macros for Excel©. J Stat Softw 7(5)

Little RJ, Rubin DB (2000) Causal effects in clinical and epidemiological studies via potential outcomes. Annu Rev Public Health 21:121–45

Lloyd S (1957) Least squares quantization in PCM. Technical report, Bell Laboratories. Published in 1982 in IEEE Transactions on Information Theory 28:128–137

Lockhart R, Taylor J, Tibshirani RJ, Tibshirani R (2014) A significance test for the lasso. Ann Stat 42:413–463

Loh W-Y (2002) Regression trees with unbiased variable selection and interaction detection. Statistica Sinca 12:361-386

Loh W-Y (2006) Logistic regression tree analysis. Pham H (ed) Handbook of Engineering Statistics, Springer, New York, pp. 537–549

Loh W-Y (2014) Fifty years of classification and regression trees. Int Statist Rev 82(3):329-348

Loh W-Y, Shih YS (1997) Split selection methods for classification trees. Statistica Sinca 7:815-840

Loh W-Y, Vanichsetakul N (1988) Tree-structured classification via generalized discriminant analysis. J Am Stat Assoc 83:715-725

Loh W-Y, Zheng W (2013) Regression trees for longitudinal and multiresponse data. Ann Applied Statist 7:495-522

Loh W-Y, He X, Man M (2015) A regression tree approach to identifying subgroups with differential treatment effects. Stat Med 34:1818-1833

Loh W-Y, Fu H, Man M, Champion V, Yu M (2016) Identification of subgroups with differential treatment effects for longitudinal and multiresponse variables. Stat Med 35(26):4837-4855

Lu Y, Black D, Genant HK, Mathur AK (2003) Study of hip fracture risk using tree structured survival analysis. Journal für Mineralstoffwechsel 10(1):11-16

Luo Q, Mehra S, Golden NA, Kaushal D, Lacey MR (2014) Identification of biomarkers for tuberculosis susceptibility via integrated analysis of gene expression and longitudinal clinical data. Front Genet 5:240

Lundberg SM, Lee S-I (2017) A unified approach to interpreting model predictions. Adv in Neural Inf Process Syst 30:4765–4774

Lundberg SM, Lee S-I (2018) Consistent individualized feature attribution for tree ensembles. Available arXiv preprint arXiv:1802.03888v3

Macnaughton Smith P, Williams W, Dale M, Mockett L (1965) Dissimilarity analysis: a new technique of hierarchical subdivision. Nature 202:1034–1035

MacQueen J (1967) Some methods for classification and analysis of multivariate observations. LeCam LM, Neyman J (eds) Proceedings of the Fifth Berkeley Symposium on Mathematical Statistics and Probability, University of California Press, 281–297

Madigan D, Raftery A (1994) Model selection and accounting for model uncertainty using Occam's window. J Am Stat Assoc 89:1535–46

Mair J, Smidt J, Lechleiutner P, Dienstl F, Puschendorf B (1995) A decision tree for the early diagnosis of acute myocardial infarction in nontraumatic chest pain patients at hospital admission. Chest 108:1502-1509

Mason L, Baxter J, Bartlett P, Frean M (2000) Boosting algorithms as gradient descent. Adv Neural Inf Process Syst 12:512–518

Mayer C, Lipkovich I, Dmitrienko A (2015) Survey results on industry practices and challenges in subgroup analysis in clinical trials. Stat Biopharm Res 7:272–282

Meinshausen N (2006) Quantile regression forests. J Mach Learn Res 7:983–999

Meinshausen N, Meier L, Bühlmann P (2009) P-values for high-dimensional regression. J Am Stat Assoc 104:1671–1681

Minka T (2002) Bayesian model averaging is not model combination. MIT Media Lab Note https://tminka.github.io/papers/minka-bma-isnt-mc.pdf

Mitchell T (1997) Machine Learning. The McGraw-Hill Companies

Monteith K, Carroll JL, Seppi K, Martinez T (2011) Turning Bayesian model averaging into Bayesian model combination. In: Proceedings of International Joint Conference on Neural Networks, pp. 2657–2663

Moodie EE, Dean N, Sun YR (2014) Q-learning: Flexible learning about useful utilities. Stat Biosci 6(2):223–243

Moodie EE, Richardson TS, Stephens DA (2007) Demystifying optimal dynamic treatment regimes. Biometrics 63(2):447–455

Murphy SA (2003) Optimal dynamic treatment regimes. J R Stat Soc Ser B 65(part 2):331–366

Murphy SA (2005) An experimental design for the development of adaptive treatment strategies. Stat Med 24(10):1455–1481

Muthén B, Brown CH, Masyn K, Jo B, Khoo ST, Yang CC, Wang CP, Kellam SG, Carlin JB, Liao J (2002) General growth mixture modeling for randomized preventive interventions. Biostatistics 3(4):459-75

Nahum-Shani I, Qian M, Almirall D, Pelham WE, Gnagy B, Fabiano GA, Waxmonsky JG, Yu J, Murphy SA (2012) Q-learning: a data analysis method for constructing adaptive interventions. Psychol Methods 17(4):478–494

Neal R, Zhang J (2006) High Dimensional classification with Bayesian neural networks and Dirichlet diffusion trees. Guyon I, Gunn S, Nikravesh M, Zadeh L (eds) Feature Extraction Foundations and Applications. Springer, New York, pp. 265–296

Nelson JC, Zhang Q, Debert W, Marangell LB, Karamustafalioglu O, Lipkovich IA (2012) Predictors of remission with placebo using an integrated study database from patients with major depressive disorder. Curr Med Res Opin 28(3):325-334

NICE (2014) Clinical guideline 175. Prostate cancer: diagnosis and treatment. January 2014. http://www.nice.org.uk/guidance/cg175

O'Kelly M. (2004) Using statistical techniques to detect fraud: A test case. Pharm Stat 3:237–246

Ondra T, Dmitrienko A, Friede T, Gradf A, Miller F, Stallard N, Posh M (2016) Methods for identification and confirmation of targeted subgroups in clinical trials: a systematic review. J Biopharm Stat 26(1):99-119

Orimaye SO, Wong JS-M, Golden KJ, Wong CP, Soyiri IN (2017) Predicting probable Alzheimer's disease using linguistic deficits and biomarkers. BMC Bioinformatics 18:34

Ouanes I, Schwebel C, Franais A, Bruel C, Philippart F, Vesin A, Soufir L, Adrie C, Garrouste-Orgeas M, Timsit JF, Misset B (2012) A model to predict short-term death or readmission after intensive care unit discharge. J Crit Care 27(4):422.e1–422.e9

Padjen I, Radner H, Öhler L, Smolen J, Aletaha D (2016) Understanding anemia in rheumatoid arthritis: The association of hemoglobin and hepcidin levels with clinical disease activity and acute phase response. Ann Rheum Dis 75:476

Patel S, Hee SW, Mistry D, Jordan J, Brown S, Dritsaki M, Ellard DR, Friede T, Lamb SE, Lord J, Madan J, Morris T, Stallard N, Tysall C, Willis A, Underwood M; the Repository Group. (2016) Identifying back pain subgroups: developing and applying approaches using individual patient data collected within clinical trials. Programme Grants for Applied Research, No. 4.10. Patel S, Hee SW, Mistry D, et al.; the Repository Group. Southampton (UK): NIHR Journals Library

Paydar K, Kalhori SRN, Akbarian M, Sheikhtaheri A (2017) A clinical decision support system for prediction of pregnancy outcome in pregnant women with systemic lupus erythematosus. Int J Med Informatics 97:239-246

Pearson K (1901) On lines and planes of closest fit to systems of points in space. Philos Mag 2 (11):559–572

Prinzie A, Van den Poel D (2008) Random Forests for multiclass classification: Random MultiNomial Logit. Expert Syst Appl 34 (3):1721–1732

Qian M, Murphy SA (2011) Performance guarantees for individualized treatment rules. Ann Stat 39:1180–1210

Quinlan JR (1986) Induction of decision trees. Mach Learn 1:81–106

Quinlan JR (1993) C4.5: Programs for Machine Learning. Morgan Kaufmann, San Mateo

Quinlan JR (2004) C5.0, www.rulequest.com

Ripley BD (1996) Pattern Recognition and Neural Networks. Cambridge University Press

Robins JM, Finkelstein DM (2000) Correcting for noncompliance and dependent censoring in an AIDS clinical trial with inverse probability of censoring weighted (IPCW) log-rank tests. Biometrics 56(3):779-788

Rosenkranz GK (2016). Exploratory subgroup analysis in clinical trials by model selection. Biom J 58(5):1217-1228

Royston P, Sauerbrei W (2004) A new approach to modelling interaction between treatment and continuous covariates in clinical trials by using fractional polynomials. Stat Med 23:2509–2525

Royston P, Sauerbrei W (2013) Interaction of treatment with a continuous variable: simulation study of power for several methods of analysis. Stat Med 32:3788-3803

Rumelhart D, Hinton G, Williams R (1986) Learning internal representations by error propagation. Rumelhart D, McClelland J (eds) Parallel Distributed Processing: Explorations in the Microstructure of Cognition, The MIT Press, Cambridge, MA. pp. 318–362

Sacchet MD, Prasad G, Foland-Ross LC, Thompson PM, Gotlib IH (2015) Support vector machine classification of major depressive disorder using diffusion-weighted neuroimaging and graph theory. Front Psychiatry 6:21

Sachs GS, Thase ME, Otto MW, Bauer M, Miklowitz D, Wisniewski SR, et al. (2003) Rationale, design, and methods of the systematic treatment enhancement program for bipolar disorder (step-bd). Biol Psychiatry 53(11):1028–1042

Sandri M, Zuccolotto P (2008) A bias correction algorithm for the Gini variable importance measure in classification trees. J Comput Graph Stat 17(3):1-18

Schnell PM, Tang Q, Offen WW, Carlin BP (2016) A Bayesian credible subgroups approach to identifying patient subgroups with positive treatment effects. Biometrics 72(4):1026-1036

Schölkopf, B, Smola A, Müller K-R (1997) Kernel principal component analysis. P of International Conference on Artificial Neural Networks: 583–588

Schulte PJ, Tsiatis AA, Laber EB, Davidian M (2014) Q-and A-learning methods for estimating optimal dynamic treatment regimes. Stat Sci 29(4):640-661

Schwarz G (1978) Estimating the dimension of a model. Ann Stat 6(2):461–464

Segal MR (1988) Regression trees for censored data. Biometrics 44(1):35-47

Segal MR (2004) Machine learning benchmarks and random forest regression. Technical report, eScholarship Repository, University of California. https://escholarship.org/uc/item/35x3v9t4

Segal M, Xiao Y (2011) Multivariate random forests. WIREs Data Mining and Knowledge Discovery 1:80–87

Seibold H, Zeileis A, Hothorn T (2015) Model-based recursive partitioning for subgroup analyses. Int J Biostat 12(1)

Seibold H, Zeileis A, Hothorn T (2016) Individual treatment effect prediction for ALS patients. Available arXiv preprint arXiv: 1604.08720

Shawe-Taylor J, Cristianini N (2004) Kernel Methods for Pattern Analysis. Cambridge University Press

Shi T, Seligson D, Belldegrun AS, Palotie A, Horvath S (2005) Tumor classification by tissue microarray profiling: random forest clustering applied to renal cell carcinoma. Mod Pathol 18 (4):547–557

Shortreed SM, Laber E, Lizotte DJ, Stroup TS, Pineau J, Murphy SA (2011) Informing sequential clinical decision-making through reinforcement learning: an empirical study. Mach Learn 84 (1–2):109–36

Sibson R (1973) SLINK: an optimally efficient algorithm for the single-link cluster method. Comput J British Comput Soc 16 (1):30–34

Simon RM, Subramanian J, Li MC, Menezes S (2011) Using cross validation to evaluate the predictive accuracy of survival risk classifiers based on high dimensional data. Briefings in Bioinformatics 1–12

Sterne JA, May M, Costagliola D, De Wolf F, Phillips AN, Harris R, et al. (2009) Timing of initiation of antiretroviral therapy in AIDS-free HIV-1-infected patients: a collaborative analysis of 18 HIV cohort studies. The Lancet 373(9672):1352–63

Stone M (1974) Cross-validatory choice and assessment of statistical predictions. J Roy Stat Soc Series B 36:111–147

Strecher VJ, Shiffman S, West R (2006) Moderators and mediators of a web-based computer-tailored smoking cessation program among nicotine patch users. Nicotine Tob Res 8(S.1):S95-S101

Strobl C (2008) Statistical Issues in Machine Learning – Towards Reliable Split Selection and Variable Importance Measures. Dissertation, Ludwig-maximilians-universität München

Su X, Tsai CL, Wang H, Nickerson DM, Li B (2009) Subgroup analysis via recursive partitioning. J Mach Learn Res 10:141–158

Su X, Zhou T, Yan X, Fan J, Yang S (2008) Interaction trees with censored survival data. Int J Biostat 4(1), 2

Sunkaria RK, Kumar V, Saxena SC, Singhal AM (2014) An ANN-based HRV classifier for cardiac health prognosis. Electron Health 7:315–330

Sutton RS, Barto AG (1998) Reinforcement Learning: An Introduction. MIT Press: Cambridge, MA

Tang F, Ishwaran H (2017) Random forest missing data algorithms. Stat Anal Data Min 00:1–14; DOI: 10.1002/sam.11348; arXiv preprint arXiv: 1701.05305

Therneau TM, Granbsch PM, Fleming TR (1990) Martingale-based residuals for survival models. Biometrika 77:147-160

Thomas M, Bornkamp B (2017) Comparing approaches to treatment effect estimation for subgroups in clinical trials. Stat Biopharm Res 9(2): 160-171

Tian X, Bi N, Taylor J (2016) MAGIC: a general, powerful and tractable method for selective inference. arXiv preprint arXiv: 1607.02630v

Tibshirani R (1996) Regression shrinkage and selection via the lasso. J R Statist Soc Series B 58 (1):267-288

Tipping ME, Bishop CM (1999) Probabilistic principal component analysis. J R Stat Soc Series B 61(Part 3):611-622

Tukey JW (1977) Exploratory Data Analysis. Pearson

van Buuren S (2018) Flexible Imputation of Missing Data. 2nd ed. Boca Raton, FL: Chapman & Hall/CRC

Vapnik V (1996) The Nature of Statistical Learning Theory. Springer, New York.

Vapnik V (2006) Estimation of Dependences Based on Empirical Data. Empirical Inference Science Afterword of 2006. Springer: New York

Varma S, Simon R (2006) Bias in error estimation when using crossvalidation for model selection. BMC Bioinformatics 7:91

Vsevolozhskaya OA, Greenwood MC, Powell SL, Zaykin DV (2015) Resampling-based multiple comparison procedure with application to point-wise testing with functional data. Environ Ecol Stat 22(1):45–59

Wager S, Hastie T, Efron B (2014) Intervals for Random Forests: The jackknife and the infinitesimal jackknife. J Mach Learn Res 15:1625-1651

Wang L, Rotnitzky A, Lin X, Millikan R, Thal, P (2012) Evaluation of viable dynamic treatment regimes in a sequentially randomized trial of advanced prostate cancer. J Am Stat Assoc 107:493–508

Wang H, Zhang X, Zou G (2009) Frequentist model averaging estimation: A review. Jrl Syst Sci & Complexity 22:732-748

Ward JH (1963) Hierarchical grouping to optimize an objective function. J Am Stat Assoc 58 (301):236–244

Watkin CJCH (1989) Learning from Delayed Rewards. Ph.D. Thesis, Cambridge University

Watkin CJCH, Dayan P (1992) Q-Learning. Mach Learn 8:279-292

Werbos PJ (1975) Beyond Regression: New Tools for Prediction and Analysis in the Behavioral Sciences, PhD Thesis Harvard University

Westfall PH, Troendle JF (2008) Multiple testing with minimal assumptions. Biometrics J 50 (5):745-55

Westfall PH, Young SS (1993) Resampling-based multiple testing: Examples and methods for p-value adjustment. Wiley: New York

White NJ, Contaifer Jr D, Martin EJ, Newton JC, Mohammed BM, Bostic JL, Brophy GM, Spiess BD, Pusateri AE, Ward KR, Brophy DF (2015) Early hemostatic responses to trauma identified with hierarchical clustering analysis. J Thromb Haemost 13:978–88

Witten IH, Frank E, Hall MA (2011) Data Mining. Practical Machine Learning Tools and Techniques. 3rd Edition. Morgan Kaufmann: Burlington, USA

Wu F, Laber EB, Lipkovich IA, Severus E (2015) Who will Benefit from Antidepressants in the Acute Treatment of Bipolar Depression? A Reanalysis of the STEP-BD Study by Sachs et al. 2007, Using Q-learning. Int J Bipolar Disord 3:7

Wu MJ, Mwangi B, Bauer IE, Passos IC, Sanches M, Zunta-Soares GB, Meyer TD, Hasan KM, Soares JC (2017) Identification and individualized prediction of clinical phenotypes in bipolar disorders using neurocognitive data, neuroimaging scans and machine learning. NeuroImage Part B, 145:254-264

Wu W, Bleecker E, Moore W, Busse WW, Castro M, Chung KF, Calhoun WJ, Erzurum S, Gaston B, Israel E, Curran-Everett D, Wenzel SE (2014) Unsupervised phenotyping of Severe Asthma Research Program participants using expanded lung data. J Allergy Clin Immunol 133 (5):1280-1288

Xu R (2013) Improvements to random forest methodology. PhD thesis, Iowa State University, Iowa, USA

Xu Y, Yu M, Zhao YQ, Li Q, Wang S, Shao J (2015) Regularized outcome weighted subgroup identification for differential treatment effects. Biometrics 71(3):645-53

Zhang B, Tsiatis AA, Laber EB, Davidian M (2013) Robust estimation of optimal dynamic treatment regimes for sequential treatment decisions. Biometrika 100(3):681–94

Zhang B, Tsiatis AA, Davidian M, Zhang M, Laber EB (2012) Estimating optimal treatment regimes from a classification perspective. Statistics 1:103–114

Zhang H (1995) Splitting criteria in survival trees. Seeber GUH, Francis BJ, Hatzinger R, Steckel-Berger G (eds) Statistical Modeling, Proceedings of the 10th International Workshop on Statistical Modeling, Springer, New York.305-314

Zhang Y, Laber EB, Tsiatis A, Davidian M (2015) Using decision lists to construct interpretable and parsimonious treatment regimes. Biometrics 71:895–904

Zhao Y, Zheng D, Rush AJ, Kosorok MR (2012) Estimating individualized treatment rules using outcome weighted learning. J Am Stat Assoc 107:1106–1118

Zhao YQ, Zeng D, Laber EB, Kosorok MR (2015) New statistical learning methods for estimating optimal dynamic treatment regimes. J Am Stat Assoc 110(510):583-598

Zheng B, Yoon SW, Lam SS (2014) Breast cancer diagnosis based on feature extraction using a hybrid of K-means and support vector machine algorithms. Expert Syst Appl 41(4):1476-1482

Zou H (2006) The adaptive lasso and Its oracle properties. J Am Statist Assoc 101(476):1418-1429

Zou H, Hastie T (2005) Regularization and variable selection via the elastic net. J R Statist Soc Series B 67(Part 2):301-320

Zou H, Hastie T, Tibshirani R (2006) Sparse principal component analysis. J Comp Graph Stat 15 (2):262–286

Chapter 7
Segmentation and Choice Models

Steven Blahut and Jeff Niemira

7.1 Online Data Collection: The Current Standard

Currently, primary data for quantitative market research are typically collected via online Internet survey. There are a variety of survey vendors who host the survey, invite participants, and collect and warehouse the resulting data. The instrument itself is developed as a text document with specific instructions to the vendor programming team to follow. These instructions may include, but are not limited to, termination and screening criteria, question skip logic, item counterbalancing and rotation, and prohibiting obviously contradictory responses.

Typically, these vendors own proprietary panels of potential respondents such as health-care providers (HCPs) or consumer/patients. HCP panels typically consist of a list of practicing physicians, physician assistants, nurse practitioners, and the like that have "opted in" (i.e., have agreed to participate in online market research). In exchange for participating, they are provided with an honoraria based on factors such as survey length and complexity, as well as specialty and the prevalence of the disease state being studied. Similarly, consumer panels are databases of disease sufferers or caregivers who have also agreed to participate in research. Members of such panels are offered compensation for their participation. Compensation varies but most often comes in the form of cash, gift cards, or points that can be redeemed for goods and services.

S. Blahut (✉) · J. Niemira
Healthcare Strategy Partners, Washington D.C., USA
e-mail: steven.blahut@quintilesims.com

© Springer Nature Switzerland AG 2020
O. V. Marchenko, N. V. Katenka (eds.), *Quantitative Methods in Pharmaceutical Research and Development*, https://doi.org/10.1007/978-3-030-48555-9_7

7.1.1 The Role of "Pre-launch" Qualitative Research

For most types of pharmaceutical market research, it is advisable to conduct a set of qualitative interviews with key stakeholders prior to launching the online survey. It is critical to ensure that the language and the content of the survey are readily understood by potential participants and that the survey is objective and measures the desired domains. This is typically done by interviewing a small but reasonably representative subset of the potential target audience either in person or via telephone. In this qualitative phase, the entire survey is inspected by the market researcher and the stakeholders, paying careful attention to wording, technical or clinical concepts, and any specific jargon. The intent is to minimize any potential confusion for online participants that could lead to erroneous responses that could negatively impact the findings.

7.1.2 Survey Complexity and Length Considerations

Complexity of the survey instrument is a key consideration of any market research. The focus of this chapter is on two of the more difficult survey types to develop—segmentation and conjoint. While either type of survey can be long and/or complex, market segmentation surveys tend to be long and conjoint surveys tend to be complex.

Survey length has a direct impact on cost—longer surveys cost more. The market research team spends more time developing them, vendors charge more to program them, and respondents are given higher honoraria (or other forms of compensation) to complete them. Therefore it is incumbent upon the research team to strike a balance of content and length. The *quantity* of data collected in a 30 min survey may not be as great as a 60 min survey, but the *quality* of the data may indeed be superior. Respondent fatigue is a very legitimate concern in longer surveys. Thoughtfulness of response tends to decline toward the end of a large instrument. This can be somewhat mitigated by rotating and randomizing the presentation of the various survey sections across the sample such that various sections are completed in different order.

Survey complexity also has cost implications. Complex conjoint and discrete choice designs are time-consuming and costly for vendors to program. Similarly, questionnaires containing complicated skip logic require careful and time-consuming review by the research team and vendors to avoid errors (which can have considerable opportunity costs).

7.1.3 "Soft-Launch" and In-Field Data Monitoring

Once the survey instrument has been programmed and vetted by the research team, it is advisable to do a "soft-launch" prior to fielding the survey. A soft launch is done by inviting a small number of potential respondents to take the survey before it is sent out to the larger group to complete. This is useful for several reasons. First, it allows the team to determine the actual length of completion based on surveys collected from a representative group of subjects. If the survey is running longer than expected, items can be altered or removed to bring it in line with the intended length. Second, it allows the team to ensure that the data being collected in the survey is being stored in a data file consistent with the vision of the analysts involved. Complex surveys involving skip logic and counterbalancing can be programmed in a manner inconsistent with programming instructions. This check of the data by the team ensures that variables, response codes, and programming logic are being properly followed when the survey goes out to the larger pool of respondents. It would be unfortunate to gather data from the entire sample only then to realize some metrics are being captured and/or stored incorrectly. Finally, it is an opportunity for the analyst to check that experimental designs created for conjoint or other exercises are being followed properly.

Once the team is satisfied that the survey and programming are being executed properly, the survey can then be fully launched. While the survey is being fielded, it is critical that the team checks daily progress to monitor length and incidence of key sample subgroups and to monitor the data for outliers and suspect responses.

7.1.3.1 Excluding Cases and Why

Online surveys are completed in a more anonymous, unmonitored setting than other types of research (such as in-person qualitative interviews). The assumption is that the vast majority of respondents of surveys of this type take it seriously and provide thoughtful honest responses. In pharmaceutical research, this is due to the fact that most often surveys are being completed by an individual who either suffers from, cares for, or treats those who suffer from a given disease or illness. However, it is still necessary to closely inspect the data for subjects who may not be providing accurate responses and flag those entries for potential exclusion. There are three effective approaches to identifying questionable cases.

Rapid Response

The easiest offenders to identify are those who finish the survey in an incredibly short amount of time. It is just not reasonable to assume that someone can finish a survey designed to be 45 min in 10 or 15 min. The datasets provided by fielding vendors should include the length of interview (LOI) for each respondent. The data of those finishing in less than half the expected time should be carefully reviewed.

"Flat Liners"

"Flat liners" refers to subjects who consistently provide the same answer over multiple questions and question batteries—even though they are meant to measure different domains. Take the example of a survey containing 50 seven-point Likert scale items covering different content (e.g., severity of disease, satisfaction with current treatment, general attitudes, etc.). It is completely reasonable to question the responses of a subject who provides the same answer across all items. These folks are obviously trying to finish the survey as fast as possible in order to obtain the honoraria without putting any real thought or effort into their responses. Often those guilty of being "rapid responders" are also "flat liners."

"Contradictors"

A well-constructed survey will include multiple items meant to measure the same construct. A good research team will reverse word some of these items. The intent is to ensure respondents are carefully reading the survey and providing thoughtful answers. Respondents who supply obviously contradictory responses to several items meant to measure the same construct are suspect, and their data should be carefully examined.

7.2   Market Segmentation

7.2.1   What Is Segmentation and What Are the Goals of Such Research?

Market segmentation has been an important part of business decision-making for decades. The first formal treatment on the subject comes from Wendell Smith (1956). The basic assumption underpinning such work is that any existing market is actually a heterogeneous collection of smaller, more homogeneous sub-markets. Each of these sub-markets, or segments, has specific beliefs, needs, attitudes, and behaviors. It is the unique composition of each segment that allows for targeted advertising, messaging, and product positioning. Essentially, segmentation creates the schematic for more efficient resource allocation in order to increase market share and thus revenue.

   In the pharmaceutical and biotech sectors, many millions of dollars are spent on research and development, clinical trials, and the approval process. Segmentation is the cornerstone of nonclinical market research guiding such activities as salesforce sizing and deployment, market targeting, message optimization, and message delivery channels. A good segmentation should provide guidance not only those segments to target (through segment-specific marketing, messaging, etc.) but also those to deprioritize, thus maximizing the impact of marketing spend.

7.2.2 Pre-launch vs. Post-Launch Segmentation

Another key consideration around segment development is when the research is being conducted. Segmentation can be done at any point along the product life cycle. Often, it is done well before launch while the product is in later phase clinical trials. In this case, the goal of the research is to identify the current landscape of the market and to identify opportunity targets for non-product-specific pre-launch marketing. Segmentation is also a valuable exercise as the product approaches launch to understand segments that have higher potential for early adoption. Segmenting at this time can also reveal groups of stakeholders who are overly loyal to existing therapies and thus may be harder to move toward a new offering. Post-launch segmentation is useful in understanding changes in stakeholder dynamics due to meaningful market events (e.g., product recalls, novel therapy entrants, changes in pricing, etc.).

7.2.3 Art vs. Science

A common misconception is that segments are discovered and not created. This belief is often held by less experienced analysts and audiences and should be dispelled as early in the process as possible. A good segmentation is the by-product of careful consideration of how it will ultimately be leveraged. For example, the goals of a segmentation that will ultimately influence salesforce allocation may look quite different than one designed to influence messaging and advertising spend. In other instances, the segmentation is a tool to help develop personas for each group in an attempt to understand each set's unique needs in terms of product or service offerings. Regional differences in the ability to conduct direct-to-consumer advertising are often an important consideration in determining how the segmentation solution will ultimately be leveraged. Some physician segmentations are totally behavioral in nature. That is, the data used to create segments is purely secondary and includes information such as prescription data (total Rx, new Rx, new to brand Rx, etc.). The resulting segmentation solution will be completely dictated by prescribing behavior and will identify high-, mid-, and low-level volume prescribers across the various products that have been used to create the segments. Other segmentations are purely "attitudinal" in nature. These can be developed for stakeholders such as physicians, patients, caregivers, or payers. Solutions of this type

are developed using completely self-explicated data from an online survey. Attitudinal segmentations are based solely on respondents' perceptions of their needs,
attitudes, and behaviors. A common approach to segmenting physicians is to
integrate the behavioral and attitudinal data to develop a more holistic segmentation
solution. Holistic segmentation requires careful consideration of the data input into
the models that develop solutions to ensure that candidate solutions do not over- or
underemphasize either type of input.

7.2.4 Top-Down vs. Bottom-Up

Segmentation solutions can be developed in an a priori or top-down approach as well
as a more "data-driven" bottom-up approach. An example of a top-down segmentation would be to create groups based on a preexisting characteristic. In physician
research, this often means specialty or prescribing volume. In patients, it is often
previous treatment or disease severity. For international research, regardless of
audience, either region or country is often considered. The schematic for such an
approach can be found in Fig. 7.1.

Often in a top-down approach, one or more of the a priori groups will be
subsegmented to identify interesting subgroups within them.

The major benefit of the top-down approach is that segments are more easily
understood and identified. Using an observable characteristic as a driving force in
segment creation is often desirable to audiences that want a more clear-cut rule for
segment membership. Segment membership can be easily identified by some easily
observable characteristic. For a purely behavioral segmentation approach, this is an
attractive feature: the five-segment solution implied in Fig. 7.2 organizes the market
in an easy to understand way. For example, segments 1 and 3 might be higher-
volume prescribers of FPs and IMs, respectively, while segments 2 and 4 are lower-
volume prescribers. Segment 5 by default is made up entirely of specialists. In many
instances, having specialists in one segment is attractive as there tend to be fewer of
them and they are often higher-volume prescribers in a given market due to their
concentration on the disease in question. Of course, any a priori group can be
segmented into subgroups regardless of whether the segmentation is behavioral,
attitudinal, or holistic in nature. However, imposing known a priori groups can lead

Fig. 7.1 Top-down
segmentation conceptual
approach

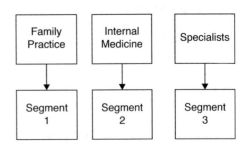

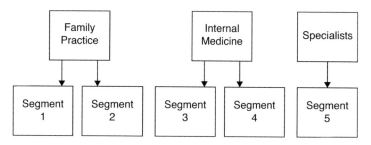

Fig. 7.2 Top-down segmentation with subsegments

to diminished inter-segment differences on other metrics not used to define the groups but meant to profile them. Attitudinal and self-stated belief metrics collected in primary research will often have fewer meaningful differences between segments when this approach is employed.

Alternatively, a "bottom-up" segmentation takes a more "data-driven" approach to segment creation. In this type of segmentation, the analyst creates segments without pre-specifying groups of segment identifiers of any kind. All available and suitable data are considered as potential segmentation inputs. This approach allows the a priori groups from a top-down segmentation to appear in any and all segments. Segments are created more organically by the various clustering algorithms that will be discussed subsequently. Segmentation solutions of this type tend to maximize difference between segments more than the top-down approach, and the resulting segments tend to be more homogeneous.

It is the scrupulous and thorough analyst that will develop and consider multiple options based on both approaches to determine an exhaustive set of candidate solutions.

7.2.5 Instrument (Survey) Development

7.2.5.1 Considerations for Online Data Collection

A typical segmentation questionnaire takes 30–45 min for respondents to complete online. This usually translates to a hardcopy of the survey in the range of 40–60 pages. The document must be explicit regarding the acceptable range of response for each item, skip patterns, and any notes for programmers to successfully transform the text document to a dynamic online survey. The actual length of the survey is a function of multiple factors:

- The number of items to be completed
- The complexity of each item
- Length and density of any text respondents are asked to review

A key consideration is respondent fatigue. While most surveys don't require that they be completed in one sitting, a long, dense instrument can compromise the quality of responses—especially toward the end. Counterbalancing of the different survey sections is often done to mitigate order bias. It is also a good idea to vary the types of questions respondents are answering. Varying the question and data collection methods within the survey can help to keep respondents engaged and lessen the likelihood of "flat liners" and "contradictors" previously mentioned.

7.2.5.2 Item Development

The goal of segmentation is to develop discrete subgroups within the data. To that end, the content of questions being asked must be carefully considered. Ideally, many or most of the questions being asked should be designed to capture divergence of opinion across the sample. A classic example from consumer goods segmentation is "Do you prefer Coke or Pepsi?" Usually people have a preexisting opinion which helps place them into like subgroups. In pharmaceutical market research with physicians, questions of this type might be "What is more important efficacy or safety?" For patients, it may be "When considering a new medication, what is more important—cost or convenience?" While these are simplified examples, the point is clear—the goal should be to include items that elicit responses across all possible options for items across the sample. The goal is to gather a wide variety of responses on as many items as possible.

There will of course be items included that may not elicit such diverse responses. For example, when it comes to price, less is almost always perceived as better. In patient populations, considering route of drug administration, oral is almost always preferred over injections or infusion. In the case where a new product offering is shared with respondents that is clearly better than the current standard of care, it would be expected that responses would be overwhelmingly positive and therefore similar. Items that produce more uniformity of response are still valuable. They can be used to profile segments and uncover "universal truths" across segments and therefore the entire market. But they will not differentiate and serve as the basis of the segmentation solution.

7.2.5.3 Data Collection Approaches

There are a variety of ways to ask questions and collect data in research of this type. As previously stated, it is advisable to incorporate several data collection techniques in the survey instrument to keep respondents engaged. Here we discuss a few of the more popular options.

Likert: Type Items

One of the most popular survey question types for capturing attitudes is the Likert item (Burnes 2008). Items of this type ask for response to a statement in the form of a quantitative answer along a numeric continuum. The most popular response scale is agreement; however, others are often used as well. Likert items can have a different number of response options, typically 5, 7, 9, or 11 (Dawes 2008). An example of a seven-point Likert item is in Fig. 7.3.

A well-crafted Likert item will typically have a neutral midpoint and an equal number of positive and negative response options on either side. It is crucial that the appropriate verbal anchors are placed on the scale to ensure proper context is given to the respondent. This is a very efficient means of data collection. Items of this type are often put into multi-item batteries to collect responses to multiple items that are representative of a similar topic or theme. However, one potential drawback of these items is that respondents have the opportunity to give the same rating to many items.

Ranking Items

Ranking items differ in that they force respondents to order a set of options from most to least on a continuum. This continuum may be desirability, importance, or anything relevant to the product or market being investigated. Items of this type are often used to determine what product features or offerings are more or less appealing to different potential segments. An example of a ranking item is in Fig. 7.4.

	Strongly Disagree			Neither Agree nor Disagree			Strongly Agree
	[1]	[2]	[3]	[4]	[5]	[6]	[7]
I often try new medications before my colleagues do	O	O	O	O	O	O	O

Fig. 7.3 Seven-point Likert item

Please rank the following product features in order of importance where 1 is most important and 4 is least important

Minimal Side Effects	
Twice a Day Dosing (BID)	
Increased Efficacy	
Cost	

Fig. 7.4 Ranking items

Items of this type can be useful to help define different unmet needs by segment. That is, the priority implied by the ranked list differs by segment. These items do not uncover the relative distance between each of the options being ranked; they provide the order in terms of priority and appeal only.

A common variant of the ranking item is the point allocation item. In this case, respondents are asked to allocate 100 points across the options giving the highest number of points to the most important and the smallest amount to the least important. Instructions are often provided that prohibit the allocation of the same amount of points to any two options so that ties are eliminated.

Forced-Choice Approaches

Forced-choice items can be similar to ranking items, but instead of ordering the options in terms of appeal or importance, the respondent is asked to choose the one most important or appealing item from the list. While items of this type provide less information than the ranking alternative, they can be used to break down the survey into different sections so as to keep respondents more engaged.

Other Approaches

Although there are many ways to collect survey data for a segmentation question-naire, one of the most common is the free response item. In items of this type, respondents are typically asked to enter a numeric response. "What percent of your patients receive Product X?" and "How many medications do you currently take?" are common examples. Another common option is the "select all that apply" technique. Here, respondents are presented with a list and asked to select each option that is pertinent to them. These are often done to quantify concomitant conditions, previous therapies, or anything that can be represented in a closed list. Open-ended/ free text questions are not ideal for segmentation as it requires recoding of text responses to make them suitable for analysis.

Some approaches are just by-products of modern programming. For example, a ranking or force-choice item can be programmed as a drag and drop exercise. Instead of respondents just entering in number rankings or clicking the most important, the exercise becomes more interactive and makes survey completion less tedious for respondents.

7.2.6 Defining the Sample

Sample frame development for segmentation is an important step that requires careful consideration. Most often in pharmaceutical market research, samples are stratified by physician specialty or patient type. Practitioners and patients require different considerations so we consider them here separately.

7.2.6.1   HCP Research

There are multiple considerations to keep in mind when developing the sample frame for physician research. Most important is to consider which specialties define the market of interest, and that therefore must be represented in the final sample. For less common diseases such as multiple sclerosis, it may be only one—neurologists. For more widespread diseases such as diabetes, there may be multiple specialties involved in treatment—family practice, internal medicine, endocrinologists, nurse practitioners, physician assistants, etc. The target market must be defined and the largest sample that budget allows must be allocated to the appropriate strata.

In the case of a single specialty, sample size may be determined by the number of physicians willing to participate in such research that can be identified. In that case, the sample may be stratified by prescribing decile, patient volume, or some other metric meant to represent productivity in the marketplace. Deciling breaks down the prescriber universe into ten groups of physicians that each prescribe 10% of the product. Higher deciles contain fewer physicians that write more prescriptions. Lower deciles contain more doctors who write relatively fewer prescriptions. Often there is a source list that identifies active physicians in the market. If there is no list available, then decile is typically unavailable and cases can be weighted based on self-reported metrics such a monthly patient volume. This list serves as the "universe" of prescribers that the segmentation is meant to represent. In most markets, the top deciles include the fewest doctors that write the most prescriptions. Conversely, the lower deciles contain many more physicians who write fewer prescriptions, on average. Table 7.1 contains a typical distribution of physician by decile in a specialty market made up of 8537 doctors.

In specialty segmentations with a universe such as the one outlined in Table 7.1, it is unlikely that a sample much more than 300 can be achieved—due to budget, time,

Table 7.1 Physicians by decile

Decile	N	Percent (%)
10	171	2.0
9	299	3.5
8	393	4.6
7	487	5.7
6	589	6.9
5	717	8.4
4	871	10.2
3	1076	12.6
2	1409	16.5
1	2527	29.6
Total	8537	100

Table 7.2 Hypothetical sample and case weights from a single specialty sample

Decile	N	Percent (%)	Self-weighting sample	Actual sample (n)	Actual percent (%)	Weight
7–10	1349	15.8	48	41	13.7	1.156
3–6	3253	38.1	114	105	35.0	1.089
1–2	3936	46.1	138	154	51.3	0.898
Total	8537	100	300	300	100	

Table 7.3 Hypothetical sample and case weights from a two-specialty sample

Specialty	Decile	N	Percent (%)	Self-weighting sample	Actual sample (n)	Actual percent (%)	Weight
OB/GYN	7–10	3644	6.3	31	35	7.0	0.895
OB/GYN	3–6	6069	10.4	52	47	9.4	1.110
OB/GYN	1–2	10,654	18.3	92	100	20.0	0.916
PCP	7–10	5509	9.5	47	53	10.6	0.894
PCP	3–6	16,070	27.6	138	117	23.4	1.181
PCP	1–2	16,214	27.9	140	148	29.6	0.942
	Total	58,160	100	500	500	100	

or response limitations. Therefore the number strata is reduced by collapsing them into a more manageable number of groups. Table 7.2 contains information about a sample and case weights that are calculated from these distributions.

The decile column shows the manner in which those groups were collapsed. Column N shows the actual number of physicians in the universe that exist in each of these new collapsed strata. If a proportional allocation of a sample of 300 was applied to these collapsed strata, the sample would be distributed as displayed in the column "self-weighting sample." The actual sample and actual percent columns contain the sample of 300 that was successfully fielded. The weight column contains the case weights for analysis. The weight is calculated as N/n. Application of this weight during analysis will allow for accurate estimates of segment sizes in the market.

In the case of a multi-specialty segmentation, a similar approach is usually followed. However, the weights are typically calculated by a multi-strata design of specialty x decile. Table 7.3 displays a hypothetical sample and weighting approach for a two-specialty sample of 500 physicians.

This approach is quite useful particularly if the resulting segmentation solution scheme is ultimately to be projected back to the source universe, as will be discussed in a subsequent section.

7.2.6.2   Patient/Caregiver Research

When segmenting patients, there are a variety of factors that may dictate sample frame development. Severity of disease and prior therapies are commonly used to create sample strata. The composition of the market in terms of these potential strata can be gleaned from epidemiological data. The sample is then developed in a way to ensure representation of the market. As with physician samples, deviations from the market reflected in the final sample are corrected through the calculation of case weights. Table 7.4 illustrates a hypothetical sample stratified by previous treatment and the calculation of the case weight to adjust for sample discrepancies.

As with physician research, the sample frame may be more complex with multiple strata. A similar approach to weight calculation would be taken for patients as well.

7.2.7   Data Preparation

Once the data are collected, there are several steps that should be taken to ensure the proper subset is chosen for segmenting. From a 45 min online survey, hundreds of variables will be collected and stored in the database. Not all of these will make for strong potential foundation variables—the set of metrics that will actually be used to create the segments. All of the collected variables will be used to profile segments from the candidate solutions. However, identifying the foundational subset is critical. For most segmentation efforts, a good set of foundation variables will number somewhere between 40 and 70 unique metrics.

In pharmaceutical market segmentation, there is often a treatment and/or diagnostic (new or otherwise) that is/are the focus of the work. There are several steps to ensure that the correct foundation variables are selected for analysis so that the resulting segments can be prioritized relative to the product(s) of interest.

Table 7.4 Hypothetical sample and case weights from a patient sample stratified by previous treatment

Prior treatments	Percent (epi data) (%)	Self-weighting sample	Actual sample (n)	Actual percent (%)	Weight
None	26.5	106	95	23.8	1.116
1	41.4	166	187	46.8	0.886
2+	32.1	128	118	29.5	1.088
Total	100	400	400	100	

7.2.7.1 Identification of Foundation Variables: Selecting the Right Subset

Key Driver/Regression Analyses

A good segmentation instrument will provide a product profile(s) of the product (s) being studied. This will be followed by a series of questions similar to "How likely would you be to prescribe this product to your patients?" or "How likely would you be to request this product from your doctor?" for physicians and patients, respectively. These direct call-to-action questions are well suited to serve as dependent measures in regression-type models to uncover what other survey items correlate highly with the desired product-specific behaviors.

Regression methods have been exhaustively explained elsewhere (e.g., Draper and Smith 1998; Hosmer et al. 2013; Pedhauzer 1997). In the key driver analysis, the goal is to uncover a set of survey items that are predictive of intent relative to the product(s) of interest. The usual pitfalls of multi-collinearity and spurious relations among independent measures must be considered and accounted for. Identification of this subset of key drivers isolates an important subset of potential foundational variables. These items will be further vetted for consideration in subsequent steps.

Factor Analytic Models

A next step in identifying the foundation variables is to organize the survey items into similar themes or domains. A good segmentation includes in its set of foundation variables those that represent numerous different domains. Factor and principal component analyses are both appropriate tools to organize the survey data into a smaller set of latent constructs (Child 2006; McDonald 1985). The two approaches are not identical (Bartholomew et al. 2008), but both are appropriate for understanding the latent structure underlying the survey data.

The factor analysis is not the segmenting algorithm, nor should it be (Stewart 1981). Rather it is a tool to help the analyst understand and organize the large set of potential foundation variables. Therefore, when the foundation variables are selected, no one theme or themes is overly represented in the set.

Distributional Analyses

Once the key drivers have been identified and the survey items have been organized into factors, the next step is to look at this distribution of response *for all candidate foundation variables.* The most efficient way to do this is to look at the histograms of all of the potential foundation variables. When inspecting these distributions, it is critical to identify those that imply a range of opinion. Multimode and uniform distributions are most appealing as they indicate that responses were not limited to

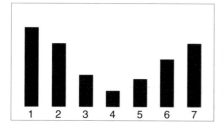
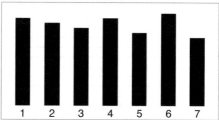

Fig. 7.5 Desirable distributions of potential foundation variables

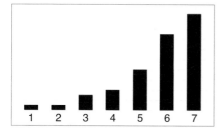
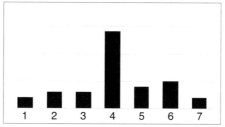

Fig. 7.6 Poor distributions of potential foundation variables

one point or end of the scale. Figure 7.5 illustrates two appealing candidates for inclusion as foundation variables.

Conversely, unimodal and highly skewed distributions are not good candidates for foundation variables as most responses are similar and thus don't imply subgroups or segments from those measures. While variables with these distributions are not good candidates for segment creation, they are useful in uncovering "universal truths," that is, attitudes or beliefs that are similar and consistent regardless of segment membership. Figure 7.6 illustrates two such distributions.

7.2.8 Segment Estimation

Once the foundation variable set has been identified, there are a multitude of clustering approaches that are available to derive segments from the data. Here, a few of the more common approaches are described in more detail.

7.2.8.1 K-Means

K-means is an algorithm that relies upon iterative refinement to arrive at the final result. It has been described in detail elsewhere (Hamerly and Elkan 2002; Hartigan and Clustering 1975; MacQueen 1967). In this approach, a pre-specified number of

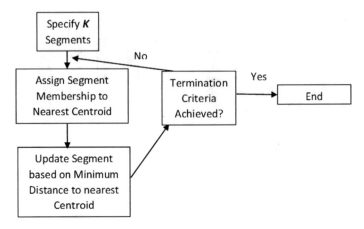

Fig. 7.7 K-means algorithm

segments K is provided to the algorithm, and each segment is defined by one of the K centroids. The initial values of each centroid can be provided by the analyst or randomly generated. The algorithm then proceeds by iterating between two steps. In step one, cases are assigned to the segment defined by the nearest centroid, typically by minimizing the squared Euclidean distance between the two. In step two, the centroids are recalculated by deriving the mean of all data assigned to each cluster centroid. The algorithm continues to repeat these steps until the termination criterion is achieved. The criteria for stopping can be the total number of iterations allowed or that no respondents change segments in the previous step. The K-means approach does not require a dependent measure to converge. Rather, it requires only a set of variables in multidimensional space segmented by their proximity to cluster centers. The approach is depicted conceptually in Fig. 7.7.

If enough iterations are specified, the algorithm will converge. However, the results may be a local rather than a global optimum. Therefore, it is advisable to run the algorithm on the foundation variable set multiple times with differing initial start values. Also, as K is specified by the analyst, multiple attempts to find adequate solutions should be run on each selected value of $K.$

The K-means approach is also very sensitive to the scale of the foundation variables used in the analysis. Therefore, it is advisable to either restrict the analysis to variables on like scales or to standardize the foundation variable set prior to analysis.

7.2.8.2   CHAID

The CHI-squared Automatic Interaction Detection (CHAID) has previously been described in detail (Kass 1980; Magidson 1994). CHAID differs from K-means in several ways. Where K-means is a descriptive approach that does not delineate between independent and dependent measures, CHAID incorporates a dependent measure on which segment creation is predicated. Additionally, the dependent and independent measures are all typically categorical in nature. That is not to imply that measures collected in a survey on an interval or ratio scale cannot be considered as foundation variables. The first step of a CHAID analysis is to categorize these variables rendering them suitable for inclusion.

CHAID is a "tree-building" approach that discovers and capitalizes on interaction effects between variables. In the initial phase of estimation, the algorithm searches for homogeneous categories within the independent measures that can be collapsed together. These categories are identified as those having high p-values in the χ^2 (for a categorical dependent measure) or F test (for a continuous dependent measure) analysis between independent and dependent measures. After the independent measure categories have been collapsed, the method then moves on to create all possible cross-tabulations for each independent measure category with the dependent measure. Given that there are a large number of statistical tests being conducted, Bonferroni adjusted p-values are calculated. The independent measure that has the lowest adjusted p-value is selected, and the groups suggested by the merging process are then used to divide the data into subgroups. The process is repeated until no independent measure has a significant p-value.

CHAID requires careful consideration when used as the sole segmentation methodology. It is important to balance the complexity of the tree. A small tree may be easy to interpret but not yield useful results. A large, complicated tree can result in many segments that are difficult to interpret and not useful for marketing applications. CHAID can, however, be a useful tool to identify foundation variables that may be useful when used in other segmentation approaches.

A related approach to segmentation called Classification And Regression Trees (CART) was developed by Breiman et al. (1984). CART is also a tree developing approach. An important distinction between CART and CHAID is that CART can incorporate both categorical and continuous independent measures. Excellent discussion of CART and related approaches can be found in Loh (2014).

7.2.8.3   Latent Class Models

Latent Class Analysis (LCA) methods have been exceedingly popular in market research and are considered the "main statistical approach to clustering and segmentation" (Wedel and Kamakura 2000). In this approach (also known as mixture models), the data in a sample are presumed to be comprised of members of two or more homogeneous segments that are mixed together in an unknown proportion. The proportion is denoted as π, with $\pi > 0$, and $\sum \pi = 1$. LCA uncovers this proportionality, thus providing the relative size of the segments in the sample.

The LCA model for continuous variables is:

$$f(y_i \mid \phi) = \sum_{s=1}^{S} \pi_s f_s(y_i|\theta_s).$$

In this representation from Vermunt and Magidson (2002), y_i are the respondents' scores on the set of observed foundation variables. S is the number of segments, and π_s is the prior probability of being in segment s. Also the distribution of y_i is assumed to be a mixture of segments specific $f_s(y_i|\theta_s)$ given the model parameter vector θ_s. The density function $f_s(y_i|\theta_s)$ can be any one of the family of exponential distributions whether they be discrete (e.g., binomial, Poisson) or continuous (e.g., normal, Dirichlet). Given that $\phi = (\pi, \theta)$, the likelihood function is:

$$L(y_i, \phi) = \prod_{i=1}^{I} f\left(\frac{y_i}{\phi}\right).$$

The likelihood can be maximized using the Newton-Raphson method (McHugh 1958) or the expectation-maximization (EM) algorithm (Dempster et al. 1977). Following Wedel and Kamakura (2000), given that an estimate of ϕ is obtained, the posterior probability p_{is} that respondent i comes from segment s can be calculated by:

$$p_{is} = \frac{\pi_s f_s(y_i|\theta_s)}{\sum_{s=1}^{S} \pi_s f_s(y_i|\theta_s)}.$$

The probabilities p_{is} are used to classify respondents into segments probabilistically.

The survey instruments developed for market research purposes almost always collect data on multiple measurement scales. LCA can accommodate these mixed measured data, that is, when the foundation variables y_i are collected as nominal, ordinal, and/or continuous. The LCA model for mixed y's from Vermunt and Magidson (2002) is:

$$f(y_i|\theta) = \sum_{s=1}^{S} \pi_s \prod_{v=1}^{V} f_s(y_{iv}|\theta_{vs}).$$

In this case, the appropriate univariate distribution function of each input y_{iv} of the foundation variables y_i can vary. For example, if y_{iv} is continuous, univariate normal or log-normal are suitable options. For other measurement scales, binomial, Poisson, or multinomial distributions are good choices.

The methods described above are like K-means segmentation in that there is no distinction made between dependent and independent measures. Should a dependent measure be required, Latent Class Regression (LCR) techniques are an attractive alternative. LCR methods also assume the sum of proportions π is equal to 1. The segments are the components weighted by π defined by unique regression equations. For example, a two-segment LCR would take the form:

$$\pi\left(\beta_{01} + \sum \beta_{j1} X_{ij1}\right) + (1 - \pi)\left(\beta_{02} + \sum \beta_{j2} X_{ij2}\right).$$

Assuming independent foundation variables ("predictors") X_j, constants β_0 and regression coefficients β_j. An excellent overview of LCR methods is presented in Wedel and DeSarbo (2002).

LCA methods have several key advantages over segmentation methods such as K-means or CHAID:

- The ability to easily incorporate mixed-mode foundation variables with no need to standardize or categorize the measures prior to analysis
- The ability, but not necessity, to have dependent measures
- The availability of multiple statistical criteria to determine the optimal number of segments (to be discussed)

7.2.9 Solution Selection Criteria

Segmenting a set of dozens of foundation measures typically produces multiple potential solutions, i.e., two, three, four, five, or more segments. Selecting the appropriate segmentation solution involves consideration of multiple factors.

7.2.9.1 Statistical Indices (Where Applicable)

LCA segmentation produces several statistical indices that offer excellent guidance as to which of the competing solutions best represent or fit the sample data. Two of the most commonly utilized are Akaike's Information Criteria (AIC) (Bozodogan 1987) and the Bayesian Information Criteria (BIC) (Schwarz 1978). When using either of these metrics, smaller values indicate a better solution. LCA models rely on maximum likelihood estimation, and the likelihood can be increased by adding additional parameters (segments) to a model. Adding segments to increase the likelihood can easily result in over-fitting the data. Both AIC and BIC penalize the assessment of model fit in terms of the number of estimated parameters. The more parameters estimated in a given model, the greater the penalty term. The Approximate Weight of Evidence (AWE) is another method of evaluating a set of competing LCA models (Celeux et al. 1997). The AWE integrates information on data-model fit as well as information on segment (mis-)classification to determine the optimal number of segments.

7.2.9.2 Managerial Implications

A good segmentation will take into account more than just the statistical indices mentioned above. That is, the choice of which segmentation solution is preferred is based on several subjective judgment factors in addition to the more objective statistics. Which subjective "metrics" is defined by the research team in response to the business needs of the client team and management? Some of the more common subjective factors include:

- Number of segments
- Segment sizes
- Segment composition
- Segment profiles
- Solution reproducibility
- Alignment with current market intelligence and established hypotheses

The number of segments is often the first subjective criteria to be evaluated. A solution that posits only two segments may not provide the desired granularity to understand the market. Conversely, a solution with eight segments may prove to be too complicated for marketers to develop segment-specific marketing materials. A good segment solution should at a minimum identify at least one target segment and also at least one that can be deprioritized. In pharmaceutical market research, an attractive solution typically has 3–6 segments.

Closely related to the number of segments, the relative size of segments is also an important criterion. Segments that are very small (<10–15% of the market being studied) may offer too little potential return on investment for the development of segment-specific marketing and reach materials. Conversely, very large segments (>35–40% of the market) can be suspect in two ways. First, a large segment may not differ meaningfully from the market as a whole, therefore defeating the purpose of segmentation. Also, a large segment is often viewed as one that contains subsegments implying that the solution itself is not desirable. That is, the large segment should have been broken down into two or more actionable subgroups. There are instances where a small or large segment may not be deleterious to a successful solution. For example, in a physician segmentation, there may be a small group of specialists that do offer a viable opportunity when considered as their own segment.

Segment composition is related to the sample frame and market that has been defined for study. In physician research, where the sample contains multiple specialties, it may be attractive to have segments that are defined by specialty (top-down segmentation). Similarly, when segmenting patients, it may be desirable to have segments defined by disease severity or previous treatment. There are also instances where a successful segmentation places respondents into groups based purely on their reported attitudes and/or behaviors. In this situation, segments are more heterogeneous in terms of observable characteristics but homogeneous in terms of wants, unmet needs, and attitudes. The decision about what segment composition constitutes a success is determined by how management intends to create materials and marketing strategy. Often it is advisable to generate candidate solutions that offer a variety of offerings in terms of segment composition. Multiple options often stimulate fertile discussion with management that ultimately lead to the selection of the most valuable segmentation solution given the intended actions/decisions being driven by the research.

Close inspection of the segment profiles across all foundation metrics is a pivotal step in selecting a segmentation solution. A profile is a summary of the means, medians, and proportions of all responses in the foundation set for each segment and overall for each solution. Often, management and marketers have opinions of what the segments "should" look like. Reviewing the profiles of a set of solutions allows the analyst and team to determine the persona of each segment and to decide which candidate solution best meets the research objectives.

The ability to accurately reproduce or predict segment membership outside of the research sample is the final criterion to consider when selecting a solution. In pharmaceutical market research, there are two widely used approaches, attitudinal and behavioral algorithms. Often both are developed, but which approach is ultimately chosen typically hinges on what data are available to develop segments.

7.2.9.3 Attitudinal Algorithms

All segmentations developed on the basis of primary survey data can and should yield an attitudinal algorithm. Attitudinal algorithms can be used to assign segment membership to individuals based on their responses to a set of items that appeared in the original survey instrument. Some attitudinal tools are used for recruitment by segment for subsequent research. Participants in qualitative research can be asked to provide their answers to the set of items prior to a focus group or interview. Attitudinal algorithms are often programmed into subsequent quantitative online research. This allows for analysis of the data and reporting of results by segment. Often the attitudinal algorithm is programmed into a company or product website. When individuals visit the website, they answer the items, are segmented, and then are presented with tailored messaging and content developed for their segment. Occasionally an algorithm is developed for use by pharmaceutical sales representatives. The sales team will ask physicians a series of questions during a visit to determine which segment that customer is in. Development of such a tool is typically done as follows. First, the analyst in concert with the research team identifies a candidate set of survey items that are suitable in terms of item content. Next, the number of desired items in the algorithm is determined. Most often these algorithms are designed to be three, five, or ten items. Commonly, either a stepwise discriminant function analysis or multinomial logit model is used to identify the best subset of predictive items. Once a candidate model is identified, it is cross-validated to ensure its functionality outside the sample.

7.2.9.4 Behavioral Algorithms

When secondary data are available such as prescription or claims data (i.e., behavioral or holistic segmentation), they can be used to create behavioral algorithms. These algorithms are built on purely secondary data and do not incorporate primary data collected in the survey instrument. Behavioral tools are most often done in physician research where prescribing data that can be linked to survey respondents are available. These models allow for segment membership to be assigned to individuals without capturing their response to survey items. This is especially appealing if a database of prescribers is available and the desire is to segment the list. Algorithms can be constructed through a variety of machine learning, regression, or other techniques.

7.3 Choice-Based Conjoint Model/DCM

Choice-based conjoint and discrete choice models provide a mathematical framework for predicting and analyzing decisions. The common theoretical justification for these models comes from utility theory and random utility maximization. These models assume that economic decisions maximize personal gain and that a latent real-valued measure, called utility, captures the ordering of personal gain. Utility is given a random component. At each decision, the subject selects the alternative which had the greatest draw from the random utility distribution. Selection of the random distribution and explanatory factors contributing to utility governs the design and form of the choice model and the experimental design on which it's estimated (Train 2002).

In pharmaceutical market research, choice modeling applies to treatment decisions made by physicians, access decisions made by regulators, coverage decisions made by payers, and request and adherence decisions made by patients. The resulting models provide a predictive framework for forecasting sales and informing product development decisions. Analysis of the underlying utility functions provides insight into stakeholders' decision-making process: What product attributes and market factors are most critical to a products success?

7.4 Choice Models

7.4.1 Goals of Such Research

Pharmaceutical market research leverages choice modeling at a few key junctures in the product development and marketing process. During product development, understanding and predicting stakeholder decisions are critical to defining the goals of a development program. These goals manifest as a target product profile (TPP), a document describing the attributes of the product the developer intends to demonstrate and strives to include on labeling and in marketing materials (FDA 2007). As the project approaches market, drug developers must understand how the product will be used, in which patient populations, and what attributes drive these market decisions. This information directs the marketing strategy to individuals most in need and content most influential to optimal patient care. Choice models inform TPP development by identifying areas of clinical need and marketing strategy by identifying the educational and access needs of the marketplace and can also be leveraged for market forecasting.

7.4.1.1 TPP Development

TPP development requires an understanding of the regulatory environment and the areas of greatest clinical need. Discussion with regulators and existing regulatory requirements and precedent will decide the majority of the TPP. The nature of regulatory decision-making, lack of access to regulators, and relative infrequency of regulatory decisions make it a poor fit for conjoint and discrete choice analysis. The critical components of the TPP, the primary endpoints, will most likely be defined prior to decision research. Choice models are best leveraged at identifying need when a product has multiple addressable patient populations and identifying attributes important in clinical practice but not necessary to clear regulatory thresholds.

Choice models can identify patients with the greatest need for a medical treatment or specific attributes of a medical treatment. This information informs whether to restrict target labeling to subset of a larger addressable population or prioritization of indications when the treatment may have clinical benefit across conditions. By estimating contribution to utility of patient attributes, choice models quantify in what patients a product has greatest perceived benefit. Interaction terms between patient attributes and the attributes of the treatment alternatives quantify what specific attributes of the medical treatment have differential perceived benefit across patients.

Choice models guiding attribute inclusion in a TPP have two common objectives, defining what elements to include in the TPP and informing achievement thresholds for the product to drive prescribing. Conjoint and discrete choice models provide information on these decisions through attribute importance in the utility functions and the predicted use decisions. Attribute important measures describe which attributes have the greatest impact on product utility. The predicted shares and shape of the utility functions can inform selection of achievement thresholds.

7.4.1.2 Patient Profiles/Drivers

After a TPP for a product has been created, drug developers must understand the market for such a product. They must know who is in that market, which patients and which physicians, and what those people need. Such choice models will focus less on the effects of product attributes on treatment decisions and more on the effect of attributes of the patient and physician and interaction between stakeholder attributes and product attributes. This leads to larger sample size requirements as these attributes are typically not controlled via an experimental design.

To identify the market, utility functions need to include patient and provider attributes. This can be accomplished by surveying physicians and soliciting patient cases. Physicians will fill out patient case forms, describing recent cases. Physicians can be expected to bring up to four or five cases in a typical 45–60 min survey. There are cases where simulated patient cases can be leveraged in a choice task, though condensing the nuances of patient cases to a simplistic profile is often impossible or ill-advised as there are many factors that physicians consider that cannot be represented this way. Physicians make separate choice decisions for each patient case across variations in the product attributes or market scenarios. Attributes of the providers and patients enter the utility functions explicitly or by estimating a mixed or mixture model and analyzing the distribution of utility functions and predicted choices by patient or provider attribute. This allows the researcher to describe the population that professed interest in using the product and which characteristics identify populations of greatest opportunity for the client brand/portfolio.

To identify the drivers and needs of the market, the same attribute important and part-worth measures used for TPP development measure the overall drivers. To assess drivers specific to a subset of the market or patient/provider characteristics associated with particular needs, the utility functions need to include interactions between patient/provider attributes and product attributes. This allows computation of importance measures for particular subsets of the market and analysis of differences in importance between subsets of the market. Mixed and mixture models can assess differences in utility functions between subsets of the market, though one must be aware of the assumptions of the latent variable or random effects distributions. For example in a mixed model, differences in utility parameters between subsets of the market suggest that the utility parameters may not be normally distributed.

7.4.1.3 Other Applications

Results from discrete choice modeling also inform business objectives outside of marketing and market research. Revenue forecasts can use the predictions of stated intended use to predict peak usage of the product. This requires conversion between the usages in the choice task, the preference share, to actual usage, the market share. This conversion should account for real-world product access restrictions not realized in the study and common over-exuberance of survey respondents for novel products. Generally market share should be between 33 and 80% of preference share. "Me too" products, more similar to other products, and products with burdensome access requirements will have a lower market share.

Discrete choice models also play a role in retrospective medical research. In retrospective medical studies, analyses correct for non-randomized treatment selection. This requires an understanding of how treatments were selected. Choice models provide such an understanding. A discrete choice model predicts the probabilities of a given patient receiving a particular treatment. In this context these predictions are called propensity scores. Analysts may weight data by the inverse of the propensity scores in a method similar to sample weighting to recreate results comparable to randomized treatment. Propensity scores can also be used to match treatment and control cases in case-control studies or used to adjust a regression analysis by including propensity as an independent variable.

Health economic research leverages discrete choice models to assess the utility of different health states. These utilities are dubbed quality-adjusted life years (QALYs) and reflect the relative utility of a year of life in a particular health condition to a year of life in good health. Making such an assessment is difficult, partially due to the abstract nature of the notion. Discrete choice models allow elicitation of the relative utility from more concrete decisions. Respondents choose between living so many years in a negative health state or a procedure that completely eliminates the negative health state but has a certain probability of death. This task is called the standard gamble. Or respondents choose between living so many years in a negative health state or a lesser number of years in good health. This task is called the time trade-off. In both cases, simple discrete choice models derive the utility functions that determine the quality adjustment associated with the negative health state (Weinstein et al. 2009).

7.4.2 Choice Model Form

To design a discrete choice or conjoint experiment, the form of the choice model must be selected. Different forms of choice models have different properties which impact sampling, experimental design, and analysis. The form of choice model should be chosen to reflect the properties of the decision-making process. Different choice models make different assumptions about substitution patterns among response options and variations in preferences between decision-makers.

7.4.2.1 Mathematical Foundation

Choice models predict a discrete outcome, y, from a set of predictors, x, and a random component ε, drawn from probability distribution $f(\varepsilon)$ over Σ. x may include attributes of the choice alternatives, attributes of the decision-maker, or attributes of the context in which the decision is made. y takes a value from a set of alternatives, S. S must be finite, collectively exhaustive, and mutually exclusive. ε captures all random variations in the decision-making process and contributions from unobserved sources.

$\forall s \in S$, define functions, $U_s(x, \varepsilon)$, such that:

$$y = s \leftrightarrow \forall t \in S, \quad s \neq t; \quad U_s(x, \varepsilon) > U_t(x, \varepsilon).$$

The selection probabilities are then:

$$P(y = s|x) = \int_{\Sigma'} f(\varepsilon)d\varepsilon,$$

$$\Sigma' \subset \Sigma | \forall t \in S, \quad t \neq s; \quad U_s(x, \varepsilon) > U_t(x, \varepsilon).$$

The function U_i is called the utility of choice alternative i. Assuming decision-makers select the option that provides themselves the greatest benefit, U_i represents the net benefit the decision-makers obtain by selecting option i. The contribution to the utility function of each attribute in x is called the part-worth of the attribute. As the model only cares about the relative magnitude of the utilities, the measure is unitless and the absolute magnitude of the utilities has no meaning. In all models discussed here, U will be linear, of the form $U_i = B_i x_i + \varepsilon_i$. What follows is an overview of models based on various selections for $f(\varepsilon)$ (Train 2002).

7.4.2.2 Logit and Multinomial Logit Models

The most common choice model is the logit ($|S| = 2$) and multinomial logit ($|S| > 2$). These arise when $f(e)$ is $|S|$ iid extreme value distributions:

$$f(\varepsilon) = \prod_{s \in S} e^{-\varepsilon_s} e^{-e^{-\varepsilon_s}}.$$

Because the utility functions can be arbitrarily scaled and $\varepsilon_s \perp \varepsilon_t \ \forall \ s \neq t$, the distribution is taken to have mean 1 and variance $\frac{\pi^2}{6}$ without loss of generality. This choice of distribution gives the selection probabilities a straightforward, closed form:

$$P(y = s|x) = \frac{e^{B_s x_s}}{\sum_{t \in S} e^{B_t x_t}}.$$

The logistic and multinomial logistic model impose a tight constraint on the substitution pattern, the independence of irrelevant alternatives (IIA). This property is demonstrated by considering the log odds ratio of the selection probabilities:

$$\log \left(\frac{P(y = s|x)}{P(y = t|x)} \right) = B_i x_i - B_j x_j.$$

Note that the ratio is independent of all alternatives $u \in S$, $u \neq s$, $u \neq t$. This implies that the relative preference for s compared to t is not affected by the presence or attributes of other alternatives. The problem with this restriction is demonstrated by the red bus/blue bus problem. Assume a commuter has a choice between commuting by car and by a red bus. Assume that the commuter has equal preference for the two options. Then a third option is added, a blue bus. The commuter does not care about the color of the bus. Intuitively, we'd expect the commuter to select car with $p(y = car) = 50\%$ and $p(y = red\ bus\ or\ y = blue\ bus) = 50\%$. IIA implies that p $(y = car) = 33\%$ and $p(y = red\ bus\ or\ y = blue\ bus) = 67\%$. A similar statement of IIA can be seen in the cross elasticities of the contributions to the utility function:

$$\frac{\partial P(y = s|x)}{\partial x_t} \frac{x_t}{P(y = s|x)} = -B_t x_t P(y = t|x).$$

Note this is independent of i, implying that a change to alternative j has the same proportional impact on all other alternatives. These properties are a consequence of assuming that the error terms on the utility functions of each alternative are independent. This property also implies that the model is biased if there is unaccounted for heterogeneity in preference. This is because any random component in the utility function for a particular attribute would imply that the errors are no longer independently and indistinguishably distributed across alternatives, as would heterogeneity in preference for particular options between respondents.

Despite these strong assumptions, logit and multinomial logits are the most common form of choice model, mostly due to their simplicity and ease of implementation. Luckily, while violations of the assumptions above will produce biased estimates, practice has shown these models to hold up well even in cases where IIA violations would be expected (Train 2002).

7.4.2.3 Probit Models

A natural selection for $f(\varepsilon)$ is the multivariate normal distribution. This leads to probit models. Given σ^2, the covariance matrix of $f(\varepsilon)$, the selection probabilities are:

$$P(y = s|x) = \int_{\Sigma'} \frac{e^{-\frac{\varepsilon^T \varepsilon}{2\sigma^2}}}{\sqrt{(2\pi)^{|S|}|\sigma^2|}} d\varepsilon,$$

$$\Sigma' \subset \mathbb{R}^{|S|} \mid \forall t\ \varepsilon_s > B_t x_t + \varepsilon_t - B_s x_s.$$

The selection probabilities have no closed form and must be evaluated by simulation or numerical methods such as Gaussian quadrature. The principal advantage of the probit model is that it permits correlations in the error terms. The general model with a full covariance matrix for $f(\varepsilon)$ permits any possible substitution pattern among the alternatives and is unbiased in the presence of unaccounted for heterogeneity in preference (Train 2002).

7.4.2.4 Nested Logit Models

The nested logit model loosens IIA for MNL models by allowing the random components of the utility functions to correlate for selected groups of alternatives. Take $P \subset \wp(S)$. Errors between utility functions for choices $\{i,j \in S \mid \exists p \in P \text{ s. t. } i, j \in p\}$ are correlated. Errors between utility functions for choices $\{i,j \in S \mid \nexists p \in P \text{ s. t. } i,j \in p\}$ are independent. In most uses, P is a partition of S. $f(\varepsilon)$ takes the form of a generalized extreme value distribution with cumulative distribution:

$$F(\varepsilon) = e^{\left(-\sum_{p \in P}\left(\sum_{s \in p} -e^{-\varepsilon_s/\lambda_p}\right)^{\lambda_p}\right)}.$$

The selection probabilities for s are:

$$P(y = s|x) = \sum_{p \in P|s \in p} \frac{e^{B_s x_s/\lambda_p}\left(\sum_{t \in p}e^{B_t x_t/\lambda_p}\right)^{\lambda_p - 1}}{\sum_{q \in P}\left(\sum_{t \in q}e^{B_t x_t/\lambda_q}\right)^{\lambda_q}}.$$

This is typically decomposed into the product of two logits:

$$P(y = s|x) = \sum_{p \in P|s \in p} \frac{e^{B_p x_p + \lambda_p IV_p}}{\sum_{q \in P}e^{B_q x_q + \lambda_q IV_q}} * \frac{e^{B_s^p x_s/\lambda_p}}{\sum_{t \in p}e^{B_t^p x_t/\lambda_p}},$$

$$IV_p = \ln\left(\sum_{s \in p}e^{B_s' x_s/\lambda_p}\right),$$

$$B_p = \bigcap_{s \in p}B_s, B_s^p = B_s \setminus B_p.$$

(Train 2002).

Ironically, the most common motivation for the nested logit model, the red/blue bus paradox, is a case of perfect correlation of errors between choice options ($\lambda_p = 0$); thus, the nested logit cannot capture the behavior.

There is an alternative formulation of the nested logit model, called the non-normalized nested logit model:

$$P(y = s|x) = \sum_{p \in P|s \in p} \frac{e^{B_p x_p + \lambda_p IV_p}}{\sum\limits_{q \in P} e^{B_q x_q + \lambda_q IV_q}} * \frac{e^{B'_s x_s}}{\sum\limits_{t \in p} e^{B'_t x_t}},$$

$$IV_p = \ln \left(\sum_{t \in p} e^{B'_t x_t} \right).$$

The name comes from the fact that contributions to the utility functions are not normalized between nests. They are scaled by λ_k, the correlation of items within the nest. This form of the model can resolve the red bus/blue bus problem. Perfect correlation isn't possible in the other form of the model because in the case of perfect correlation, it is impossible to normalize the utility functions. The non-normalized nested logit is not consistent with the random utility maximization. The typical interpretation of utility functions and part-worths is inappropriate for this model. In general, the first formulation of the nested logit is preferred, though inconsistency with random utility maximization does not preclude the model from accurately reflecting a decision process. The appropriate model formulation can be determined empirically with the model selection methods discussed in Sect. 7.4.7. It is important to be aware that both of these models are referred to as nested logit in software documentation. Analysts should be aware which method is implemented by their choice of statistical software package (Heiss 2002; Silberhorn et al. 2008).

7.4.2.5 Random Effects MNL Models

Mixed models add a random component to the part-worths in the MNL model, α, drawn from probability distribution, $g(\alpha)$ over Ω:

$$B_{jk} = B_j + \alpha_{jk},$$

$$P_k(y = i|x, \alpha) = \frac{e^{B_{jk} x_i}}{\sum\limits_{j \in S} e^{B_{jk} x_j}},$$

$$P(y = i|x) = \int_{\Omega} P_k(y = i|x, \alpha) g(\alpha) d\alpha.$$

Generally, k represents the survey respondent or patient case. The conceptual basis for the model is that part-worths may vary between individuals. The random component of the part-worths captures this variation. In the random effects MNL model, IIA still holds within the choices of each respondent or patient case. The model can capture any substitution pattern in the overall population (Train 2002).

7.4.2.6 Mixture MNL Models

Mixture models predict choice probabilities as a weighted sum of a set of MNL models with different part-worths. The model is formulated as a latent class model. There is a latent variable, $c \in C$. A multinomial logit model predicts the choices given c:

$$P_c(y = i|x, c) = \frac{e^{B_{jc}x_i}}{\sum_{j \in S} e^{B_{jc}x_j}},$$

$$P(y = i|x) = \sum_{c \in C} P_c(y = i|x)P(c).$$

Conceptually, each stakeholder in the market is a member of some class c. Each class uses a different utility function. It is equivalent to a random effects MNL model where $g(\alpha)$ has finite support (Hess et al. 2006).

7.4.2.7 Ordered Logit and Probit Models

The ordered logit and probit models are variations on the standard logit and probit models. They apply when responses are ordinal in nature, such as Likert-like scales or levels of formulary coverage. In such cases, assume that each response represents a range of the utility of the object being evaluated. For the formulary coverage example, assume a payer uses a four-tiered formulary. The payer will reimburse the product proportional to the utility of product to the payer. If the utility is below a threshold, v_1, then the product will not be covered; if the utility is between v_1 and v_2, it will be in tier 4; if the utility is between v_2 and v_3, it will be in tier 3; etc. The probability of each coverage tier is:

$$P(Tier = Not\ Covered) = F(v_1 - U)$$
$$P(Tier = 4) = F(v_2 - U) - F(v_1 - U)$$
$$P(Tier = 3) = F(v_3 - U) - F(v_2 - U)$$
$$P(Tier = 2) = F(v_4 - U) - F(v_3 - U)$$
$$P(Tier = 1) = 1 - F(v_4 - U)$$

If the errors on the utility are normal, then F is the cumulative normal function and the model is called an ordered probit. If the errors on the utility are logistic, then F is the logistic function and the model is called an ordered logit.

7.4.3 Sample Considerations

Determining the sampling strategy involves determining the population of interest. This definition requires an initial understanding of the decision-making process in the particular market and the goals of the research.

7.4.3.1 Stakeholders

Most often the population of interest is the physicians who treat the condition or conditions addressed by the product. Assuming reasonable market access, for most pharmaceutical products, the physician asserts the greatest influence on product use. For patient profile and driver research, the physician is best informed about the medical properties of available treatments and how those match to the clinical needs of the patients. For TPP development, physician decisions influence what secondary endpoints most affect treatment choice and what administrative and dosing options facilitate product use and physicians know which patients seem most appropriate for a potential product.

The other common study populations are patients and payers. Patients should be included in research when product attributes related to the patient experience (e.g., dosing, administration, and convenience) are expected to play a large role in treatment decisions or if diagnosis or treatment requires initiative from the patients (as with erectile dysfunction or restless leg syndrome). Payers should be included in research if prediction and understanding of the impact of coverage and out-of-pocket costs to patients are a research goal.

7.4.3.2 Sample Size

Discrete choice research requires sufficient sample sizes to acquire reasonable estimates of the choice model parameters. Sample size calculation for these models is difficult. The errors on the parameter estimates and predictions depend on the parameter values. The amount of information in each elicited decision depends on the nature of the choice task, the number of options presented, and the number and overlap of the attributes of those options. The homogeneity of the study population also impacts the accuracy of model estimates.

A number of rules have been proposed for determining the minimal sample size for discrete choice studies. A good ad hoc rule of thumb is to have 20 respondents view each choice task. This corresponds to at least 20 respondents per model degree of freedom. Another rule of thumb states:

$$N > \frac{500c}{ta},$$

where c is the largest number of levels of a single attribute; t is the number of choice tasks; and a is the number of alternatives. This equation assumes general attributes, present on all alternatives. The nature of the pharmaceutical market means such a property rarely presents in actual market decisions. Products are too clinically nuanced and claims about products too strictly regulated to reduce all products in a space to the same concise set of attributes and levels. But, the equation is applicable to driver studies where the choice task presented need not reflect the decisions presented in the marketplace.

Errors on the parameters of the utility function can be calculated directly for MNL models or for more complex models via data simulation. This requires knowledge of the experimental design and a prior estimate of the model parameters. Given a probability distribution over the model parameters and experimental design, datasets of survey results for various sample sizes and strategies can be simulated. Inspecting plots of errors for various sampling strategies informs selection of the appropriate sample design (de Bekker-Grob et al. 2015; Lancsar and Louviere 2008).

7.4.3.3 Subpopulations

Beyond sample size, having sufficient sample of certain subpopulations may be important to producing accurate choice models and addressing research goals. Standard logit and multinomial logit models assume homogeneity of preference across the study population. Large deviations from this assumption result in omitted variable bias in the resulting model estimates. To include an attribute of the respondent in the choice model, a sufficient number of respondents must possess that attribute and the experimental design should be balanced across the attribute. While probit, mixed, and mixture models can address bias from omitted or unobserved properties of the decision-maker, analysis of the differences between subpopulations requires sufficient sample from the subpopulation.

The required sample size within a subpopulation depends on the nature of the hypothesized differences between the subpopulation and the rest of the sample. A simple hypothesis is a difference in brand preference. Such a hypothesis can be modeled by the addition of a two-level parameter to each alternative's utility function. Assuming every brand appears in each choice task, the rule of thumb mentioned above suggests a minimum sample size of 20. This assumes that sampling and design constraints allow the researcher to incorporate the attribute of the decision-maker into the design without impacting the design's efficiency. Violations of this assumption will require a larger subsample. Rarely can a respondent attribute enter the experimental design efficiently, and sample sizes of at least 30 or 40 are advisable in most studies. A complex hypothesis that a subpopulation could differ on any component of the utility function results in a fully interacted model. This would require a sample from the subpopulation sufficient to estimate the entire model.

7.4.3.4 Design Complexity

Different choice models and experimental designs require different sample sizes. More complex decision models and more complex experiments require larger sample sizes. Design complexity takes many forms. The simplest metric for complexity is the number of parameters in the choice model. This typically corresponds to the number of attributes tested and the number of levels, i.e., the variations in description or performance each attribute may take. Additional parameters also enter the choice model if different products have different attributes that contribute to their utility. Having the same attributes on multiple products in the choice set simplifies the choice model by allowing each choice task to contribute multiple measurements of the same parameter.

A related type of complexity enters the model by the number of response options. Additional response options may reduce sample size by effectively increasing the number of measurements provided by each choice task. In a two-option task, each choice task provides a measurement of the relative utility of option A to option B. Adding a third option yields two additional measurements, A to C and B to C. Despite this, in the context of prescribing decisions, additional choices commonly increase the design complexity. Rarely are medical treatments describable by the same set of attributes, so adding options typically adds attributes and attribute levels.

A difficult to parametrize design space introduces a different type of complexity. This manifests as combinations of attribute levels that cannot be presented together. An example would be testing cancer treatments with both progression-free survival (PFS) and overall survival (OS) contributing to product utility. PFS cannot exceed OS. This restriction introduces correlation in the independent variables of the experimental data, reducing the efficiency of the design.

7.4.4 Data Collection/Survey Design Considerations

Survey instruments may elicit preferences in a number of ways. Conjoint analysis uses preferences elicited directly, as opposed to inferred through analysis of choice behavior. Discrete choice modeling uses decision behaviors to derive utility functions. Hybrid approaches combine the two, constructing an aggregate utility measure from preferences elicited directly and using this aggregate measure in the utility functions in the discrete choice model.

7.4.4.1 Conjoint

Conjoint is a broad term, used to describe any technique that derives a preference ranking from a set of configurations of attributes and levels. In common conjoint analysis, respondents evaluate products or product attributes independently. These evaluations are combined to derive a ranking of products and product configurations. Preference elicitation tasks take the form of a rating scale or ranking. When evaluations of full or partial configurations are collected, linear or ordinal models are used to derive the contributions of individual attributes to the utility. When derived from a model, utility contributions are dubbed derived or revealed preferences; when given directly, they are referred to as stated preferences. Studies often collect both stated and derived preference.

In a typical conjoint survey, respondents first complete an exercise assigning an importance to each attribute, typically via constant sum allocation. Then, for each attribute, respondents rate each level, typically on a Likert-like scale. These are the stated importances and performances. Respondents then evaluate a set of partial or complete product configurations, either through rating scale, ranking, or choice task. Regressing attribute level preferences against the choice of the configurations yields the derived importance of the attributes.

Conjoint analysis requires fewer respondents and shorter surveys than discrete choice modeling. Because preference is collected directly, it can be done more concisely. Deriving utility functions from observations of behavior requires completion of a greater number of tasks and imposes restrictions on the nature of those tasks. Conjoint analysis is more speculative than more rigorous discrete choice modeling. It does not yield parameters that represent an interpretable value of some behavioral theory. Authors have advocated using different terminology for methods using the RUM theory, though use of the term in literature is mixed (Louviere et al. 2010).

Max-Diff

A popular and useful conjoint task is the max-diff exercise. A max-diff exercise produces a ranking of a set of items from a set of simpler ranking tasks on a subset of the items. Respondents are shown a series of subsets of the full item set. For each subset, respondents select the most and least appealing item. Responses are combined to derive a ranking of the full set by fitting a choice model to the responses, usually a multinomial logit or random effects multinomial logit. Max-diff exercises allow rankings to be obtained when the full item set is too large to expect respondents to accurately complete a full ranking exercise.

7.4.4.2 Discrete Choice

Discrete choice uses selections from a finite set of options to derive preferences and the utility functions that define preferences. Respondents are presented with descriptions of a set of options and asked to select one. Design of the decision presented in the survey should reflect decisions made in the actual market. In pharmaceutical market research, this typically means patient case collection and eliciting treatment decisions for each collected patient case. Discrete choice models may also be fit to actual market decisions when such data is available. Discrete choice analysis requires larger sample sizes and longer surveys but provides more robust and interpretable results to conjoint analysis.

Allocations

Instead of selecting a single option in a choice task, allocations can serve as the dependent measure in a discrete choice model. In such situations respondents state their intended choice selection for the next 10 or 20 market decisions, or the distribution of selection over some period of time as a percentage. Estimation of the model in this situation requires inference about the number of decisions actually represented by the allocation. In practice this value determines the variance of the selection, how much variation in responses would be observed if the same respondent were repeatedly asked the same allocation question. Determination of this value is at the discretion of the analyst. Giving each task a weight greater than 20 often leads to over-fitting. An intuitive selection is to use the number of response options as the number of decisions represented in each allocation.

Allocations are not an ideal method of elicitation but are often necessary. Market stakeholders rarely make decisions in such a manner. More often the market presents decisions discretely. Physicians decide the treatment of each patient independently; they do not look at their patient pool and allocate them to treatments en masse. Allocations may lead to different results from repeated discrete choices through behavioral phenomena like diversification bias (Read and Loewenstein 1995). That said, presenting physicians with sufficient information to make decisions reflective of how they would do so in the market is often infeasible. Physicians cannot select a product without sufficient details about the patient. Collecting patient cases and decisions about those patient cases greatly increases the length and expense of a survey. By using an allocation exercise, physicians consider their entire patient pool and the proportion of those patients suitable for each treatment option, alleviating the need to present or collect patient details in the survey instrument.

7.4.4.3 Hybrid Methods

Researchers may combine conjoint and discrete choice methods to compromise between the logistical simplicity of conjoint methods and theoretical rigor of discrete choice. The typical method constructs utility measures using conjoint analysis. These measures incorporate the effects of multiple product, patient, or physician attributes and represent their contribution to utility as a single value. This aggregate measure becomes the independent variable in the discrete choice model. This simplifies the discrete choice model by reducing the number of parameters, thus requiring fewer respondents and fewer choice tasks. The aggregate utility measure is typically the sum of the Likert-like scale ratings multiplied by the stated importance of the attribute. Other derivations of the aggregate utility are possible, such as the predicted preference from a full- or partial-profile max-diff exercise.

7.4.4.4   Number of Choice Tasks

The number of choice task that can be completed by each respondent depends on the complexity of choice task. Generally, a single respondent can be expected to complete up to 8 complex tasks, or as many as 20 for simple choice tasks, though it's rare to get more than 20 due to budgetary restrictions on survey length (Johnson 2000).

7.4.5   Efficient Designs

Anyone who has performed many regression analyses has encountered poor or inestimable models due to correlation in the independent measures. In discrete choice analysis, the analyst controls the distribution of some of the independent measures through the design of the survey instrument. A survey, designed to minimize the error of estimates of choice model parameters, achieves greater precision and can incorporate greater complexity, with less data. Less ambitiously, good experimental design ensures identification of the choice model.

7.4.5.1   Attribute and Levels

The first step of creating the experimental design is to determine the parameters of the choice model. The list of parameters is dubbed the attributes. The tested values of these attributes are the levels. Some attributes are clinical properties of the pharmaceutical product, for example, the efficacy, safety, or dosing. The levels are the values of these attributes, for example, the efficacy attribute in an oncological therapy may have values of 7, 8, or 9 months of PFS. Descriptors of the respondent, physician, patient case, or market situation may also be attributes. The full set of attributes and range of levels that the choice model will be able to assess defines the domain of the discrete choice experiment. Knowing the domain, form of choice model, and type of choice exercise establishes the data requirements for estimating the choice model over the domain. Experimental design creates a data collection process that ensures the collected data matrix, X, meets those requirements.

The data matrix can be manipulated in different ways. Parameters fall into three categories, those determined by the survey design, those determined by the sample design, and those that cannot be controlled.

The researcher may choose parameters determined by survey design directly. These are the attributes of the description of the situation and options that the survey presents to respondents to set up a choice task. Because of how much control the researcher has over these parameters, experimental design focuses heavily on them.

Parameters determined by sample design are attributes of the respondent or patient cases collected from the respondent. Researchers have some control over these. The sample can be stratified to ensure a certain number of observations at each value. If survey design varies between respondents, survey versions can be balanced within values of these parameters. Feasibility and cost of sample collection severely limit the extent of manipulation of the data matrix on these parameters.

The final group consists of respondent-level effects that cannot be controlled for but whose effect should be considered in the experimental design.

It is also important to consider what is not in the data matrix. Omitted variables will affect the quality of results. The effect of variables that were not included in the model but which may contribute to choices should be considered. The experimental design can be constructed to mitigate the effect of omitted variable bias.

7.4.5.2 Measures of Design Efficiency

The most common measure for evaluating the design is D-efficiency. The D-efficiency is proportional to the determinant of Fisher information matrix. This is a natural target for optimization as covariance of the probability distribution on the parameter estimates is proportional to the inverse Fisher information matrix.

The Fisher information matrix is calculated from the data matrix, X, and depends on the form of choice model. X is a m x n matrix, where m is the number of model parameters and n is the number of choices. Let χ_i be the ith parameter. Let x_s be the subspace of parameters included in U_s. For linear models the Fisher information matrix is:

$$\frac{X^T X}{\sigma^2}.$$

The determinant of this matrix is maximized when the component vectors are orthogonal.

Optimizing designs for the linear model or starting from a design optimized for the linear model and modifying simplifies the experimental design process. A design that identifies the model in the linear case will always identify the MNL model (Kuhfeld 2005).

7.4.5.3 Design Optimization

The general problem of finding the design that maximizes D-efficiency is equivalent to finding the maximum volume submatrix of the data matrix associated with showing every possible combination of attributes and levels. This problem is NP-hard, meaning absolute optimization is not computationally feasible for most designs. Instead sufficiently optimized experimental designs are found by using a combination of look-up tables of known optimal designs and heuristic search algorithms such as simulated annealing or the Fedorov exchange algorithm. For modestly sized experimental domains, heuristic search can be performed over the full design space. For larger domains, computation time can be reduced by starting with a known optimal design for a design space that is a superset of the desired design space, removing the elements that are outside the desired design space, and using the result as the search space for the heuristic optimization algorithm. For very large domains, partitioning the design space, finding sufficiently optimal designs for the subspaces, and combining them can reduce computation time. For certain configurations of the Fisher information matrix, combining optimized solutions over subspaces produces optimal or near-optimal results. This method can also give the errors on the model parameters a more desirable structure (Zwerina et al. 1996; Nguyen and Miller 1992).

7.4.5.4   Blocking

Blocking is the practice of defining a set of or subsets of the experimental design such that within subset D-efficiency is maximized. It is equivalent to adding a categorical predictor to the design that minimally reduces D-efficiency. The most common use of blocking is to mitigate missing variable bias from respondent attributes or respondent-specific effects by ensuring the estimates of the other parameters are as independent as possible from the missing variables.

7.4.6   Estimation

7.4.6.1   Maximum Likelihood and Gradient Descent

MNL, nested logit, and ordered logit models are typically estimated by employing a gradient descent algorithm to maximize the log-likelihood. A similar approach is taken for probit and ordered probit models, with the additional complication that the likelihood function has no closed form. Thus the integral and its gradient must be approximated, either through simulation or numerical methods. This puts a practical limit on the complexity of probit models, specifically on the number of response options and the number of non-zero terms in the covariance matrix of the errors on the utility functions.

7.4.6.2   Expectation-Maximization (EM) Algorithm

For mixture models, the most common method of estimation is the EM algorithm. Each respondent is initially assigned to a class. A choice model is fit to the data of each class, the expectation step. The probability of class membership given these models is computed for each respondent, the maximization step. Choice models are fit for each class, using the responses weighted by the probability of class membership. The process is repeated until convergence.

The EM algorithm has poor convergence properties, often taking many iterations to converge. The algorithm converges to local, not global, optima. The process should be repeated using different initial class assignments and the best final result used as the estimate.

7.4.6.3 Hierarchical Bayesian Approaches

Random effects MNL models are typically estimated by hierarchical Bayesian estimation. The posterior distribution of the model parameters is sampled via Markov chain Monte Carlo. The method requires the selection of a prior for the distribution, $g(\alpha)$. In the case where $g(\alpha)$ is multivariate normal, the priors are iid normal for the mean of $g(\alpha)$ and inverse-Wishart for the covariance of $g(\alpha)$. A common choice is to have the priors on the means be normal distributions with a mean of 0 and variance of 1 and for the prior on the covariance to be inverse-Wishart with scale I and degrees of freedom equal to the number of model parameters plus 2. Models can be improved and estimated with less data if priors are set more intelligently, leveraging existing information about the decision process. This estimation method produces a sample from the posterior distribution of the parameter estimates, not point estimates for those parameters. The theoretically correct method for computing predictions is to take the mean of the predictions of all sampled models. This is computationally difficult. A more common method is to take the mean (or median) posterior estimates for each parameter and use those values as the point estimates. Likewise, the model may be estimated by $g(\alpha)$ as defined by the posterior parameter estimates that define $g(\alpha)$ or by using the empirical estimate of $g(\alpha)$, the posterior estimates of the draws from $g(\alpha)$ observed in the sample. The latter is preferred because it is robust to misspecification of $g(\alpha)$, though in cases where the distribution of model parameters across the population is accurately distributed by the choice of $g(\alpha)$, the former is more accurate.

7.4.7 Model Selection

7.4.7.1 Statistical Criteria

A number of statistical measures have been developed to evaluate the fit of discrete choice models. The simplest is the log-likelihood. This is the log of the probability of the observed data given the fitted model. Greater log-likelihood indicates better model fit. The values are not comparable between models nor datasets. To standardize the value somewhat, McFadden proposed a pseudo-R^2 statistic based on the likelihood:

$$Pseudo - R^2 = 1 - \frac{LL_M}{LL_0},$$

where LL_M is the log-likelihood of the fitted model and LL_0 is the log-likelihood of an intercept-only model. The value has a minimum of 0. It tends to be smaller than OLS R^2; a benchmark range is that a pseudo-R^2 of >0.2 is an excellent model fit.

A related procedure for comparing two models is the likelihood ratio test. The test statistic is the ratio of the log-likelihoods of the two models being compared:

$$\frac{LL_M}{LL_0},$$

where LL_M is the log-likelihood of the proposed model and LL_0 is the log-likelihood of the null model. The statistic is distributed chi-square with degrees of freedom equal to the degrees of freedom of the proposed model minus the degrees of freedom of the null model.

Two statistics that are essentially log-likelihoods penalized for model complexity are Akaike's information criterion (AIC) and Bayesian information criterion (BIC):

$$BIC = \ln{(n)}k - 2LL,$$
$$AIC = 2k - 2LL,$$

where K is the number of parameters in the model; n is the sample size; and LL is the log-likelihood. For both statistics, the model with the lower value is preferred. BIC applies a greater penalty to complex models than does AIC. Both are widely used, and the smaller the statistic, the better the fit.

7.4.7.2 Iteration and Estimation Constraints

Often choice models may be improved by iterative model selection methods such as forward or backward inclusion. In cases where certain part-worths are known to contribute either positively or negatively to utility, it is beneficial to complete this process by hand. Removing attributes from the utility functions which have no or little influence or whose estimated contribution is nonsensical improves the estimates of the other part-worths.

Models estimated by maximum likelihood do not easily permit constraints on the estimates of the part-worths. As such this process is completed post hoc, by iteratively removing part-worths from the model or by treating separate attribute levels as a single level.

Bayesian approaches allow greater flexibility in this area. One approach is to restrict the estimates of the part-worths by modifying the priors. For a parameter where the contribution of utility must be positive, a log-normal prior enforces this constraint or, in the case of a random effects MNL, assuming that the individual level part-worths are distributed log-normal. Another approach is to constrain the parameter estimates within the MCMC algorithm, either by resampling restricted draws or tying mis-ordered values. This approach should be used with caution, as it often leads to flat estimates due to the incongruity between the sampled values and the proposed distribution for $g(\alpha)$. To circumvent this, one can use the unrestricted estimates when evaluating $g(\alpha)$ but the restricted estimates when calculating the log-likelihood. This can be thought of as using a peculiar, nonlinear utility function. Finally, the naïve method of simply tying mis-ordered values after estimation performs surprisingly well in practice though it is difficult to justify statistically (Johnson 2000).

7.4.8 Sensitivity Analysis and Attribute Importance

Beyond providing predictions of decisions, discrete choice models can be analyzed to describe the drivers for decisions. The properties of the drivers are described by the models' sensitivity to the attributes and the attribute importance.

The model sensitivity is the magnitude of the change in the predicted decision as each attribute is changed. For MNL and probit models, this is well captured by the part-worths. A more generalizable measure that works when the model does not have a single parameter defining the contribution of each attribute to the utilities is the change in the probability of a decision between two values of an attribute. The nonlinear nature of the models implies that this measure will vary across the model domain. Typically, a base case, the most likely combination of attribute levels, is chosen. The change in probability as each attribute changes is assessed at this point. Alternatively, one could report an average of the change across the model domain.

The importance of an attribute is the impact an attribute has on the decision relative to the other modeled attributes. It is commonly expressed as the range of the sensitivities for each attribute, normalized to sum to 1. It is difference in choice probability between the most and least preferred level of each attribute divided by the sum of said differences across all the attributes. Similar to the sensitivities, this measure may vary across the domain of the model. Typically, the importance is reported for a base case.

7.5   Summary and Conclusion

The concepts and approach outlined in this chapter represent some of the more widely used approaches to segmentation and choice models in the biopharma industry. Both segmentation and choice models are critical to the successful development and marketing of new products. They are also widely used to investigate the impact of market events on previously launched in-line products as well. As more and larger dataset become available for analysis, these approaches will no doubt continue to evolve to accommodate them.

References

Bartholomew, D. J., Steele, F., Galbraith, J., & Moustaki, I. Analysis of multivariate social science data. (2nd ed.). Taylor & Francis, 2008.

Bensmail, H., Celeux, G., Raftery, A. E., & Robert, C. P. Inference in model-based cluster analysis. Statistics and Computing volume (1997): 7, 1-10.

Bozodogan, H. "Model selection and Akaike's information criteria (AIC): The general theory and its analytical extensions." Psychometrika (1987): 52, 345.

Breiman, L., Freidman, C. J., Olshen, R. A., & Stone, C. Classification and regression trees. Monterey, CA: Wadsworth, 1984.

Child, D. The essentials of factor analysis, 3rd edition. Bloombury Academic Press, 2006.

Dawes, J. "Do data characteristics change according to the number of scale points used? An experiment using 5-point, 7-point, and 10-point scales ." International Journal of Market Research (2008): 50, 61-77.

de Bekker-Grob, E. W., Donkers, B., Jonker, M. F., & Stolk, E. A. "Sample size requirements for discrete-choice experiments in healthcare: a practical guide." The Patient-Patient-Centered Outcomes research (2015): 8, 373-384.

Dempster, A. P., Laird, N. M., & Rubin, D. B. "Maximum likelihood from incomplete data via the E-M algorithm." Journal of the Royal Statistics Society: Series B 39, 1-38 (1977).

Draper, N. R. & Smith, H. Applied regression analysis. New York: Wiley, 1998.

FDA. Draft guidance for industry review staff, target product profile-a strategic development process tool. 2007.

Hamerly, G. & Elkan, C. Alternatives to the k-means algorithm that find better clusterings. Proceedings of the eleventh international conference on information and knowledge management. 2002.

Hartigan, J. A. Clustering Algorithms. New York: Wiley, 1975.

Heiss, F. Specification(s) of nested logit models. Manhaim, Germany: Mannheimer Forschunginstitut Okonomie und Demographischer Wandel, 2002.

Hess, S., Bierlaire, M., Polak, J.: Discrete mixtures models. Paper presented at the 6th Swiss Transport Research Conference (Ascona, Switzerland). http://www.strc.ch/conferences/2006/Hess_Bierlaire_602 Polak_STRC_2006.pdf (2006). Accessed March 2017.

Hosmer, D. W., Lemeshow, S., & Sturdivant, R. X. Applied logistic regression, 3rd edition. New York: Wiley, 2013.

Johnson, R. R. Monotonicity constraints in choice-based conjoint with hierarchical bayes. Research paper. 2000.

Kass, G. V. "An exploratory technique for investigation large quantities of categorical data." Applied Statistics (1980): 29, 119-127.

Kuhfeld, Warren F. Marketing research methods in SAS. Experimental Design, Choice, Conjoint, and Graphical Techniques. Cary, NC, SAS-Institute TS-722 (2005).

Lancsar, E. & Louviere, J. "Conducting discrete choice experiments to inform healthcare decision making." Pharmacoeconomics (2008): 28, 661-677.

Loh, W-Y. "Fifty years of classification and regression trees." International Statistical Review (2014): 82, 329-348.

Louviere, J., Flynn, T. N., & Carson, R. T. "Discrete choice experiments are not conjoint analysis." Journal of choice modelling (2010): 3, 57-72. . Web.

MacQueen, J. B. Some methods for classification and analysis of multivariate observations. Proceedings of 5th Berkeley Symposium on Mathematical Statistics and Probability. Berkeley, CA: University of California Press, 1967. 1, 281–297.

Magidson, J. "The CHAID approach to segmentation modeling: CHi-squared Automatic Interaction Detection." Bagozzi, R. Advanced Methods of Marketing research. New York: Wiley, 1994.

McDonald, R. P. Factor analysis and related methods. Hillsdale, NJ: Erlbaum, 1985.

McHugh, R. B. "Note on 'Efficient estimation and local identification in latent class analysis'." Psychometrika (1958): 23, 273-274.

Nguyen, Nam-Ky, and Alan J. Miller. "A review of some exchange algorithms for constructing discrete D-optimal designs." Computational Statistics & Data Analysis 14.4 (1992): 489-498.

Pedhauzer, E. J. Multiple regression in behavioral research: Explanation and prediction. Ft. Worth, TX: Harcourt Brace, 1997.

Read, D., & Loewenstein, G. "Diversification bias: Explaining the discrepancy in variety seeking between combined and separated choices." Journal of Experimental Psychology: Applied (1995): 1, 34-49. . Web.

Schwarz, G. E. "Estimating the dimension of a model." Annals of Statistics (1978): 6, 461-464.

Silberhorn, H., Bortug, Y., & Hilderbrandt, L. "Estimation with the nested logit model: specifications and software particularities." OR Spectrum (2008): 30, 635-653.

Stewart, D. W. "The application and misapplication of factor analysis in marketing research." Journal of Marketing Research (1981): 18, 51-62.

Train, K. E. Discrete Choice Models with Simulation. Cambridge, MA: Cambridge University Press, 2002.

Vermunt, J. K. & Magidson, J. "Latent class cluster analysis." Hagenaars, J. A. & McCutcheon, A. L. Applied Latent Class Analysis. Cambridge: Cambridge University Press, 2002. 89-106.

Wedel, M. & Kamakura, W. A. Market Segmentation Conceptual and Methodological Foundations 2nd Edition. Norwell, MA: Kluwers, 2000.

Wedel, M. & DeSarbo W. S. Market Segment Derivation and Profiling Via a Finite Mixture Model Framework, Marketing Letters (2002): 13 (1), 17–25

Wendell R. Smith. Product Differentiation and Market Segmentation as Alternative Marketing Strategies Journal of Marketing (1956):Vol. 21, No. 1, pp. 3.

Weinstein, M. C., Torrance, G., & Mcguire, A. QALYs: The basics. Value in Health (2009). Web.

Zwerina, Klaus, Joel Huber, and Warren F. Kuhfeld. "A general method for constructing efficient choice designs." Durham, NC: Fuqua School of Business, Duke University (1996).

Chapter 8
Modern Analytic Techniques for Predictive Modeling of Clinical Trial Operations

Vladimir V. Anisimov

8.1 Introduction

Statistical design and operation of multicenter clinical trials over time are affected by the uncertainties in input information, a natural stochasticity in patient enrollment and screening processes and various events' appearances.

There are different interconnected stages of trial design and operation including patient enrollment planning/prediction, choosing randomization scheme and statistical models for analyzing patient responses, monitoring/predicting various operational characteristics including enrollment performance on different levels, the number of events of various types, detecting unusual data patterns, etc.

The complexity of contemporary clinical trials and multistate hierarchic structure of operational processes require developing novel analytic techniques for efficient modeling and forecasting different characteristics. Some controversies in the analysis of multicenter clinical trials are considered by Senn (1997, 1998).

Typically, a sample size is defined by the number of patients that have to be randomized to the trial to have enough information for statistically relevant conclusions about the properties of the drug. Thus, one of the tasks is to design the trial in such a way (choose countries and centers in countries) that the required number of patients will be reached within a planned time.

Forecasting patient enrollment is one of the bottleneck problems as uncertainties in enrollment substantially affect randomization process, trial time completion, supply chain, and associated costs. Using Poisson processes with fixed rates to describe the enrollment process is an accepted approach (Carter et al. 2005; Senn 1997, 1998). However, in real trials the enrollment rates in different centers vary and to mimic this variation Anisimov and Fedorov (2005, 2007a, b) introduced a model (so-called Poisson-gamma model referred to as a PG model), where the variation in

V. V. Anisimov (✉)
Center for Design and Analysis, Amgen Inc., London, UK

© Springer Nature Switzerland AG 2020
O. V. Marchenko, N. V. Katenka (eds.), *Quantitative Methods in Pharmaceutical Research and Development*, https://doi.org/10.1007/978-3-030-48555-9_8

rates is modeled using a gamma distribution. This model can be described in the framework of the empirical Bayesian approach where the prior distribution of the rates is a gamma distribution with parameters that are evaluated either using historical data or data provided by study managers (Anisimov 2011a). Anisimov and Fedorov (2007b) also described the Bayesian technique for calculating the posterior gamma distribution of the rates at any interim time using real enrollment information. Later on, Gajewski et al. (2008, 2012) independently considered a similar Bayesian model for modeling enrollment but using one clinical center.

Note that the use of Poisson-gamma mixed models and an associated negative binomial distribution has a long history, for example, Bates and Neyman (1952), for describing the variation of positive variables in modeling flows of various events.

To account for wider realistic scenarios, the technique developed in Anisimov and Fedorov (2005, 2007a, b) (see also Anisimov 2008) was extended further to capture the situations where clinical centers can be initiated with random delays and also can be closed earlier (Anisimov 2011a). A PG model was also used in Mijoule et al. (2012) to consider some extensions related to other distributions of the enrollment rates and sensitivity analysis, and in Bakhshi et al. (2013) for the evaluation of parameters of a PG model using meta-analysis of historical trials.

There are also other models considered in the literature for modeling patient enrollment (see survey Barnard et al. 2010). Most of the papers by other authors are mainly dealing with predicting the global enrollment and there are two basic directions. One is using mixed Poisson processes where the global rate is modeled using different approaches, see Deng et al. (2014); Gajewski et al. (2008); Tang et al. (2012); and Williford et al. (1987). Another one uses Brownian or fractional Brownian motions, Lai et al. (2001) and Zhang and Lai (2011).

However, as these papers are dealing with the modeling enrollment on global level, there are some limitations. Specifically, these approaches typically require rather large number of centers and patients (to use some approximations) and cannot be applied on the individual level, e.g., to distinguish enrollment performance in different centers/countries; create forecasts on country/region levels, etc. Moreover, at study start-up and early stages, these techniques also may not be appropriate, as in general at these stages there are small numbers of active centers and patients recruited.

From another side, a PG model is designed on the individual center level and also can be used on the next levels (using different approximations); thus, it is not limited to restrictions above. Therefore, this model is rather flexible and can be applied to the vast majority of trials at different stages.

A brief review of the papers related to these directions is provided in Heitjan et al. (2015), and some additional discussion mainly related to the use of analytic models with random parameters is given in Anisimov (2016b).

It is worth to mention a very important direction in randomized clinical trials dealing with the properties of different randomization schemes. Randomization is an essential part of a trial design, and the choice of randomization affects the power of statistical tests and the amount of drug supply required to satisfy patient demand. The properties of various types of randomization schemes are studied by many authors. As this direction requires a special attention which is not in the scope of a current chapter, we refer readers to the book by Rosenberger and Lachin (2013) and also the earlier paper (Lachin 1988) with references therein. The properties of imbalance caused by permuted-block randomization using a Poisson-gamma enrollment model are studied in (Anisimov 2011c; Anisimov et al. 2017). Another way of randomizing patients to different treatments and maintaining balance between treatment arms is minimization, e.g., Senn et al. 2010.

There is also a large part of clinical trials (event-driven) where a sample size is defined by the number of some clinical events that is required to have enough information for reliable statistical conclusions about the parameters of patient responses, e.g., oncology and cardiovascular trials. For these trials, one of the main tasks is predicting not only the number of enrolled patients but mainly the number of events that will happen for these patients and time to reach this number.

A useful review of different approaches for event-driven trials is provided in Heitjan et al. (2015). However, for predicting the number of events over time and time to stop trial, the authors of papers cited there mainly use Monte Carlo simulation technique. Therefore, as the natural step in modeling trial operation, Anisimov (2011b) developed an analytic technique (based on closed-form expressions) for predictive modeling of the event's counting process together with patient enrollment in ongoing event-driven multicenter trials. In the chapter, this methodology is developed further to forecasting the multiple events at start-up and interim stages. Some approaches to optimal trial design accounting for enrollment and follow-up stages and to risk-based monitoring and detection unusual event patterns are also proposed.

As the next step in modeling trial operation, to model more complicated hierarchic processes on the top of enrollment including follow-up patients, various events (clinical and nonclinical, AE), patient's visits, and related costs, a new methodology based on using so-called evolving stochastic processes is developed (Anisimov 2016a). This methodology can serve as some general framework to model various types of operational processes related to patient enrollment and event processes. In the chapter, this methodology is extended to modeling different events during a follow-up period and calculating predictive distributions of the number of counts. A few examples are considered.

8.2 Predictive Patient Enrollment Modeling

A large clinical trial usually involves a large number of patients who have to be recruited by many clinical centers typically in different countries.

Consider a clinical trial where the patients are recruited by different clinical centers and then, after a screening period, they are randomized to different treatments according to some randomization scheme. At trial design and interim stages, it is crucial to predict how many patients will be recruited in total and also predict the time when a certain number of patients (sample size) will be reached.

For operational purposes and to verify specific trial goals and planned schedule, it is also important to predict and monitor enrollment in particular regions, in particular, to detect centers/countries with unusually low or high enrollment which is one of the purposes of data management and risk-based monitoring (RBM).

Most of clinical trials use so-called competitive enrollment (no restrictions on the number of patients to be recruited in particular centers/regions). Nevertheless, sometimes due to some geographical or population reasons, the teams may use restrictive enrollment, e.g., in some countries/regions it might be set the upper (or low) thresholds (say, to enroll not more (or less) patients than a given number). However, adding some restrictions may substantially increase the enrollment stopping time and put trial deadline goals at risk (Anisimov et al. 2003). Therefore, in this chapter the focus is on competitive enrollment. Note that some results can be extended to the trials with restrictive enrollment as well.

8.2.1   Poisson-Gamma Enrollment Model

Let us formalize the basic model, which will be used for predictive enrollment modeling and also as a baseline model for forecasting event process and other operational characteristics.

There are three major uncertainties in patient enrollment. This first one is dealing with the stochasticity of enrollment process in each clinical center, the second one is associated with the variation in enrollment rates between different centers, and the last one is related to center's initiation delays.

In the framework of a Poisson-gamma (PG) model introduced in Anisimov and Fedorov (2005, 2007b) and further extended in Anisimov (2011a), it is proposed to model the process of patient's enrollment in different centers using Poisson processes with some rates, model variation in enrollment rates using a gamma distribution, and model delays in centers initiation also using some probability distributions, e.g., uniform, gamma.

The formal construction is defined as follows. Denote by $\Pi_\lambda(t)$ an ordinary homogeneous Poisson process with a given rate λ. This means, for any $t > 0$,

$$\Pr(\Pi_\lambda(t) = k) = \frac{e^{-\lambda t}}{k!}(\lambda t)^k, \quad k = 0, 1, 2, ..$$

Denote also by $\Pi(a)$ a Poisson random variable with parameter a. Assume that the enrollment rate λ_i in center i has a gamma distribution with some parameters (α,β)—shape and rate parameters—and probability density function:

$$f(x, \alpha, \beta) = \frac{e^{-\beta x}\beta^\alpha x^{\alpha-1}}{\Gamma(\alpha)}, x > 0,$$

where $\Gamma(\alpha)$ is a gamma function. Suppose that center i is initiated at time u_i, which can be also some random variable.

Denote by $n_i(t)$ the number of patients enrolled in center i in time interval $[0, t]$ (enrollment process in center i). Then this process can be represented as

$$n_i(t) = \Pi_{\lambda_i}\left([t - u_i]_+\right),$$

where by definition $[a]_+ = \max(0, a)$.

Thus, $n_i(t)$ is a nonhomogeneous in time doubly stochastic Poisson process (Cox process), Cox and Isham (1980), with cumulative rate at time t, $\lambda_i[t - u_i]_+$.

Consider some useful relations. The process $\Pi_\lambda(t)$ where rate λ has a gamma distribution with parameters (α, β) is a Poisson-gamma (PG) process (Bernardo and Smith 2004) with parameters (t, α, β). Denote by PG(t, α, β) a PG random variable with parameters (t, α, β) (it has the same distribution as the process $\Pi_\lambda(t)$) and by Pg(k, t, α, β) its probability mass function. Then

$$\mathrm{Pg}(k, t, \alpha, \beta) = \Pr(\Pi_\lambda(t) = k) = \frac{\Gamma(\alpha + k)}{k!\Gamma(\alpha)} \frac{t^k \beta^\alpha}{(\beta + t)^{\alpha + k}}, k = 0, 1, 2, .. \qquad (8.1)$$

For $t = 1$, $\Pi_\lambda(1)$ corresponds to a doubly stochastic Poisson variable with gamma distributed rate λ, thus, we omit t and use notation PG(α, β). According to Johnson et al. (1993: 199), $\Pi_\lambda(t)$ has a negative binomial distribution, and the following relation is true:

$$\mathrm{Pg}(k, t, \alpha, \beta) = \Pr\left(Nb\left(\alpha, \frac{\beta}{\beta + t}\right) = k\right), \qquad (8.2)$$

where $Nb(\alpha, p)$ denotes a random variable which has a negative binomial distribution with size α and probability p:

$$\Pr(Nb(\alpha, p) = k) = \frac{\Gamma(\alpha + k)}{k!\Gamma(\alpha)} p^\alpha (1 - p)^k, k = 0, 1, ..$$

Then in the case where u_i is given, for $t > u_i$ the process $n_i(t)$ is a PG process with parameters $(t - u_i, \alpha, \beta)$ and $\Pr(n_i(t) = k) = \mathrm{Pg}(k, t - u_i, \alpha, \beta)$, $k = 0, 1, 2, ..$

If u_i is a random variable, the distribution of $n_i(t)$ can be written in the integral form and in general cannot be derived in terms of simple formulae. Therefore, for general cases we can use some approximations that will be discussed further.

Consider some region I that indicates a subset of sites with indexes $i \in I$. Denote by $n(I, t)$ the number of patients enrolled in this region in time interval $[0,t]$. Define the global cumulative enrollment rate in the region in time interval $[0,t]$ as:

$$\Lambda(I, t) = \sum_{i \in I} \lambda_i [t - u_i]_+. \qquad (8.3)$$

According to properties of a Poisson process, the process $n(I, t)$ is a nonhomogeneous doubly stochastic Poisson process with cumulative rate $\Lambda(I, t)$. Therefore, the enrollment process in any region (also globally) can be represented as a doubly stochastic Poisson process where the cumulative rate has an explicit representation in the terms of weighted sum of gamma distributed random variables. Thus, the distribution of the enrollment process on different levels can be modeled and predicted using properties of a PG model and different types of approximations. For example, in regions with large number of centers, the process $n(I, t)$ can be approximated by a normal distribution, and it is possible to calculate in the closed form the predictive mean and bounds for the enrollment process over time and correspondingly to evaluate the predictive mean and bounds for the enrollment time. This approach is realized in (Anisimov 2011a). For an individual center, the relation (8.1) gives the explicit formula for distribution of the enrollment process in this center. In general, we need to account for delay u_i and use $[t - u_i]_+$ instead of t. Note also that the cumulative rate $\Lambda(I, t)$ in (8.3) as a sum of gamma distributed variables in general does not have a gamma distribution. However, for fixed times of initiation u_i the rate $\Lambda(I, t)$ can be approximated by a gamma distributed variable with aggregated parameters (Anisimov 2011a).

Thus, a PG model allows to model enrollment behavior at different levels of trial hierarchy. Note that Carter et al. (2005) also considered rates of Poisson processes as random variables but using a uniform distribution. However, this approach has some limitations as it assumes that rates are bounded in some interval. Moreover, the analysis of real trials shows that the empirical distributions of the rates are rather far from uniform distribution and heavy tailed.

This statement is supported by Fig. 8.1, which shows a histogram of the empirical rates for a real case study with 100 centers. For this study, the duration of enrollment in centers varies from 1 till 398 (in days), and the number of enrolled patients varies from 0 till 22. Figure 8.1 shows rather typical behavior of empirical rates for rather large studies.

Consider now in more detail the implementation of a PG model for modeling and forecasting patient enrollment. There are two basic stages in predicting patient enrollment and various events:

1. Start-up (baseline) prediction before trials starts and therefore there is no real trial data available yet.
2. Interim prediction where it is possible to use real trial data and perform reforecasting of trial operational behavior for the remaining period with the purpose to update trial deadlines.

At both stages, the advanced predictive techniques can use a PG model; however, input data may have different formats, and the model parameters will be evaluated differently.

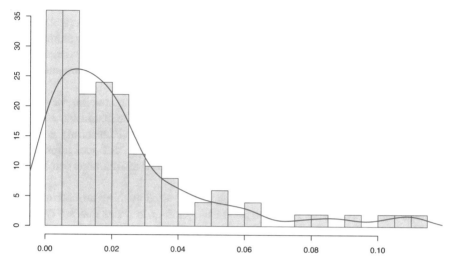

Fig. 8.1 Histogram of the enrollment rate for real case study. Continuous line is the empirical density

8.2.2 Trial Start-Up Stage

This stage may also include an early stage of the trial with not so many centers initiated and not so many patients recruited yet. Typically, during this stage, the basic input information that is provided by clinical teams for enrollment prediction includes the following key elements:

1. A total planned number of randomized patients to be enrolled (sample size)
2. An expected number of screened patients and screening duration
3. A list of initially planned regions and countries to be involved into the study
4. A planned number of centers to be initiated in each country and some information about the schedule of initiation
5. The expected enrollment rates in centers or countries (this may include screening/enrollment rates and dropout probabilities)

This information has many uncertainties. In particular, at the start-up stage usually the exact schedule of center's initiation is not known, and the screening/enrollment rates and dropout probabilities are also not known. Therefore, one of the main problems at this stage is how to account for these uncertainties, evaluate trial enrollment feasibility, and forecast the enrollment time (time to stop enrollment). There is no universal approach since a solution may depend on input data format and data availability.

One approach can be to use data from similar historic studies (similar therapeutic indication, inclusion/exclusion criteria, etc.) conducted in the same regions. Then potentially this information can be used to create the initial trial enrollment design.

Specifically, the enrollment rates for a new trial can be treated as random variables with a prior distribution where parameters can be evaluated using historical data in these regions and some prior information. As the rates are positive, it is natural to use a gamma distribution. For a new trial, we can also assume that the centers in the regions are initiated in time according to some distributions where parameters are estimated using historical data.

As usually teams for each country/region may provide some time intervals where a given number of centers are planned to be initiated, then at the first instance we can assume that the times of center's initiation are distributed uniformly in these intervals (Anisimov et al. 2007; Anisimov 2009). If some historical information about center's initiation dates is available, other types of distributions can be also used, e.g., gamma, beta, or empirical.

However, the historical information should be used with some caution. The analysis of real trials shows that the point estimators of the rates that are typically used in the form k_i/τ_i, where k_i is the number of patients enrolled in center i and τ_i is the enrollment window, may substantially differ in the same centers for different trials even for very similar therapeutic area and indication. One reason for this is a random fluctuation of the enrollment. However, the estimators of parameters of a PG model behave rather stable, e.g., Bakhshi et al. (2013) and Minois et al. (2017). Therefore, it can be proposed to use a PG model for both historical and new trials and, instead of estimating the enrollment rates in given sites using point estimators, to estimate the variability in enrollment rates using a PG model and then aggregate recruitment in the region or for the whole trial. In this case, the estimators of the parameters of a PG model for historical trials can be used as prior estimators of the enrolment model for the new trial, Minois et al. (2017).

Note that during the start-up stage there can be rather long transient period until most of the centers will be initiated. Thus, the total number of patients and centers may not be too large. Therefore, during this period it is important to account for the process of centers initiation and the methods based on modeling enrollment in the individual centers are much more preferable compared to models based on the global prediction. Thus, it is natural to use at this stage a PG enrollment model. This model is very flexible as it provides the opportunity to model the enrollment on different levels (center, country, region, trial) and has many additional features, e.g., predicting with credibility bounds, predicting probability to complete in time, evaluate effects of changing the number of centers, etc. One of the additional advantages of a PG model is that most of these characteristics can be calculated using closed-form expressions; thus, there is no need to use Monte Carlo simulation.

If there is no information from similar trials, then we can use the planned/ expected rates provided by clinical teams weighted with some expert estimators. These data can be used as sample statistics for evaluating the prior parameters of a PG model (on country or regional level). Some discussion on using baseline estimates of rates at the trial start-up was provided in Anisimov et al. (2007) and Anisimov (2011a). Bakhshi et al. (2013) investigated a PG model further and suggested the empirical way to set the prior parameters by using a meta-analysis.

Note that at start-up and early stages other approaches based on models for global enrollment, e.g., using Poisson models with mixed global gamma distributed rate, Gajewski et al. (2008, 2012), and Brownian (Lai et al. 2001) or fractional Brownian (Zhang and Lai 2011) motions, may not be appropriate as in general at these stages there is a small number of active centers and patients recruited.

Let us provide a formalization of a PG model at the start-up stage and how it can be used for modeling and predicting enrollment at different levels.

8.2.2.1 Enrollment Prediction at Trial Start-Up Stage

Typically, at the trial start-up stage clinical teams have some historic information about the enrollment performance of similar clinical trials in these sites or regions and may use also the expert estimates. Therefore, by analyzing the historical rates, the teams may provide the expected means and standard deviations of the enrollment rates for the planned trial (on center or country level) that can be used to estimate the prior parameters of the rates used in prediction. The same is related to the times of site's initiation.

Assume that this information is available and consider a slight generalization of a PG model compared to the initial setup in Anisimov and Fedorov (2005, 2007b). Suppose that at the trial start-up the following data are available in each center:

m_i—Mean enrollment rate
s_i^2—Variance of enrollment rate
u_i—Center initiation time which can be a random variable with some given distribution

In the framework of a PG model, we assume that the enrollment rate λ_i in center i has a gamma distribution with some parameters (α_i, β_i). According to the properties of a gamma distribution, these parameters can be expressed via mean and variance as $\alpha_i = m_i^2/s_i^2$, $\beta_i = m_i/s_i^2$. Thus, the enrollment process $n_i(t)$ in center i is a PG process with cumulative rate at time t, $\lambda_i[t - u_i]_+$.

For a doubly stochastic Poisson process $\Pi(\Lambda(t))$ with cumulative rate at time t, $\Lambda(t)$,

$$E[\Pi(\Lambda(t))] = E[\Lambda(t)], \quad Var[\Pi(\Lambda(t))] = E[\Lambda(t)] + Var[\Lambda(t)]. \quad (8.4)$$

These relations can be used for evaluation the mean and the variance of the enrollment processes in different centers/regions. Then these values can be used for enrollment forecasting using some approximations.

Let us first calculate the mean and the variance of the enrollment process $n(t)$ in one center. Assume that the enrollment rate is λ and the time of center initiation is τ, which is a random variable with cumulative distribution function $G(x) = \Pr(\tau \leq x)$. Then the process $n(t)$ is a doubly stochastic Poisson variable with cumulative rate $\Lambda(t) = \lambda_i[t - \tau]_+$. Define the following functions:

$$m(t) = \int_0^t x dG(x)$$
$$b^2(t) = \int_0^t x^2 dG(x)$$

(8.5)

It is easy to calculate that

$$E[\Lambda(t)] = E[\lambda](tG(t) - m(t)), E[\Lambda^2(t)] = E[\lambda^2](t^2G(t) - 2tm(t) + b^2(t))$$ (8.6)

As $Var[\Lambda(t)] = E[\Lambda^2(t)] - (E[\Lambda(t)])^2$, then

$$E[n(t)] = E[\Lambda(t)],$$ (8.7)

$$Var[n(t)] = E[\Lambda(t)] + Var[\Lambda(t)] = E[\Lambda(t)] + E[\Lambda^2(t)] - (E[\Lambda(t)])^2.$$ (8.8)

According to relation (8.3), the cumulative rate in any region is a sum of independent individual rates. Thus, the mean and the variance of $\Lambda(I, t)$ can be computed as sums of individual means and variances using relations (8.5)–(8.8). Therefore, in the cases where it is possible to calculate the functions (8.5) in a closed form, the mean and the variance of $\Lambda(I, t)$ can be also computed in the closed form.

Consider now several important cases. Assume first that the time of center initiation is deterministic ($\tau = u$), and the enrollment rate λ has mean m and variance s^2. Then

$$E[\Lambda(t)] = m(t - u), t > u, \text{ and zero if } t \leq u,$$

$$Var[\Lambda(t)] = s^2(t - u)^2, t > u, \text{ and zero if } t \leq u,$$

and the mean and the variance of $n(t)$ are calculated according to (8.7), (8.8).

Consider now some region I with $N(I)$ centers and assume that for center i the values: m_i, the mean enrollment rate; s_i^2, the variance of enrollment rate; and u_i, site initiation time, are given. Denote by $\Lambda(I, t)$ a cumulative rate in region I, and put:

$$E(I, t) = E[\Lambda(I, t)], S^2(I, t) = Var[\Lambda(I, t)].$$

Then

$$E(I, t) = \sum_{i \in I} m_i[t - u_i]_+, S^2(I, t) = \sum_{i \in I} s_i^2[t - u_i]_+^2.$$ (8.9)

These expressions can be used to calculate the mean and the variance of the enrollment process $n(I, t)$ in region I according to (8.7), (8.8). Consider now the case when time of initiation τ is a random variable. Typically, at the start-up stage clinical teams may provide a planned schedule of center initiation knowing for some countries/regions only the time intervals where a given number of centers are planned to be initiated. In this case, in the absence of other information, it is natural to use a uniform distribution for times of center's initiation in these intervals.

Another way can be to use a gamma distribution for initiation times where the parameters can be evaluated using historical data or some prior information.

Assume that the time of center initiation in interval $[a, b]$ has a uniform distribution. Denote by $M(t, a, b, m)$ and $S^2(t, a, b, m, s^2)$, the mean and the variance of the cumulative enrollment rate $\Lambda(t)$ in this center. In Anisimov et al. (2007) and Anisimov (2009), the following result was proved:

$$M(t, a, b, m) = \begin{cases} 0, & \text{if} \quad t \le a \\ \dfrac{m(t-a)^2}{2(b-a)}, & \text{if} \quad a < t \le b \\ mt - \dfrac{m(a+b)}{2}, & \text{if} \quad t > b \end{cases} \tag{8.10}$$

$$S^2(t,a,b,m,s^2) = \begin{cases} 0, & \text{if} \quad t \le a \\ \dfrac{m^2(t-a)^3(4b-a-3t)}{12(b-a)^2} + \dfrac{s^2(t-a)^3}{3(b-a)}, & \text{if } a < t \le b. \\ \dfrac{(m^2+s^2)(b-a)^2}{12} + s^2\left(t - \dfrac{a+b}{2}\right)^2, & \text{if} \quad t > b \end{cases} \tag{8.11}$$

Thus, in the case where for each center i in region I the mean rate m_i, SD s_i and the interval of center initiation $[a_i, b_i]$ are given, the mean and the variance of the cumulative rate $\Lambda(I, t)$ are calculated as follows:

$$E[\Lambda(I,t)] = E(I,t) = \sum_{i \in I} M(t, a_i, b_i, m_i), \tag{8.12}$$

$$Var[\Lambda(I,t)] = S^2(I,t) = \sum_{i \in I} S^2(t, a_i, b_i, s_i^2). \tag{8.13}$$

Consider now the case where a center initiation time has a gamma distribution. Assume that a center is initiated in interval $[a, \infty)$ and the time τ of initiation has the form $\tau = a + \eta$, where η has a gamma distribution with parameters (ψ, θ), and the enrollment rate λ has a mean m and variance s^2. Denote by $F(t, \psi, \theta)$ a cumulative distribution function of a gamma distribution with parameters (ψ, θ). Then it is possible to prove the following result:

Lemma 8.1 In the expression (8.5),

$$m(t) = aF(t - a, \psi, \theta) + \frac{\psi}{\theta} F(t - a, \psi + 1, \theta), \quad t > a, \text{ and zero for } t \le a.$$

$$b^2(t) = a^2 F(t - a, \psi, \theta) + 2a\frac{\psi}{\theta} F(t - a, \psi + 1, \theta)$$
$$+ \frac{\psi(\psi + 1)}{\theta^2} F(t - a, \psi + 2, \theta), \quad t > a, \text{ and zero for } t \le a.$$

Using these expressions we can calculate in each center $E[\Lambda(t)]$ and $Var[\Lambda(t)]$ using relations (8.6), and then calculate in any region I, $E[\Lambda(I, t)]$, and $Var[\Lambda(I, t)]$ by summing by all centers in the region the individual means and variances.

Similar expressions for $m(t)$ and $b^2(t)$ can be derived for the case when a center initiation time has a beta distribution. Note that a beta distribution is similar to the uniform one; however, it shifts the probability weight to the beginning or end of the interval. To use a beta distribution, we should know some specific prior information.

Denote by $\beta(p, q)$ a random variable that has a beta distribution in interval $[0, 1]$ with parameters (p, q). Assume that the time τ of center initiation has a beta distribution in interval $[a, b]$, so we can represent τ as $\tau = a + (b - a)\beta(p, q)$. Denote by $B(t, p, q)$ a cumulative distribution function of $\beta(p, q)$ (for $t \in (0, 1)$ this is an incomplete beta function). Then

$$P(\tau \le t) = B\left(\frac{t - a}{b - a}, p, q\right).$$

For the ease of notation denote $z = (t - a)/(b - a)$. Let us introduce the following functions:

$$Q_1(z, p, q) = E\big[\beta(p, q)[z - \beta(p, q)]_+\big],$$
$$Q_2(z, p, q) = E\big[\beta^2(p, q)[z - \beta(p, q)]_+\big],$$

for $z > 0$ and set $Q_1(z, p, q) = 0$, $Q_2(z, p, q) = 0$ for $z \le 0$. Using integral transformations, we can derive the following relations:

$$Q_1(z, p, q) = \frac{p}{p + q} B(z, p + 1, q),$$

$$Q_2(z, p, q) = \frac{p(p + 1)}{(p + q)(p + q + 1)} B(z, p + 2, q).$$

Now using similar considerations as above, we can prove the following statement:

Statement. If the time of center initiation has a beta distribution, in the expression (8.5), $m(t) = aB(z, p, q) + (b - a)Q_1(z, p, q)$, $b^2(t) = a^2B(z, p, q) + 2a(b - a)$ $Q_1(z, p, q) + (b - a)^2 Q_2(z, p, q)$, where $z = (t - a)/(b - a)$.

Using these formulae and relations (8.6)–(8.8), the mean and the variance of the enrollment process can be computed analytically in any region. In the next section, the technique for calculating the approximations of the predictive mean and bounds of the enrollment process and of the enrollment time using the expressions for mean and the variance of the cumulative rate is provided.

8.2.2.2 Enrollment Prediction at Trial Start-Up Stage in Any Region

Consider some region I with cumulative rate at time t, $\Lambda(I, t)$ and denote $E(I, t) = E[\Lambda(I, t)]$, $V^2(I, t) = E[\Lambda(I, t)] + Var[\Lambda(I, t)]$. According to (8.4), these functions represent the mean and the variance of the enrollment process $n(I, t)$ in this region and can be computed for rather general cases of centers initiation as shown above.

Denote by $N(I)$ the number of centers in region I. If $N(I)$ is rather large (in general it may be enough to have $N(I) > 10$, but for a good approximation and estimation parameters, it is advisable to have $N(I) \geq 20$), then the process $n(I, t)$ for any $t > 0$ can be approximated by a normal random variable with mean $E(I, t)$ and variance $V^2(I, t)$. Thus, the predictive $(1 - \delta)$–confidence interval for $n(I, t)$ can be approximated as

$$\left(E(I, t) - z_{1-\frac{\delta}{2}} V(I, t), E(I, t) + z_{1-\frac{\delta}{2}} V(I, t) \right),$$

where z_a is an a-quantile of a standard normal distribution.

Let us define an approximate upper Q-bound for the process $n(I, t)$ as

$$Z(Q, t) = E(I, t) + z_Q V(I, t). \tag{8.14}$$

This means that with probability Q the value $n(I, t)$ is below $Z(Q, t)$, so $Z(Q, t)$ can serve as an upper bound. Correspondingly, an approximate low P-bound for the process $n(I, t)$ is

$$Z(1 - P, t) = E(I, t) + z_{1-P} V(I, t).$$

This means, with probability P the value $n(I, t)$ is above $Z(1 - P, t)$. These formulae allow us to evaluate the predictive intervals for time to reach a region target as times of crossing by the line bounds the horizontal line $Y = L(I)$, where $L(I)$ is the enrollment target in the region.

Consider now a global enrollment process with mean and variance functions $(E(t), V^2(t))$ calculated as in (8.12), (8.13) where summation is taken across all centers. In Anisimov (2011b) it was proved that the interval of crossing the horizontal line $y = n$ by the curves $E(t) + z_{1-\frac{\delta}{2}} V(t)$ and $E(t) - z_{1-\frac{\delta}{2}} V(t)$ can serve as an approximate $(1 - \delta)$-predictive interval for a global enrollment time.

Consider now prediction in not so large regions. If $N(I) < 10$, a normal approximation may not perform well. In this case it is possible to use another type of approximation. Consider the case where the times of centers initiation u_i are deterministic. Then the cumulative rate $\Lambda(I, t)$ is a sum of gamma distributed variables that have in general different distributions. Therefore, $\Lambda(I, t)$ in general does not follow a gamma distribution. Nevertheless, in Anisimov (2011a) it was proposed to approximate $\Lambda(I, t)$ by a gamma distributed variable with the same mean and variance as of $\Lambda(I, t)$. This approximation in some sense is similar to the Welch-Satterthwaite approximation that was originally used to approximate the linear combinations of independent chi-square random variables. An exhaustive Monte Carlo simulation shows that this approximation works perfectly well even for rather small values of $N(I)$ about 3–5. This means the following result:

Lemma 8.2 Consider some region I with $N(I)$ centers and assume that for center i the values: m_i, – the mean enrollment rate; s_i^2, – the variance of enrollment rate; u_i, – center initiation time, are given.

Then for any time $t > 0$, the cumulative rate $\Lambda(I, t)$ defined in (8.3) can be approximated by a gamma distributed random variable with parameters $(A(I, t), B(I, t))$, where

$$A(I,t) = \frac{E^2(I,t)}{S^2(I,t)}, B(I,t) = \frac{E(I,t)}{S^2(I,t)}, \tag{8.15}$$

and functions $E(I, t)$ and $S^2(I, t)$ are defined in (8.9). Correspondingly, the process $n(I, t)$ can be approximated by a PG process with parameters $(1, A(I, t), B(I, t))$.

Relation (8.2) allows using in calculations in R standard formulae for a negative binomial distribution, e.g., for a PG variable $PG(t, \alpha, \beta)$, the standard functions for distributions look as

$$\Pr(PG(t, \alpha, \beta) = k) = \mathrm{dnbinom}\left(k, \mathrm{size} = \alpha, \mathrm{prob} = \frac{\beta}{\beta + t}\right),$$

$$\Pr(PG(t, \alpha, \beta) \le k) = \mathrm{pnbinom}\left(k, \mathrm{size} = \alpha, \mathrm{prob} = \frac{\beta}{\beta + t}\right),$$

$$Q(P, t, \alpha, \beta) = \mathrm{qnbinom}\left(P, \mathrm{size} = \alpha, \mathrm{prob} = \frac{\beta}{\beta + t}\right),$$

where $Q(P, t, \alpha, \beta)$ is a P-quantile of $PG(t, \alpha, \beta)$ variable which is defined as the first integer L such that $Pr(PG(t, \alpha, \beta) \le L) \ge P$.

These formulae can be used in R-tools to evaluate numerically the predictive distributions and bounds of the process $n(I, t)$ using relations (8.15) and also for the global process.

The advantage of this methodology is that it is based on the derived closed-form expressions, and computation time is negligible.

8.2.3 Enrollment Reforecasting at Interim Stage

At the interim stage, it is natural to use real data and re-estimate parameters of the model with the purpose to adjust them to real data and improve accuracy of prediction of the remaining enrollment. It is typically assumed that there is already some number of active centers that have enrolled a reasonable number of patients (enough to use statistical estimation). Note that the methods and results may depend on trial goals and data availability.

There can be also other tasks at the interim stage including evaluating enrollment performance, risk-based monitoring other operational characteristics, detecting center/country outliers, etc. These results will be discussed further after analysis of the interim stage.

Consider a general framework that is using here. Assume that there are N active centers, and the enrollment processes in different centers are modeled using PG processes. Without loss of generality, we can assume that all centers belong to the same pool of centers (have the same parameters of a PG enrollment model). Otherwise, the centers can be divided on clusters where within each cluster we can assume the homogeneity of centers.

Therefore, assume that all rates λ_i have a prior gamma distribution with the same parameters (α, β). Suppose that at interim time t_1 the following data are available:

k_i—The number of patients recruited in center i, and
v_i—The duration of active enrollment in center i up to time t_1.

Using data (k_i, v_i), $i = 1, .., N$, the parameters (α, β) can be estimated using maximum likelihood technique (Anisimov and Fedorov 2007b; Anisimov 2011a). Following these papers, the log-likelihood function up to a constant has the form:

$$L(\alpha, \beta) = \sum_{i=1}^{N} \ln \Gamma(\alpha + k_i) - N \ln \Gamma(\alpha) + N\alpha \ln \beta - \sum_{i=1}^{N} (\alpha + k_i) \ln (\beta + v_i) + C,$$

and ML estimators can be found using numerical optimization. Note that according to a general theory of ML, the estimators are asymptotically normal:

$$\left(\widehat{\alpha}, \widehat{\beta}\right) \approx (\alpha, \beta) + \frac{B\mathcal{N}(0, 1)}{\sqrt{N}},$$

where $\mathcal{N}(0, 1)$ stands for a standard normal random variable.

Thus, at large N the error of estimation is practically negligible. However, to have a good accuracy of estimation, it is recommended to have at least 20 centers with 30–40 recruited patients in total. The estimation technique also works for smaller values; however, in these cases the error in estimation and its impact on the accuracy of prediction can be evaluated separately. Discussion of this technique may have a special interest but is outside of the scope of this chapter.

As different centers have initially different enrollment rates, the next step is to adjust the estimated prior rates to real interim data. In Anisimov and Fedorov (2007b), an empirical Bayesian approach was proposed (see also Anisimov 2011a). As Poisson and gamma are conjugate distributions, it is a known fact that given data (k_i, v_i) in center i the posterior rate $\widetilde{\lambda}_i$ also has a gamma distribution with parameters $(\alpha + k_i, \beta + v_i)$.

Therefore, it is proposed to model the future enrollment process in center i by a doubly stochastic Poisson process with posterior rate $\widetilde{\lambda}_i$, which is also a PG process.

Denote by $\tilde{n}(I,t) = n(I,t_1 + t) - n(I,t_1), t > 0$, the remaining incremental predictive enrollment process in region I. If all centers in region I will continue to recruit until stopping recruitment globally, then $\tilde{n}(I,t)$ is a doubly stochastic Poisson process with posterior cumulative rate:

$$\tilde{\Lambda}(I,t) = t \sum_{i \in I} \widetilde{\lambda}_i,$$

which in general does not have a gamma distribution.

In what follows, we use for simplicity the notation (α, β) for ML estimators instead of $\left(\widehat{\alpha}, \widehat{\beta}\right)$. There are simple formulae for calculating the posterior mean and variance of the individual rates:

$$E\left[\widetilde{\lambda}_i\right] = \frac{\alpha + k_i}{\beta + v_i}, \quad Var\left[\widetilde{\lambda}_i\right] = \frac{\alpha + k_i}{(\beta + v_i)^2}, \qquad (8.16)$$

Denote

$$\tilde{E}(I) = \sum_{i \in I} \frac{\alpha + k_i}{\beta + v_i}, \quad \tilde{S}^2(I) = \sum_{i \in I} \frac{\alpha + k_i}{(\beta + v_i)^2}. \qquad (8.17)$$

Then, the mean and the variance of the posterior cumulative rate are

$$E\left[\tilde{\Lambda}(I,t)\right] = \tilde{E}(I)t, \quad Var\left[\tilde{\Lambda}(I,t)\right] = \tilde{S}^2(I)t^2. \qquad (8.18)$$

Therefore, basing on results of Sect. 8.2.2.2, the posterior remaining predictive enrollment process $\tilde{n}(I,t)$ in any region I can be modeled using either a normal approximation (for rather large $N(I)$), or using a PG process with parameters $\left(t, \tilde{A}(I), \tilde{B}(I)\right)$ where the parameters are calculated as follows:

$$\tilde{A}(I) = \frac{\tilde{E}^2(I)}{\tilde{S}^2(I)}, \tilde{B}(I) = \frac{\tilde{E}(I)}{\tilde{S}^2(I)}. \qquad (8.19)$$

For both approaches, the predictive mean and bounds of the number of patients recruited over time can be computed using closed-form expressions as shown in Sect. 8.2.2.2. Correspondingly, the predictive bounds for the time to reach region target or total sample size can be evaluated using either Q-bounds for the process $n(I,t)$ and normal approximation (8.14), or quantiles of a PG distribution and relations (8.18), (8.19).

The derivations above assume that there are N active centers that will continue to recruit until stopping the global enrollment. However, in real trials this is a typical situation where at interim time not all centers are initiated yet and some new ones may be initiated in the future.

For these cases, when the center's initiation times are deterministic, the technique for predicting future enrollment process is developed in (Anisimov 2011a). Consider now a typical situation when a clinical team has some planned schedule of center's initiation on, say, monthly basis. In general, this means that there are N_2 new centers that are scheduled to be initiated in given time intervals (a_i, b_i) with mean and SD of the rates (m_i, s_i), $i = 1, .., N_2$. Thus, if no other information is provided, it is natural to assume that the times of initiation have a uniform distribution in corresponding intervals. Denote by $\tilde{\Lambda}(N_2, t)$ a global cumulative enrollment rate for these N_2 centers. The mean and the variance of this rate can be computed using formulae (8.12), (8.13). The global rate for all centers including active centers and those to be initiated is

$$\tilde{\Lambda}(N, N_2, t) = \tilde{\Lambda}(N, t) + \tilde{\Lambda}(N_2, t), \tag{8.20}$$

where $\tilde{\Lambda}(N, t)$ is the posterior global cumulative enrollment rate in N active centers. Thus, the mean and the variance of the global rate can be directly calculated.

Therefore, for predicting the remaining enrollment process accounting for new centers to be initiated, it is possible to use the same technique as explained above using either a normal approximation or approximation via a PG process. Note that the latter approximation can also be applied to the case of many centers. Calculations show that in this case both approximations practically coincide; therefore, using a PG approximation is more universal.

The technique developed above allows us to evaluate the predictive bounds of the remaining enrollment time using low and upper predictive bounds for the enrollment process.

However, it is interesting to note that it is also possible to evaluate directly the distribution of the remaining enrollment time for the case when the number of active centers will remain the same until the end of enrollment. This idea was first noted for the case when the centers are initiated at the same time in (Anisimov and Fedorov 2007b), for a general case using a PG approximation for remaining enrollment process in Lemma 2.2 (Anisimov 2011a), and then later on in (Gajewski et al. 2012) for a special case of one center.

Let us define a Pearson type VI distribution (Johnson et al. 1994: 381) with parameters (n, c, d) and probability density function:

$$p(x, n, c, d) = \frac{1}{B(n, c)} \frac{x^{n-1} d^c}{(x + d)^{n+c}}, x \geq 0,$$

where $B(n, c)$ is a beta function.

It is shown above that if the number of active centers remains the same, then under rather general conditions the global posterior cumulative rate $\tilde{\Lambda}(N, t)$ of the remaining enrollment process can be approximated by a gamma random variable with mean $\tilde{E}t$ and variance $\tilde{S}^2 t^2$, where $\left(\tilde{E}, \tilde{S}^2\right)$ are calculated using relation (8.17) by summing across all centers. Thus, the global remaining enrollment process is approximated by a PG process with parameters $(t, \tilde{A}, \tilde{B})$, where the values $(\tilde{A}, \tilde{B})$ are calculated for all centers using relations (8.19) with values $\left(\tilde{E}, \tilde{S}^2\right)$. Then, according to considerations in Anisimov and Fedorov (2007b), the remaining enrollment time is approximated by a Pearson type VI distribution with parameters $(n_R, \tilde{A}, \tilde{B})$ where n_R is the remaining number of patients left to recruit.

There are no standard formulae in R for calculating characteristics of Pearson type VI distribution. Note that there is a special package PearsonDS available from CRAN, which computes various characteristics. However, for practical reasons it might be simpler to use the approach based on computing predictive bounds for the predictive enrollment process as shown in Sect. 2.2.2.

Consider now a very important notion of the probability of success (PoS) (probability to complete enrollment before planned time). Denote by $n(t)$ the global enrollment process, by n the enrollment target (sample size), by Ω the enrollment time—time to reach the enrollment target—and by T_{pl} the planned enrollment time.

Note that for any $t > 0$,

$$\Pr(\Omega \le t) = \Pr(n(t) \ge n). \tag{8.21}$$

Thus, PoS is the probability $\Pr(n(T_{pl}) \ge n)$. The right part in (8.21) can be evaluated using different approaches. Assume first that the number of centers and the predictive number of patients are large enough to use a normal approximation for $n(t)$. Then for any $t > 0$,

$$\Pr(\Omega \le t) \approx \Phi\left(\frac{E(t) - n}{V(t)}\right),$$

where $E(t)$, $V^2(t)$ are the mean and the variance functions of the global enrollment process $n(t)$, and $\Phi(x)$ is the cumulative distribution function of a standard normal distribution with parameters $(0,1)$. Thus,

$$PoS = \Phi\left(\frac{E(T_{pl}) - n}{V(T_{pl})}\right) \tag{8.22}$$

This relation implied the following criterion of successful enrollment completion:

Criterion: the trial will complete enrollment in time with probability P if the following relation is true:

$$E(T_{pl}) \ge n + z_P V(T_{pl}), \tag{8.23}$$

where z_P is a P-quantile of a standard normal distribution.

In the following sections, it will be shown how this relation can be used for adaptive enrollment adjustment and creating optimal enrollment design.

Consider now the case when the number of centers N is not very large, say, less than 20. Denote the mean and the variance of the global cumulative predictive rate at time t by $E(t)$ and $S^2(t)$. Consider the approximation of this rate at time T_{pl} by a gamma random variable with mean $E(T_{pl})$ and variance $S^2(T_{pl})$. This approximation is valid under rather general assumptions as discussed in Sect. 8.2.2.2. Then the value $n(T_{pl})$ can be approximated by a PG random variable with parameters (A, B), where

$$A = \frac{E^2(T_{pl})}{S^2(T_{pl})}, B = \frac{E(T_{pl})}{S^2(T_{pl})}.$$

Thus, in R language, for calculation PoS in (8.21), we can use the function:

$$PoS = 1 - \text{pnbinom}\left(n - 1, \text{size} = \frac{E^2(T_{pl})}{S^2(T_{pl})}, \text{prob} = \frac{E(T_{pl})}{E(T_{pl}) + S^2(T_{pl})}\right),$$

where pnbinom(k, size $=$ a, prob $=$ p) is the function in R that computes the cumulative probability distribution function of a negative binomial distribution $Nb(a, p)$ with size a and probability p defined in Sect. 8.2.1.

At interim time t_1 in calculations, we need to consider the remaining incremental process and the remaining number of patients n_R instead of n.

These results form a general methodology for modeling, predicting and reforecasting enrollment processes at different stages and in different regions.

8.2.4   Interim Assessment of Enrollment Performance and Risk-Based Monitoring

Different centers and countries have initially different enrollment rates and therefore may perform differently. The question of a paramount interest is to analyze the enrollment performance of different centers/countries at the interim time and detect the unusual data patterns and outliers (units that either low or high enrolling) with the purpose to make some decisions, e.g., investigate more closely the causes of the unusual behavior, send monitors, etc.

Note that a typical approach used in practice for detecting outliers in some cohort of variables $\{X_i\}$ is to evaluate the sample mean $E = E[\{X_i\}]$ and the variance $S^2 = Var[\{X_i\}]$ in the cohort and then use the following rule:

- If for some j, $X_j > E + ZS$ (or correspondingly $X_j < E + ZS$), then X_j is considered as an outlier, where Z is typically chosen as some quantile of a normal distribution or just as values 1, 2, and 3.

However, this rule is actually based on the assumption that the values X_i have a normal distribution. Nevertheless, many of characteristics related to enrollment and event's appearance are very far from normal distribution. The examples are the enrollment rates and the times till particular events, say, till the arrival of the first patient. In these examples, the empirical estimator of the rate as the ratio of the number of patients enrolled and the enrollment time has a Poisson-gamma distribution. The time till first arrival has a Pareto distribution. Both distributions are heavy tailed, and the latter distribution even may not have the theoretical mean or variance. Thus, using the rules based on normal assumptions may lead to biased results and statistically not valid conclusions.

Therefore, the methods of the analysis and data monitoring should be model-based and oriented on the type of data.

8.2.4.1 Interim Assessment of Center's Enrollment Performance

Consider two different approaches for detecting the unusual center's enrollment performance and selecting low and high enrolling centers. The first approach uses P-values, another one uses quantiles of a PG model. Assume that at interim time t_1 the following data are available:

k_i—The number of patients recruited in center i

v_i — The duration of active enrollment in center i up to time t_1

P-values Consider the hypothesis H_0: all centers belong to the population with the same parameters of a PG enrollment model. Denote by (α, β) the parameters of a PG model estimated using these data and maximum likelihood technique. Then, given v_i the number of patients recruited in center i has a PG distribution with parameters (v_i, α, β) (see (8.1)). Thus, for testing this hypothesis we can define the upper and low P-values as follows:

$$P_{Upp}(k_i, v_i, \alpha, \beta) = \Pr(PG(v_i, \alpha, \beta) \geq k_i), \qquad (8.24)$$

$$P_{Low}(k_i, v_i, \alpha, \beta) = \Pr(PG(v_i, \alpha, \beta) \leq k_i). \qquad (8.25)$$

By selecting different thresholds that may depend on sample size and data, we can select the sets of centers with P-values less than a given value. Centers with small upper P-values reflect high enrolling centers. Correspondingly, centers with small low P-values reflect low enrolling centers.

Numerical example Consider a study with $N = 50$ centers, all centers are initiated in a 2-month period deterministically using a pseudo-uniform distribution. Time of interim assessment of enrollment performance is 6 months. Assume that the first 42 centers have the mean enrollment rate $m_1 = 0.05$ patients per day, the next 4 centers are low enrolling with mean rate $m_2 = m_1/6$, and the remaining 4 centers are high enrolling with mean rate $m_3 = 4m_1$. Suppose that the enrollment process in

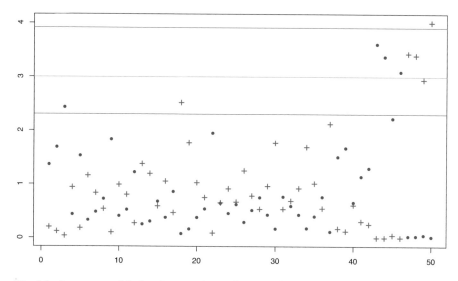

Fig. 8.2 Assessment of the interim center's enrollment performance, P-values

each of the first 42 centers is a PG process with the same parameters: shape $\alpha = 2$ and rate $\beta = \alpha/m_1 = 40$. In the unusual eight centers, the enrollment process follows a Poisson process with rate which is a mean enrollment rate. To get the interim data, the number of patients in each center is simulated according to either a PG process (in the first 42 centers) or a Poisson process.

Then for one simulated sample we get a set of data (k_i, v_i), where v_i are given and k_i are simulated. ML estimators of a PG model for all 50 centers are (1.704, 24.228). P-values for these data in log scale $(-\log(\text{P-value}))$ are shown in Fig. 8.2, where for each center, the crosses (red) show upper P-values, and the rectangles (blue)—low P-values. Horizontal separation lines correspond to $-\log$ of probabilities (0.02, 0.05, 0.1). Thus, it is visible that low enrolling centers 43,..,46 have rather small low P-values (three of them have low P-values less than 0.05). Correspondingly, high enrolling centers are also clearly detected with upper P-values less or about 0.05. Other centers are within typical variation where for two centers (3 and 18) the low P-value for the 3rd one and the upper P-value for the 18th one are less than 0.1 which can be explained by a random fluctuation.

The most critical centers are center 50 that has the best performance with enrollment window 160 days and 38 patients enrolled and center 43 that has the worst performance with enrollment window 177 days and 0 patients enrolled. This approach is realized in R using relations (8.2), (8.24), (8.25) and standard formulae for a negative binomial distribution.

2D classification using PG quantiles Another approach uses quantiles of a PG distribution and can create a visual 2D classification of the centers.

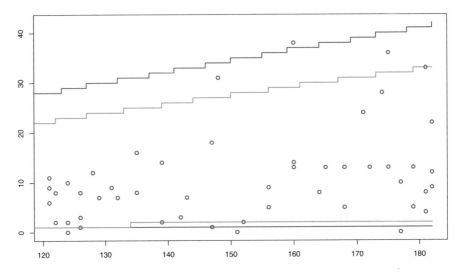

Fig. 8.3 Assessment of the interim center's enrollment performance, 2D classification

Denote by $Q(P, t, \alpha, \beta)$ a P-quantile of $PG(t, \alpha, \beta)$ distribution. Let us select rather small critical levels ε_H and ε_L for high and low enrolling centers, respectively. Then criterion to detect high and low enrolling centers has the following form:

1. If $k_i > Q(1 - \varepsilon_H, \alpha, \beta, v_i)$ then center i is high enrolling
2. If $k_i < Q(\varepsilon_L, \alpha, \beta, v_i)$ then center i is low enrolling

To create 2D classification on the plane (z, n), the upper curve $Q(1 - \varepsilon_H, \alpha, \beta, z)$ and the low curve $Q(\varepsilon_L, \alpha, \beta, z)$ for $z = 1, 2, 3, ..$ are created together with the points (v_i, k_i) for each center. Then the points over the upper curve correspond to high enrolling centers and the points below the low curve correspond to low enrolling centers. This is shown in Fig. 8.3. The upper quantiles are calculated for $\varepsilon_H = 0.02$, 0.05. The low quantiles are calculated for $\varepsilon_L = 0.05, 0.1$. Note that using the same probability thresholds we select the same centers using either P-values or 2D classification. So this is a matter of preference which method to choose for risk-based monitoring of center's enrollment performance.

8.2.4.2 Interim Assessment of Country's Enrollment Performance

Consider now an approach for detecting the countries with unusual center's enrollment performance. This approach is based on the approximation of the enrollment processes in countries by PG processes and computing P-values for these approximations. As typically country may include not so many centers, we use PG approximation instead of a normal one.

Assume that the interim data (k_i, v_i) are given and denote by (α, β) the parameters of a PG model estimated using these data and maximum likelihood technique. Put for simplicity $m = \alpha/\beta$, $s^2 = \alpha/\beta^2$ (the mean and the variance of the prior gamma distributed rate).

Consider some country J and define the aggregated country mean and variance of the rate:

$$E(J) = m\sum_{i\in J} v_i, S^2(J) = s^2 \sum_{i\in J} v_i^2.$$

Let $k(J) = \sum_{i\in J} k_i$ be the number of patients recruited in country J.

Lemma 8.3 The distribution of $k(J)$ can be approximated by a PG distribution with parameters $(A(J), B(J))$, where

$$A(J) = \frac{E^2(J)}{S^2(J)}, B(J) = \frac{E(J)}{S^2(J)} \qquad (8.26)$$

Indeed, the global enrollment rate $\Lambda(J)$ in country J up to the interim time has the form:

$$\Lambda(J) = \sum_{i\in J} \lambda_i v_i.$$

It is easy to see that the mean and the variance of $\Lambda(J)$ are $E(J)$ and $S^2(J)$. In Lemma 8.2, it was proved that $\Lambda(J)$ can be well approximated by a gamma random variable with parameters (8.26). This proves the lemma.

Basing on this result, we can apply a similar technique as in Sect. 8.2.4.1 and calculate the upper and lower P-values for country J similar to relations (8.24) and (8.25) as follows:

$$P_{Upp}(J) = \Pr(PG(A(J), B(J)) \geq k(J)),$$
$$P_{Low}(J) = \Pr(PG(A(J), B(J)) \leq k(J)).$$

8.3 Optimal Trial Design

8.3.1 Optimal Enrollment Design at Start-Up Stage

This section deals with the optimal enrollment design accounting for different performance of centers in different countries, cost and time constraints, and the probability of success.

In general, it can be different criteria of optimality depending on team goals and various constraints. Typically, the costs of centers initiation and monitoring in different countries/regions vary, and the enrollment rates also can vary. Therefore, the one of the questions of a paramount interest is which countries to choose and how many centers in these countries to select to satisfy trial goal.

Consider the following input data:

-   A set of all possible countries that can be chosen for this study: $\{1, 2, .., J\}$
-   The expected mean enrollment rates per center in different countries $\{m_j, j = 1, .., J\}$
-   The variances of enrollment rates in countries $\left\{s_j^2, j = 1, .., J\right\}$ (for simplicity it is assumed that the mean rate and the variance for all centers in each country are the same, but this assumption can be easily relaxed)
-   Some planned set of restrictions on the number of centers in countries W, e.g., the minimal or maximal numbers of centers in countries
-   Cost per selecting one center in country j, $\{C_j, j = 1, .., J\}$
-   Cost of running one center per unit of time in country j, $\{c_j, j = 1, .., J\}$ (for simplicity it is assumed that the costs per different centers in one country are the same)
-   Cost per one enrolled patient in different countries $\{q_j, j = 1, \ldots, J\}$

Assume for simplicity that all centers in country j are initiated in time interval (a_j, b_j) according to a uniform distribution, $j = 1, .., J$. Let n be the total number of patients to be recruited and T be the expected (planned) duration of enrollment.

Consider the following problem: find an optimal allocation of counties/centers that maximizes the probability of success given certain restrictions on the number of centers and that the total trial cost does not exceed a given threshold C_{total}.

Suppose for simplicity that for all j, $b_j < T$ and the total number of centers N is large enough to use a normal approximation for the global enrollment process.

Let us evaluate the costs of trial operation in time interval $[0, T]$.

Assume that we have chosen some subset of centers $\{N_j, j = 1, .., J\}$ from countries $\{1, .., J\}$. Then the mean and the variance of the global cumulative rate in country j in interval $[0, T]$ using relations (8.10), (8.11) are calculated as

$$E[\Lambda(j, T)] = E(j, T) = N_j m_j \left(T - \frac{a_j + b_j}{2} \right),$$

$$Var[\Lambda(j, T)] = S^2(j, T) = N_j \left(\frac{\left(m_j^2 + s_j^2 \right) (b_j - a_j)^2}{12} + s_j^2 \left(T - \frac{a_j + b_j}{2} \right)^2 \right).$$

The mean and the variance of the global cumulative rate for all countries are calculated as

$$E(T, N_j, j = 1, .., J) = \sum_{j=1}^{J} E(j, T); \, S^2(T, N_j, j = 1, .., J) = \sum_{j=1}^{J} S^2(j, T).$$

The average operational cost including the initiation and running N_j centers in country j in time interval $[0, T]$ is

$$C(j,T) = N_j\left(C_j + c_j\left(T - \frac{a_j + b_j}{2}\right)\right).$$

Correspondingly, the average cost per enrolled patients in country j in time interval $[0, T]$ is $q_j E(j, T)$. Thus, the global average operational cost is

$$R(T, N_j, j = 1, .., J) = \sum_{j=1}^{J} (C(j, T) + q_j E(j, T)).$$

Denote

$$V^2(T, N_j, j = 1, .., J) = E(T, N_j, j = 1, .., J) + S^2(T, N_j, j = 1, .., J).$$

Note that maximizing the probability function $\Phi(f(x))$ is equivalent to maximizing the function $f(x)$. Therefore, we come to the following result:

Lemma 8.4 The optimal allocation of centers $\{N_j, j = 1, ..., J\} \in W$ in countries that maximizes PoS given that the global cost does not exceed a certain level and allocation restrictions is a solution of the following optimization problem:

- Find

$$\max_{\{N_j, j=1,...,J\} \in W} \frac{E(T, N_j, j = 1, .., J) - n}{V(T, N_j, j = 1, .., J)},$$

- Given

$$R(T, N_j, j = 1, .., J) \le C_{total},$$

$$\{N_j, j = 1, .., J\} \in W.$$

It can be also other formulations of the trial optimal design. For example, we can consider a dual problem:

- Minimize total cost $R(T, ..)$ given some restrictions on $\{N_j\}$, and that PoS is no less than a given probability P_0.

Another opportunity can be to impose some stochastic restrictions. As for any center's allocation $\{N_j, j = 1, ..., J\}$ the trial cost depends on the recruitment time $\tau(n, N_j, j = 1, .., J)$, we can also consider a problem to maximize PoS given that the total cost does not exceed some threshold with a given probability. This leads to the following optimization problem:

- Find

$$\max_{\{N_j,\,j=1,..,J\}} \frac{E\left(T,N_j,j=1,..,J\right)-n}{V\left(T,N_j,j=1,..,J\right)},$$

- Given

$$\Pr\left(R\left(\tau\left(n,N_j,j=1,..,J\right),N_j,j=1,..,J\right)\leq C_{total}\right)\geq P_0.$$

$$\left\{N_j,j=1,..,J\right\}\in W$$

The choice of the optimization problem depends on team and trial goals. These optimization problems can be solved numerically using the methods of constrained nonlinear optimization or discrete search. Similar optimization problems can be formulated for interim enrollment design.

8.3.2 Optimal Adaptive Enrollment Adjustment at Interim Stage

This section deals with the optimal enrollment adjustment accounting for predictive study performance and provides a technique for solving the following problem: if study is going not as planned how to adjust the number of centers to reach a trial goal with a given probability and minimal costs.

Let us keep notation of Sect. 8.2.3. Assume that the recruitment in trial is slower than expected and consider the following problem: what is the minimal number of new centers that have to be initiated to make PoS no less than a given level P_S.

Let N_{max} be the maximum number of new centers that potentially can be initiated in the future. Assume that these centers can be initiated in given time intervals (a_i,b_i) after the interim time t_1 with mean and variance of the rates $\left(m_i,s_i^2\right), i = N+1,..,N+N_{max}$. Consider another time scale to account for the remaining time after the interim time t_1. This means, $t \to t + t_1$.

Denote by $W = \{i_1,i_2,\ldots,i_{N_2}\}$ some subset of N_2 new centers out of potential N_{max} centers. Let us define for this subset the mean and the variance of the enrollment rate as

$$E(i_1, i_2, \ldots, i_{N_2}, t) = \sum_{i \in W} M(t, a_i, b_i, m_i),$$

$$S^2(i_1, i_2, \ldots, i_{N_2}, t) = \sum_{i \in W} S^2\left(t, a_i, b_i, m_i, s_i^2\right).$$

Consider the mean and the variance of posterior enrollment rate for N centers active at interim time t_1:

$$\tilde{E}(N, t) = \sum_{i=1}^{N} M(t, a_i, b_i, m_i),$$

$$\tilde{S}^2(N, t) = \sum_{i=1}^{N} S^2\left(t, a_i, b_i, m_i, s_i^2\right).$$

Note that in these formulae the mean and the variance (m_i, s_i^2) of the rates for centers active at interim time are considered as posterior characteristics calculated using interim data and estimated parameters as in (8.16). For new N_2 centers the values (m_i, s_i^2) can be evaluated using historical data and experience of study teams. However, if there is no other information, it is advisable to assume that these centers have the same prior parameters as the active centers. This means, for new centers we can use relations $m_i = \frac{\alpha}{\beta}, s_i^2 = \frac{\alpha}{\beta^2}$.

For the global rate $\tilde{\Lambda}(N, W, t)$ using a given subset W of new centers and (8.20) we get

$$E\left[\tilde{\Lambda}(N, W, t)\right] = \tilde{E}(N, t) + E(i_1, i_2, \ldots, i_{N_2}, t),$$

$$Var\left[\tilde{\Lambda}(N, W, t)\right] = \tilde{S}^2(N, t) + S^2(i_1, i_2, \ldots, i_{N_2}, t).$$

Consider the variance of the global enrollment process:

$$V^2(N, W, t) = E\left[\tilde{\Lambda}(N, W, t)\right] + Var\left[\tilde{\Lambda}(N, W, t)\right].$$

Denote by n_R the number of patients left to recruit at the interim time and by T_R the planned remaining recruitment time. Then according to (8.22), PoS has the form:

$$PoS = F(W) = \Phi\left(\frac{\tilde{E}(N, T_R) + E(W, T_R) - n_R}{\sqrt{\tilde{S}^2(N, T_R) + S^2(W, T_R) + \tilde{E}(N, T_R) + E(W, T_R)}}\right). \quad (8.27)$$

The right part in (8.27) is the function of subset W. Assume that there is some target function (cost) associated with this subset, $C(W)$. Using relation (8.23) we can formulate the following result:

Lemma 8.5 The optimal set of new centers that have to be added to minimize function $C(W)$ and keep PoS no less than P_S is a solution of the following optimization problem:

- Find

$$\min_W C(W),$$

- Given

$$\tilde{E}(N, T_R) + E(W, T_R) \geq n_R$$

$$+ z_{P_S} \sqrt{\tilde{S}^2(N, T_R) + S^2(W, T_R) + \tilde{E}(N, T_R) + E(W, T_R)}. \quad (8.28)$$

In particular, if we are only interested to minimize the number of new centers that can be initiated in the natural order $\{1, 2, .., N_{max}\}$, then we can set $C(W) = length(W)$. Then the solution will provide the minimal number of new centers that have to be added to make PoS no less than P_S. A solution can be easily found numerically using a recurrent procedure: start from $N_2 = 1$. If (8.28) is true, stop. Otherwise, set $N_2 = N_2 + 1$ and repeat step.

In the sections above the advanced analytic methodology for predictive patient enrollment modeling, risk-based monitoring trial performance and optimal design and adjustment enrollment associated processes are developed. The next section is devoted to modeling the event's counts on the top of enrollment process.

8.4 Modeling Event's Counts in Event-Driven Trials

This section includes the analysis of the advanced models and techniques for modeling counts of non-repeated clinical events, specifically events in oncology trials. The models include predicting event's counts at the trial start-up stage, reprojection at the interim stage and also risk-based data monitoring, and analysis of centers performance including detection of units with high/low number of events.

Consider an ongoing clinical trial where the patients are recruited by different clinical centers. Upon registration, a patient takes a prescribed treatment and then is followed-up until the occurrence of particular events or treatment reactions. Typical example is an oncology trial.

The problem is to predict the number of particular events that may happen over time accounting for ongoing enrollment, and also predict the time when the total number of events will hit some prescribed level (sample size). A general methodology for interim predicting event's counts together with ongoing enrollment with applications to oncology studies is developed in (Anisimov 2011b). Here this methodology is extended to cover the initial trial design and also to risk-based monitoring and detecting centers with unusual number of events.

Consider first the case of one clinical center. Assume that the patients arrive according to a nonhomogeneous doubly stochastic Poisson process with instantaneous possibly random rate at time t, $\lambda(t)$. Suppose first that there is only one type of events A. Denote by τ_A the time it takes until the event A happens (starting from zero point) and let $p_A(x) = \Pr(\tau_A \leq x)$ be its cumulative distribution function. In Anisimov (2011b) the following result is proved.

Lemma 8.6 The predictive number of events A in interval $[0, t]$ for the newly recruited patients in this center has a mixed Poisson distribution with parameter (possibly random):

$$\int_0^t \lambda(u) p_A(t - u) du. \tag{8.29}$$

Consider a special important case when enrollment follows a homogeneous doubly stochastic Poisson process in some interval and time until event has an exponential distribution. Denote the following function:

$$d(t, a, b) = \begin{cases} 0, & t \leq a \\ t - a, & a < t \leq b. \\ b - a, & t \geq b \end{cases}$$

Lemma 8.7 Assume that a center is active only in a fixed time interval $[a, b]$, $\lambda(t) = \lambda$ for $t \in [a, b]$ and zero otherwise (λ can be random), and time till event A has an exponential distribution with parameter μ_A. Then the predictive number of events A in interval $[0, t]$ in this center has a mixed Poisson distribution with parameter $\lambda q(t, a, b)$, where

$$q(t, a, b) = d(t, a, b) - \frac{1}{\mu_A} e^{-\mu_A(t-a)} \left(e^{\mu_A d(t,a,b)} - 1 \right). \tag{8.30}$$

In relations above, we can also consider a random effect model for event rates by assuming that μ_A has a gamma distribution with some parameters. However, for simplicity we restrict our attention to the case when μ_A is deterministic as using random rates will involve more complicated calculations. Another point is that typically in oncology trials the events happen rather rare, thus, adding extra parameters will lead to additional errors in estimation. Moreover, the variation in enrollment rates is mainly caused by differences in enrollment in different centers, but for event rates the variation can be caused by the differences between patients.

Consider now more general situation when there are two types of events, where another event L means that patient is lost to follow-up. In what follows, assume that the rates of these events are μ_A and μ_L correspondingly, which are deterministic values.

Denote by $p_A(t, L)$ the probability that in time interval $[0, t]$ the event A will happen before the event L and by $p_L(t, A)$ the probability that the patient in time interval $[0, t]$ will be lost to follow-up. Using properties of exponential distribution it is easy to calculate that

$$p_A(t, L) = \frac{\mu_A}{\mu}(1 - e^{-\mu t}); \quad p_L(t, A) = \frac{\mu_L}{\mu}(1 - e^{-\mu t}), \tag{8.31}$$

where $\mu = \mu_A + \mu_L$. Using Lemma 8.7 and the properties of exponential random variables, we can prove the following result. Denote by $k(t, A)$ and $k(t, L)$ the predictive number of events A and L in the interval $[0, t]$, respectively.

Lemma 8.8 Assume that a center is active only in a fixed time interval $[a, b]$, $\lambda(t) = \lambda$ for $t \in [a, b]$ and zero otherwise where λ has a gamma distribution with parameters (α, β), and there are two types of events, A and L with rates μ_A and μ_L, respectively.

Then for any $t > 0$, the vector $(k(t, A), k(t, L))$ has a two-dimensional PG distribution of the form:

$$\Pr(k(t, A) = k, k(t, L) = j) = \frac{\Gamma(\alpha + k + j)}{\Gamma(\alpha)k!j!} \frac{\beta^\alpha q_A^k(t, a, b) q_L^j(t, a, b)}{(\beta + q_A(t, a, b) + q_L(t, a, b))^{\alpha + k + j}} \tag{8.32}$$

where

$$q_B(t, a, b) = \frac{\mu_B}{\mu} \left(d(t, a, b) - e^{-\mu(t-a)} \left(e^{\mu d(t,a,b)} - 1 \right) / \mu \right), \tag{8.33}$$

with $\mu = \mu_A + \mu_L$, and $B = A$ or $B = L$, respectively.

In particular, each of the variables $k(t, A)$ and $k(t, L)$ has a PG distribution of the form (8.1) where we should put $t = q_A(t, a, b)$ or $t = q_L(t, a, b)$, respectively. If λ is deterministic, then the variables $k(t, A)$ and $k(t, L)$ are independent and have Poisson distributions with parameters $\lambda q_A(t, a, b)$ and $\lambda q_L(t, a, b)$, respectively. Proof is given in Appendix 8.1.

The results of Lemma 8.8 form the basis for creating predictions of the event's counts at start-up stage. Note that even for a deterministic λ, in spite of the fact that the marginal distributions have Poisson distributions, the processes $k(t, A)$ and $k(t, L)$ over time are not Poisson processes. For the analysis of the incremental behavior and constructing interim predictions, we need to consider a joint distribution of the number of events together with ongoing enrollment.

Denote by $n(t)$ the predictive number of patients recruited in interval $[0, t]$. Consider a joint distribution of the process $Z(t) = (n(t), k(t, A), k(t, L))$.

Lemma 8.9 Assume that the assumptions of Lemma 8.8 are valid. Then, conditionally on λ, the process $Z(t)$ is a continuous time Markov process.

A full description of three-dimensional distributions of $Z(t)$ is rather complicated. Therefore, consider marginal distributions that are of the most interest and can be used in predictive formulae.

Consider a transition interval $[t_1, t_2]$. Suppose for simplicity that the center is active in this interval, that means, $a \leq t_1$, $t_2 \leq b$. Other situations can be easily considered as well.

Denote $\Delta = t_2 - t_1$. Assume that at time t_1, $(n(t_1), k(t_1, A), k(t_1, L)) = (n_1, i_1, j_1)$, where $i_1 + j_1 \leq n_1$.

As the enrollment process is a PG process with rate λ, then the number of new patients that arrive in the interval $[t_1, t_2]$ is a PG variable $Pg(\Delta, \alpha, \beta)$ (see (8.1)). If λ is deterministic, this is a Poisson variable $\Pi(\lambda\Delta)$.

The number of new events A and L that will happen in this interval is a sum of two parts. The first part includes the events that may happen for $n_1 - i_1 - j_1$ patients in trial without events that are at risk at time t_1. For each of these patients the events A and L may happen with probabilities $p_A(\Delta, L)$ and $p_L(\Delta, A)$, respectively (8.31). Therefore, a two-dimensional vector of the number of new events, A and L, is represented as a multinomial random variable $Mn(n_1 - i_1 - j_1, p_A(\Delta, L), p_L(\Delta, A))$, where we use two components, and by definition:

$$\Pr(Mn(n, p, q) = (i, j)) = \frac{n!}{i! j! (n - i - j)!} p^i q^j (1 - p - q)^{n-i-j}. \tag{8.34}$$

Another part of new events is related to the events that may happen for the new patients that arrive in this interval $[t_1, t_2]$. As stated in Lemma 8.8, for the number of new events A and L, we can use representations:

$$k(\Delta, A) = \Pi(\lambda q_A(\Delta)); k(\Delta, L) = \Pi(\lambda q_L(\Delta));$$

where the functions $q_A(\Delta)$ and $q_L(\Delta)$ according to (8.33) have the form:

$$q_B(\Delta) = \frac{\mu_A}{\mu} \left(\Delta - \left(1 - e^{-\mu\Delta} \right)/\mu \right), B = A, L. \tag{8.35}$$

and the vector $(k(\Delta, A), k(\Delta, L))$ has a two-dimensional PG distribution.

Thus, the two-dimensional increment in the number of new events A and L in interval $[t_1, t_2]$ can be represented as

$$Mn(n_1 - i_1 - j_1, p_A(\Delta, L), p_L(\Delta, A)) + (k(\Delta, A), k(\Delta, L)). \tag{8.36}$$

If λ is deterministic, then the values $k(\Delta, A)$ and $k(\Delta, L)$ are independent.

This expression can be used for interim predicting the number of future events. If the number of centers is rather large for using a normal approximation, then the marginal mean and variance of this incremental value can be computed and used in predictive formulae. For not very large numbers, the marginal distributions in (8.36) can be computed numerically.

8.4.1 Design of the Event-Driven Trial at Start-Up Stage

Consider the initial trial design. Assume that there are N centers planned to be initiated. Suppose that the main goal is to reach a given number $\nu(A)$ of clinical events A. For this purpose typically it can proposed the following setup: perform a patient enrollment during some period of time T, then stop enrollment, follow-up the enrolled patients, and wait until the total number of events will reach $\nu(A)$.

Let us provide the technique for predicting the number of events accounting for ongoing enrollment on global and region levels.

Consider some region I and assume that in center $i \in I$ the enrollment rate λ_i is possibly some random variable with mean m_i and variance s_i^2, and center initiation time u_i is given. Assume also that all centers will continue to recruit until stopping time T. Suppose that the rates of events A and L, μ_A and μ_L, are some given constants that do not depend on the center.

Denote by $n(I, t)$ the number of patients enrolled in region I in time interval $[0, t]$ and by $k(I, B, t)$ the number of events B, where $B = A$ or $B = L$, respectively.

According to (8.33), for a generic event B define the following (in general random) function:

$$\Sigma(I, B, t, T) = \sum_{i \in I} \lambda_i q_B(t, u_i, T).$$

Put

$$E(I, B, t, T) = \sum_{i \in I} m_i q_B(t, u_i, T), \tag{8.37}$$

$$S^2(I, B, t, T) = \sum_{i \in I} s_i^2 q_B^2(t, u_i, T). \tag{8.38}$$

The results above imply the following lemma.

Lemma 8.10 For the trial design above, the predictive number $k(I, B, t)$ of events B in region I in time interval $[0, t]$ has a doubly stochastic Poisson distribution with parameter $\Sigma(I, B, t, T)$. Correspondingly,

$$E[k(I, B, t)] = E(I, B, t, T), \ Var[k(I, B, t)] = S^2(I, B, t, T) + E(I, B, t, T).$$

The same result is valid for the global number of events $k(B, t)$, where in the relations above a summation should be taken by all centers.

This result allows us to predict the number of events A or L over time with predictive bounds. The bounds can be calculated using similar technique developed in Sect. 8.2.2.2. That means, for not very large N we can use the approximation of $\Sigma(I, B, t, T)$ by a gamma random variable using relation (8.15) and quantiles of a Poisson or PG distributions. For rather large $N \geq 20$, we can use a normal approximation for $k(I, B, t)$ and relations (8.37), (8.38).

Consider now various opportunities of constructing an optimal design. A crucial point here is to determine the optimal duration of the enrollment T. If T is not very large, the number of patients enrolled in the trial will be also not very large, so it will take longer to reach the number of events needed. From another side, if T is rather large, presumably too many patients can be enrolled and the number of events may happen even before the end of enrollment period. This may lead to extra costs and possible regulatory problems.

To illustrate wide opportunities, consider rather simple enrollment setting: all centers are initiated simultaneously at trial start-up and have the same parameters (m, s^2) of the enrollment rates. Assume that there is only one type of events A and denote $\mu_A = \mu$. Consider also for simplicity the design for averaged characteristics: evaluate the average trial duration T_A (time to reach on average the number of events $\nu(A)$) given that the enrollment duration is T.

For this scenario the total mean number of events at time t is $E(A, t, T) = Nmq_A(t, 0, T)$, where according to (8.33),

$$q_A(t, 0, T) = \min(t, T) - e^{-\mu t}\left(e^{\mu \min(t,T)} - 1\right)/\mu.$$

Thus, the average trial duration T_A is a solution in t of the equation:

$$Nmq_A(t, 0, T) = \nu(A).$$

If $Nmq_A(T, 0, T) < \nu(A)$, then $T_A > T$ and a solution can be easily found as

$$T_A = \left[\log\left(e^{\mu T} - 1\right) - \log(\mu) - \log\left(T - \frac{\nu(A)}{Nm}\right)\right]/\mu.$$

If $Nmq_A(T, 0, T) > \nu(A)$, then there is no solution in the region $\{t > T\}$. Thus, $T_A < T$ and can be found as a solution of nonlinear equation $Nm(t - (1 - e^{-\mu t})/\mu) = \nu(A)$. As the derivative of the left hand side part is positive, a solution is unique.

Example Consider a numerical example. Assume that there are $N = 40$ centers, $m = 0.01$ patients per center per day, $\mu = m/6$ event's rate per patient, and the planned number of events to reach $\nu(A) = 50$. Consider several scenarios for different values of the duration of enrollment T. Calculations show that for values $T = 7, 8, 10, 12, 14$ (in months) the predictive average total numbers of patients enrolled are 84, 96, 120, 144, and 168, and the average trial durations are 651, 565, 480, 445, and 434 (in days), respectively. Thus, the duration of enrollment substantially affects the total trial duration.

Consider now an optimization problem. Let us introduce the potential costs. Assume that C_1 is the cost (per day) of running enrollment stage, C_2 is the cost at the follow-up stage (after stopping enrollment), C_3 is the cost (per day) of excess the planned trial time T_E. Then the average cost function has the following form:

$$W(T) = C_1 T + C_2 [T_A - T]_+ + C_3 [T_A - T_E]_+,$$

where $[a]_+ = \max(0, a)$.

Let us take a desired threshold for study duration $T_E = 450$ days. Then for several scenarios, the values of optimal T minimizing $W(T)$ and T_A are

1. For $C_1 = 7$, $C_2 = 1$, $C_3 = 10$, the optimal $T = 335$, and $T_A = 455$
2. For $C_1 = 5$, $C_2 = 1$, $C_3 = 10$, the optimal $T = 353$, and $T_A = 447$
3. For $C_1 = 2$, $C_2 = 1$, $C_3 = 10$, the optimal $T = 404$, and $T_A = 435$
4. For $C_1 = 1.5$, $C_2 = 1$, $C_3 = 10$, the optimal $T = 415$, and $T_A = 434$

Thus, if the cost of enrollment stage is not very high, it might be more efficient to consider a longer enrollment stage in order to reach the number of events sooner.

Note that this is the design on average. There are many other opportunities to consider stochastic setting, e.g., using predictive distributions for trial duration consider similar criteria as in Sect. 8.3, e.g., find an optimal T given some restrictions on the number of centers and costs, maximize probability to complete trial in time, minimize costs, etc. Particular setting of the optimal problem may essentially depend on trial goals and different restrictions.

It can be also another design in event-driven trial: define initially a given number of patients n, perform the enrollment stage until n patients will be enrolled, and then, if still the number of events $\nu(A)$ is not reached, follow-up the enrolled patients and wait until the total number of events will reach $\nu(A)$.

Note that for the purpose of the analysis of the averaged design, this design is nearly equivalent to the previous design. However, for creating predictions during the enrollment stage, this setup is more complicated for analytic investigation as the enrollment stage has a random duration. However, this design can be reduced to the previous one by considering a deterministic duration of enrollment stage $T(n)$, where $T(n)$ is the average time to reach n patients to be enrolled. In large trials the relative error in the approximation of enrollment time by the averaged time is rather small. Thus, this approach provides rather good approximation and keeps very nice analytic properties of the design and various opportunities for optimization.

8.4.2 Risk-Based Monitoring in Event-Driven Trials at Interim Stage

In this section we develop the technique for analyzing the performance of different centers and detecting unusual data patterns (centers with too high or too low number of events).

Consider the trial at interim time t_1. Assume that there can be two types of events, A or L, and the following data are available:

k_i—The number of patients recruited in center i
v_i—The duration of active enrollment in center i up to time t_1

For each patient it is known the exposure time for this patient and the type of event if it happens (or no events).

Assume that the enrollment follows a PG model with the same parameters for all centers. Assume also that the rates of events μ_A and μ_L are the same for all patients and centers.

Consider first the procedure of estimating parameters. Denote by (α, β) the parameters of a PG model estimated using enrollment data and ML technique as described in Sect. 8.2.3. For estimating rates μ_A and μ_L let us rearrange the event data in the following way.

Consider three groups of patients:

- Group O: no events, n_O patients, durations of follow-up periods z_k
- Group A: the event A happened, n_A patients, durations of follow-up periods x_i
- Group L: patients are lost to follow-up, n_L patients, durations of follow-up periods y_j

Denote

$$\Sigma_1 = \sum_{k=1}^{n_O} z_k + \sum_{i=1}^{n_A} x_i + \sum_{j=1}^{n_L} y_j.$$

Then the log-likelihood function has the form:

$$L(\mu_A, \mu_L) = -(\mu_A + \mu_L)\Sigma_1 + n_A \log (\mu_A) + n_L \log (\mu_L),$$

and ML estimators are

$$\mu_A = \frac{n_A}{\Sigma_1}; \mu_L = \frac{n_L}{\Sigma_1}. \tag{8.39}$$

Consider now a hypothesis H_0: the parameters of enrollment and event models in all centers are (α, β) and (μ_A, μ_L), respectively.

Lemma 8.11 Given hypothesis H_0 and data (k_i, v_i) in center i, the vector of the number of events $(k(i, A, v_i), k(i, L, v_i))$ that happened up to interim time t_1 has a multinomial distribution (see (8.34)) $Mn(k_i, p(v_i, A), p(v_i, L))$, where for $B = A$ or $B = L$,

$$p(v, B) = \frac{\mu_B}{\mu} (1 - (1 - e^{-\mu v})/\mu v), \tag{8.40}$$

with $\mu = \mu_A + \mu_L$.

In particular, the marginal distribution of the variable $k(i, B, v_i)$, for $B = A$ or $B = L$, is a binomial distribution with parameters $(k_i, p(v_i, B))$.

Proof is given in Appendix 8.2. Lemma 8.11 equips us with the technique for testing an unusual behavior of the number of events prior to interim time using P-values.

Lemma 8.12 Assuming a hypothesis H_0 and given enrollment data (k_i, v_i) in center i, the number of events $(k_A(i), k_L(i))$ and estimated event's rates (μ_A, μ_L), the upper and low P-values for the actual number of events B are calculated as follows:

$$P_{Upp}(i, B) = \Pr(Bin(k_i, p(v_i, B)) \geq k_B(i)), B = A, L$$
$$P_{Low}(i, B) = \Pr(Bin(k_i, p(v_i, B)) \leq k_B(i)), B = A, L$$

These values can be computed in R using standard functions for binomial distribution:

$$\Pr(Bin(k, p) \leq n) = pbinom(n, size = k, prob = p),$$
$$n = 0, 1, \ldots, k.$$

By selecting different thresholds, we can select the sets of centers with small P-values for both types of events. In particular, centers with small upper P-values for event L reflect the case of high number of lost to follow-up patients.

8.4.3 Forecasting in Event-Driven Trials at Interim Stage

Consider now forecasting of the number of events. Assume that at the interim time t_1 there can be two types of events, A and L, and there are N active centers with the following data:

k_i—The number of patients recruited in center i
v_i—The duration of active enrollment in center i up to time t_1

Let also event data be divided in three groups of patients:

- Group O: no events, n_O patients, durations of follow-up periods z_k
- Group A: the event A happened, n_A patients, durations of follow-up periods x_i
- Group L: patients are lost to follow-up, n_L patients, durations of follow-up periods y_j

Assume that the enrollment follows a PG model with the same parameters for all centers and the rates of events μ_A and μ_L are the same for all patients and centers.

Denote by (α, β) the parameters of a PG model estimated using enrollment data and ML technique as described in Sect. 8.2.3 and by μ_A and μ_L the estimated event rates (8.39).

Consider some region I with $N(I)$ active centers where the numbers of events in three groups defined above are $n_O(I), n_A(I)$, and $n_L(I)$, correspondingly. Denote by $k(I, t, A)$ the predictive number of events A in region I in time interval $[t_1, t_1 + t]$. Put also $T_1 = [T - t_1]_+$, the remaining enrollment duration at the interim time. Furthermore, given data (k_i, v_i) in center i, define for each active center the posterior rate $\widetilde{\lambda}_l$ which has a gamma distribution with parameters $(\alpha + k_i, \beta + v_i)$. Assume also that it can be some number of new centers $N_2(I)$ that are planned to be initiated in the future at given times $t_1 + u_i$ where the enrollment rates λ_i have the expected mean and variance m_i and s_i^2. Let also $v_R(A) = v(A) - n_A$ be the remaining number of events A and T_R be the remaining duration of the trial (to reach in total $v(A)$ events).

Theorem 8.1   The predictive number of new events A, $k(I, t, A)$, that will happen in region I in time interval $[t_1, t_1 + t]$ can be represented as a convolution of two independent random variables:

$$k(I, t, A) = \Pi(\Sigma(I, t, A, T_1)) + Bin(n_0(I), p_A(t, L)), \tag{8.41}$$

where

$$\Sigma(I, t, A, T_1) = \sum_{i \in I, active} \widetilde{\lambda}_i q_A(t, 0, T_1) + \sum_{i \in I, new} \lambda_i q_A(t, u_i, T_1), \tag{8.42}$$

with function $q_A(t, a, b)$ defined in (8.33), where the first sum is taken across all active centers in I, and the second sum is taken across new centers, and $p_A(t, L)$ is defined in (8.31).

Correspondingly, the probability to complete trial in time is

$$\Pr(k(T_R, A) \geq v_R(A)). \tag{8.43}$$

Here $k(t, A)$ is the predictive total number of events A in time interval $[t_1, t_1 + t]$ which is represented as in (8.41) where in calculations the sums are taken across all centers.

The proof follows from results of Lemmas 8.6, 8.8, and 8.9.

Note that the variable $\Pi(\Sigma(I, t, A, T_1))$ can be approximated by a PG variable using similar considerations as in Lemma 8.2, where the mean and the variance of posterior rates $\widetilde{\lambda}_l$ in active centers are given in (8.16) and in the new centers $m_i = \frac{\alpha}{\beta}, s_i^2 = \frac{\alpha}{\beta^2}$. Therefore, the distribution of $k(I, t, A)$ can be approximated by the convolution of two independent random variables as in (8.41), PG and binomial.

From another side, the mean and the variance of $k(I, t, A)$ in (8.41) can be computed directly as the means and variances of the values $\widetilde{\lambda}_i$ and λ_i are known. Thus, for rather large number of events, we can use a normal approximation and derivations similar to Sect. 8.2.2.2 for evaluating the mean and predictive bounds for the number of events A over time and also for the probability to complete the trial in time (8.43).

Analytic representations (8.41), (8.42) also open wide opportunities for the analysis of the adaptive trial adjustment (e.g., how many centers to add if the time to complete trial is rather long) and for creating an optimal design by minimizing costs given some restrictions and probability to complete.

8.5   Modeling Trial Operational Characteristics

To model other types of events (e.g., repeated events) and more complicated hierarchic operational characteristics let us first describe an innovative methodology for modeling evolving processes on the top of enrollment. This methodology covers modeling repeated events associated with patients, patient's visits, number of patients in follow-up period, costs analysis, etc. (Anisimov 2016a).

Let us introduce a construction of the evolving stochastic process that was defined first for other stochastic models in (Anisimov 1991). This class of processes can be used as some general framework to describe various types of operational processes related to patient enrollment.

Assume that upon arrival each patient generates a stochastic process describing the evolution of some operational characteristics, future visits, different events associated with this patient, etc. To formalize this model, consider for center i a sequence of patient's arrival times $\{t_{1i} \leq t_{2i} \leq \ldots\}$ and define a family of stochastic processes $\{\xi_{ki}(t, \theta), t \geq 0, k = 1, 2, \ldots\}$ where the process $\xi_{ki}(t, \theta)$ is associated with k-th patient, and θ is some unknown parameter. These processes are jointly independent at different i and k with distributions not depending on k. For example, $\xi_{ki}(t, \theta)$ can be a Poisson process with unknown rate θ of some events during the follow-up period, or a point process of follow-up visits. More examples are given below.

Various operational characteristics can be represented as sums of evolving processes, for example, the total number of particular events in a site, the number of AE, screen failures, etc. Define in center i the evolving process as

$$Z_i(t) = \sum_{k:t_{ki} \leq t} \xi_{ki}(t - t_{ki}, \theta). \tag{8.44}$$

On global (study) level the evolving process is defined as $Z(t) = \sum_i Z_i(t)$.

In this way, we can represent various operational characteristics and, in particular, the evolution of different type events. Parameter θ can represent some unknown parameters and has to be estimated using trial data. In the following exposition we will omit θ for simplicity.

Consider several examples where the evolving process describes the number of particular events that may happen for the newly recruited patients in event-driven trials.

Example 8.1 Modeling one type of events A in event-driven trials.

Consider one center i and the model of event's appearance described in Lemma 8.6. Define the process $\xi_{ki}(t)$ as follows:

$$\xi_{ki}(t) = 0, \quad t < \tau_{ki}(A) \text{ and } \xi_{ki}(t) = 1, \quad t \geq \tau_{ki}(A),$$

where the variables $\tau_{ki}(A)$ are jointly independent and have the same distribution as τ_A. Then the process $Z_i(t)$ represents the number of events A in center i in time interval $[0, t]$.

Example 8.2 Modeling two types of events in event-driven trials.

Consider the model of appearance of events A and L described in Lemma 8.8. Define the process $\xi_{ki}(t)$ as follows:

Let $\{x_{ki}(t), t \geq 0\}$ be a family of jointly independent right-continuous Markov chains in continuous time with three states $\{0, A, L\}$, where the states A and L are absorbing and the transition rates from 0 to A and from 0 to L are μ_A and μ_L, respectively.

To model a two-dimensional vector $(k(t, A), k(t, L))$ of the number of events A and L in interval $[0, t]$, we define a two-dimensional process:

$$\xi_{ki}(t) = (\chi(x_{ki}(t) = A), \chi(x_{ki}(t) = L)),$$

where $\chi(B)$ is the indicator of event B: $\chi(B) = 1$ if B happened, and $\chi(B) = 0$ otherwise. Denote by τ_{ki} a time of transition of $x_{ki}(t)$. Then $\xi_{ki}(t) = (0, 0)$ while $t < \tau_{ki}$, and for $t \geq \tau_{ki}$, $\xi_{ki}(t) = (1, 0)$, or $\xi_{ki}(t) = (0, 1)$ depending on whether the transition happened to state A or L. Then the process $Z_i(t)$ represents the vector $(k(t, A), k(t, L))$ in center i.

Consider now rather general representation of multiple events. Assume that there can be multiple events $A_1, A_2, \ldots, A_K$, and the evolution of events appearance for one patient is described by some generic multistate right-continuous process $x(t)$ where the states $A_1, A_2, \ldots, A_K$ are absorbing, and the processes $x_{ki}(t)$ are jointly independent and have the same distributions for different patients. Define K-dimensional process:

$$\xi_{ki}(t) = (\chi(x_{ki}(t) = A_1), \chi(x_{ki}(t) = A_2), \ldots, \chi(x_{ki}(t) = A_K)).$$

Then the process $Z_i(t)$ in (8.44) represents the vector of the number of events $(k(t, A_1), k(t, A_2), \ldots, k(t, A_K))$ that may happen in center i in time interval $[0, t]$.

In this general setting, it is also possible to extend the results of Lemma 8.8 and derive similar to (8.32) the representation of the joint predictive distribution for the vector $(k(t, A_1), k(t, A_2), \ldots, k(t, A_K))$ as K-dimensional PG distribution.

The following rather general result is valid.

Lemma 8.13 Assume that the enrollment in center i follows a doubly stochastic Poisson process with rate $\lambda(t)$ and for the process of event's evolution $x(t)$ the transition probabilities

$$Q(0, A_k, t) = Pr(x(t) = A_k \mid x(0) = 0), \quad k = 1, \ldots, K$$

can be calculated where 0 is the initial state of $x(t)$.

Then the vector $(k(t, A_1), k(t, A_2), \ldots, k(t, A_K))$ in center i has a K-dimensional doubly stochastic Poisson distribution with a vector parameter $(g(t, A_1), \ldots, g(t, A_K))$, where according to (8.29)

$$g(t, A_k) = \int_0^t \lambda(u) Q(0, A_k, t - u) du, \quad k = 1, \ldots, K. \tag{8.45}$$

In particular, if the rate $\lambda(u)$ is deterministic, then components of the vector $(k(t, A_1), k(t, A_2), \ldots, k(t, A_K))$ are independent and follow Poisson distributions with parameters (8.45).

Note that multiple events can appear in different therapeutic areas, e.g., oncology studies, multiple sclerosis, etc. For particular models of events appearance, the process $x(t)$ can be described as a Markov chain and transition probabilities can be derived in a closed form.

For example, in (Anisimov 2011b) for the case of oncology trials with three types of events, recurrence, death, and lost to follow-up, a Markov chain with six states is considered, and formulae for transition probabilities are derived and used in predictive modeling.

For calculating the mean and the variance of the evolving process in a closed form, we can use the following result. Assume for simplicity that some center is active in interval [0,T], the enrollment rate is λ which can be also random, and the evolving process in one center $Z(t)$ is constructed according (8.44) using a generic process $\xi(t)$. Denote $A(t) = E[\xi(t)]$, $B^2(t) = E[\xi^2(t)]$. The following lemma follows directly from Lemma 2.1 (Anisimov 2016a).

Lemma 8.14 For any $t > 0$,

$$E[Z(t)] = E[\lambda] \int_0^{\min(t,T)} A(t - u) du, \tag{8.46}$$

$$Var[Z(t)] = E[\lambda] \int_0^{\min(t,T)} B^2(t - u) du + Var[\lambda] \left(\int_0^{\min(t,T)} A(t - u) du \right)^2.$$

This result can be used for creating predictive intervals at rather large number of centers basing on normal approximation. It is interesting to note that under rather general conditions it is also possible to calculate a moment generating function (MGF) of $Z(t)$. Let us define a MGF of $\xi(t)$,

$$f(\psi, t) = E[\exp(\psi \xi(t))],$$

where we assume that this function exists in some region $\psi \leq \psi_0$ for any $t > 0$.

Theorem 8.2 Assume that some center is active in interval [0,T], the enrollment rate is λ which can be also random, and the evolving process $Z(t)$ in this center is constructed according (8.44) using a generic process $\xi(t)$. Then for any $t > 0$, the MGF of $Z(t)$ has the form:

$$E[\exp(\psi Z(t))] = E[\exp(-\lambda \min(t, T)(1 - \phi(\psi, t, T)))] \qquad (8.47)$$

where

$$\phi(\psi, t, T) = \frac{1}{\min(t, T)} \int_0^{\min(t, T)} f(\psi, t - u)du.$$

If λ has a gamma distribution with parameters (α, β), then

$$E[\exp(\psi Z(t))] = \beta^\alpha(\beta + \min(t, T)(1 - \phi(\psi, t, T)))^{-\alpha}. \qquad (8.48)$$

Proof is given in Appendix 8.3.

Note that in the case where the process $Z(t)$ takes integer values in the space $\{0, 1, 2, \ldots\}$, it is more convenient to use a probability generating function (PGF) $G(z, t) = E[z^{Z(t)}]$, $|z| \leq 1$. There is a simple relation $G(z, t) = M(\log(z), t)$ where $M(\psi, t)$ is a MGF.

Let us illustrate these results using a model for predicting the number of repeated events associated with follow-up patients in one center.

Example 8.3 Repeated events.

Consider one center that is initiated at time 0 and assume that the enrollment follows a PG process with gamma distributed rate λ. Suppose that upon arrival each patient generates a Poisson process of some events A with a constant rate μ. These can be some clinical or operational events. Denote by $Y(t)$ the total number of events in time interval $[0, t]$. Then the process $Y(t)$ can be represented as the evolving process where the generic process $\xi(t)$ is a homogeneous Poisson process with rate μ.

Note that in spite of rather simple formulation, it is not possible to derive simple formulae for the distribution of $Y(t)$. However, it is possible to derive an expression for a PGF which can be used to calculate probabilities via calculating the n-th order derivatives. Another opportunity is using a normal approximation for a large number of centers.

Consider first a normal approximation and use Lemma 8.14. Then the functions $A(t)$ and $B^2(t)$ are

$$A(t) = E[\xi(t)] = \mu t, \, B^2(t) = E[\xi^2(t)] = \mu t + \mu^2 t^2$$

Using formulae (8.46), it is easy to calculate that

$$E[Y(t)] = \frac{m\mu t^2}{2}, \ Var[Y(t)] = m\left[\frac{\mu t^2}{2} + \frac{\mu^2 t^3}{3}\right] + s^2 \frac{\mu^2 t^4}{4},$$

where $m = E[\lambda]$, $s^2 = Var[\lambda]$.

Thus, for predictive number of events A in N centers at large N, we can use a normal approximation with mean $NE[Y(t)]$ and variance $NVar[Y(t)]$.

Now let us derive a MGF of the process $Y(t)$ in one center. Assume for simplicity that the rate λ is deterministic. Using notation of Theorem 8.2 where we omit T, we get

$$f(\psi, t) = E[\exp(\psi\xi(t))] = \exp(\mu t(e^\psi - 1)),$$

$$\phi(\psi, t) = \frac{1}{\mu t(e^\psi - 1)}\left(e^{\mu t(e^\psi - 1)} - 1\right),$$

and

$$E[\exp(\psi Y(t))] = \exp(-\lambda t(1 - \phi(\psi, t))).$$

Then a PGF has the form

$$P(z, t) = E\left[z^{Y(t)}\right]$$

$$= \exp\left(-\lambda t\left(1 - \frac{1}{\mu t(z-1)}\left(e^{\mu t(z-1)} - 1\right)\right)\right). \tag{8.49}$$

Using the formula for PGF, it is possible to calculate the probability distribution using relations $Pr(Y(t) = 0) = P(0+, t)$ and

$$Pr(Y(t) = k) = \frac{1}{k!}\frac{\partial^k P(z, t)}{\partial z^k}\bigg|_{z=+0}, \ k = 1, 2, \ldots$$

In our example it is easy to see that

$$Pr(Y(t) = 0) = \exp(-\lambda t(1 - (1 - e^{-\mu t})/\mu t)). \tag{8.50}$$

Correspondingly, calculating the first derivative and putting $z = 0$ we get

$$Pr(Y(t) = 1) = \frac{\lambda}{\mu}(1 - e^{-\mu t} - \mu t e^{-\mu t})$$

$$\times \exp(-\lambda t(1 - (1 - e^{-\mu t})/\mu t)). \tag{8.51}$$

Other probabilities can be also calculated step-by-step or evaluated using numerical algorithms of calculating higher derivatives. However, on this way we can reliably calculate only a few probabilities for not very large values of k.

Using (8.49) it is also possible to analyze an approximate behavior of $Y(t)$ for small number of events. Indeed, assume that μt is rather small which means that the events happen rather rare. Then

$$P(z,t) \approx \exp\left(-\frac{\lambda \mu t^2}{2}(1-z)\right).$$

This PGF corresponds to a Poisson process with rate $\lambda \mu t^2/2$.

Thus, at small μt and not so large λt (usual enrollment rate), the value $\lambda \mu t^2$ is also rather small, and the probability distribution of $Y(t)$ is approximated as follows:

$$\Pr(Y(t)=0) \approx 1 - \lambda \mu t^2/2, \Pr(Y(t)=k) \approx \frac{(\lambda \mu t^2)^k}{k!}, k=1,2,\ldots$$

These relations are in agreement with (8.50) and (8.51).

This is rather unusual result which shows that for this model the number of events is growing over the time proportionally to t^2 in both cases of large and small $\lambda \mu t^2$.

Note that the results of this example can be extended to the case when center is active only in interval $[0, T]$, the rate λ has a gamma distribution, and each patient has a fixed follow-up period U. However, the formulae will be more complicated as the result will depend on the relations between t, T and U. Interested readers can try to derive these formulae themselves.

Some other examples on using evolving processes to model the number of follow-up and lost patients, multiple patient's visits and operational costs associated with visits are given in (Anisimov 2016a).

8.6 Discussion

The chapter is focused on the development and discussion of different techniques for predictive analytic modeling and forecasting clinical trials operation including patient enrollment and screening processes, event's modeling in event-driven trials, risk-based monitoring of some operational characteristics including enrollment performance and detecting the unusual event's patterns.

For modeling and predicting operational processes associated with patient enrollment a new methodology that uses evolving stochastic processes is proposed. This provides rather general and unified framework to describe wide range of operational processes including follow-up patients, various associated events including dropout, different patient's visits, and related costs. Some examples on calculating predictive distributions of the number of events that appear during the follow-up period are considered.

The background technique uses a PG model for modeling enrollment, which is extended further to model other processes constructed on the top of enrollment. This technique has several advantages compared to other approaches used for global enrollment modeling. It accounts for multicenter's effects, different times of opening and closing centers; allows predicting the mean and credibility bounds for the number of recruited patients (on different levels, center/country/global) and for time to complete enrollment; and also can predict probability to complete a trial in time.

The developed technique also allows an optimal interim adaptive adjustment: if enrollment is going not as planned, evaluate the optimal set of new centers needed to be added with the purpose to complete enrollment in time with a given confidence accounting for time constraints and minimizing costs.

This technique has also several other features that are available only in the stochastic framework, e.g., supporting risk-based monitoring and evaluating center/country enrollment performance using probabilistic thresholds based on P-values and quantiles for corresponding PG distributions.

It is essential to note that all basic characteristics can be calculated or approximated using closed-form expressions. Thus, there is no need to use Monte Carlo simulation. The availability of formulae has many advantages as it allows investigating the functional dependences on different parameters (number of centers, rates, center's delays, etc.) and, thus, analyzing in real time the impact of various factors and finding the optimal solutions. This would be hard to achieve using simulation.

Note also that during the course of clinical trial, the enrollment and other processes at different levels are in general nonhomogeneous doubly stochastic hierarchic processes where the global and individual parameters depend on processes of initiation and closing centers. These types of dependences are captured by a PG model, and this feature profitably differentiates a PG model from other models that are used mainly for global prediction: using global Poisson models in Deng et al. (2014), Gajewski et al. (2008), and Williford et al. (1987), and Brownian and fractional Brownian motions in Lai et al. (2001) and Zhang and Lai (2011).

Therefore, the methodology developed in the chapter opens very wide opportunities to modeling various operational characteristics of clinical trials and improving the efficiency of clinical trial operations.

Acknowledgments The author would like to thank Dr. Olga Marchenko for her kind invitation to write this chapter and also to express his sincere gratitude to the Referee for careful reading and many useful comments and suggestions that lead to the improvement of the presentation.

Appendix

Appendix 8.1: Proof of Lemma 8.8

Given λ, at time t the total number of both events, A and L, according to Lemma 8.7 has a Poisson distribution with parameter $\lambda q(t, a, b)$ in the form (8.30) where we should put $\mu_A = \mu$. According to properties of a Poisson process, given some event happen, this event will be A or L with probabilities μ_A/μ or μ_L/μ. Thus, the values $k(t, A)$ and $k(t, L)$ are independent and have Poisson distributions with parameters $\lambda q_A(t, a, b)$ and $\lambda q_L(t, a, b)$, respectively, and we get the second part of the statement with relations (8.33).

Assume now that λ has a gamma distribution with parameters (α, β). Then the vector $(k(t, A), k(t, L))$ has a mixed two-dimensional Poisson distribution with vector parameter $(\lambda q_A(t, a, b), \lambda q_L(t, a, b))$ that is

$$\Pr(k(t, A) = k, k(t, L) = j)$$

$$= E\left[\exp\left(-\lambda(q_A(t, a, b) + q_L(t, a, b)) \frac{(\lambda q_A(t, a, b))^k}{k!} \frac{(\lambda q_L(t, a, b))^j}{j!}\right)\right]. \qquad (8.52)$$

According to (8.1) the following relation is true:

$$E\left[\exp\left(-\lambda t\right)\frac{(\lambda t)^k}{k!}\right] = \frac{\Gamma(\alpha + k)}{k!\Gamma(\alpha)} \frac{t^k \beta^\alpha}{(\beta + t)^{\alpha + k}}, k = 0, 1, 2, \ldots$$

This relation together with (8.52) implies (8.32).

Appendix 8.2: Proof of Lemma 8.11

The patients arrive to a center according to a PG process. For a Poisson process $\Pi_\lambda(v)$, it is known (Snyder and Miller 2012: 62) that given $\Pi_\lambda(v) = k$, the arrival times have the same distribution as the order statistics of k independent variables t_i with the common uniform distribution in interval $[0, v]$. This result does not depend on λ, thus, it is also true for a random λ. Furthermore, if the patient arrived at time t_i that has a uniform $[0, v]$ distribution, then using (8.31) we get that the probability to have event B in interval $[0, v]$ is

$$p(v, B) = \frac{\mu_B}{\mu} \frac{1}{v} \int_0^v \left(1 - e^{-\mu(v-x)}\right) dx.$$

This implies (8.40). Therefore, the total number of events B has a binomial distribution $Bin(k, p(v, B))$. Correspondingly, as each time it may happen either event A or L, then the joint distribution of the number of events A and L is a multinomial distribution.

Appendix 8.3: Proof of Theorem 8.2

By construction:

$$E[\exp(\psi Z(t))] = E\left[\exp\left(\psi \sum_{k:t_k \le t} \xi_k(t - t_k))\right)\right]$$

$$= E\left[\sum_{n=0}^{\infty} E[\exp\left(\psi \sum_{k=1}^{n} \xi_k(t - t_k))|\Pi_\lambda(\min(t,T)) = n\right]\right.$$

$$\left. \times \Pr(\Pi_\lambda(\min(t,T)) = n|\lambda)\right].$$

Given $\Pi_\lambda(v) = n$, the arrival times have the same distribution as the order statistics of n independent variables t_k with the common uniform distribution in interval $[0, v]$ (Snyder and Miller 2012: 62). Thus,

$$E\left[\exp\left(\psi \sum_{k=1}^{n} \xi_k(t - t_k)) \mid \Pi_\lambda(\min(t,T)) = n\right] =$$

$$= E\left[\exp\left(\psi \sum_{k=1}^{n} \xi_k(t - U_k(\min(t,T)))\right)\right],$$

where $U_k(a)$ are independent and uniformly distributed in $(0, a)$ variables. Note that

$$E[\exp(\psi \xi_1(t - U_1(\min(t,T)))] = \phi(\psi, t, T).$$

Thus,

$$E\left[\exp\left(\psi \sum_{k=1}^{n} \xi_k(t - U_k(\min(t,T)))\right)\right] = \phi^n(\psi, t, T).$$

As

$$\Pr(\Pi_\lambda(\min(t,T)) = n \mid \lambda) = \exp(-\lambda \min(t,T)) \frac{(\lambda \min(t,T))^n}{n!}$$

then

$$E[\exp(\psi Z(t))] = E\left[\sum_{n=0}^{\infty} \phi^n(\psi, t, T) \exp(-\lambda \min(t,T)) \frac{(\lambda \min(t,T))^n}{n!}\right].$$

Taking sum, we get the expression (8.47). This completes the main part of the proof. For the case when λ is gamma distributed, the relation (8.48) follows from (8.1) for $k = 0$ by putting instead of t the value $\min(t, T)(1 - \phi(\psi, t, T))$.

References

Anisimov V (1991) Limit theorems for evolving accumulation processes. *Theory of Probability and Mathematical Statistics* 43:5–11.

Anisimov V, Fedorov V, Jones B (2003) Optimal design of multicenter trials with random enrollment. *GSK BDS Technical Report*, TR 2003-03.

Anisimov V, Fedorov V (2005) Modeling of enrollment and estimation of parameters in multicenter trials. *GSK BDS Technical Report*, TR 2005-01.

Anisimov V, Fedorov V (2007a) Design of multicenter clinical trials with random enrollment, in book "*Advances in Statistical Methods for the Health Sciences*", Series: Statistics for Industry and Technology, Balakrishnan, N.; Auget, J.-L.; Mesbah, M.; Molenberghs, G. (Eds.) Birkhäuser, Ch. 25, 387–400.

Anisimov V, Fedorov V (2007b) Modeling, prediction and adaptive adjustment of recruitment in multicenter trials. *Statistics in Medicine* 26(27): 4958–4975.

Anisimov V, Downing D, Fedorov V (2007) Recruitment in multicenter trials: prediction and adjustment. In *mODa 8 - Advances in Model-Oriented Design and Analysis*, eds. J. Lopez-Fidalgo, J.M. Rodriguez-Diaz and B. Torsney, Physica-Verlag, 1–8.

Anisimov V (2008) Using mixed Poisson models in patient recruitment in multicenter clinical trials, *Proc. of the World Congress on Engineering*, v. II, 1046–1049.

Anisimov V (2009) Predictive modeling of recruitment and drug supply in multicenter clinical trials. In: *Proc. of the Joint Statistical Meeting*, Biopharmaceutical Section, Washington, DC, American Statistical Association, August: 1248–1259.

Anisimov V (2011a) Statistical modeling of clinical trials (recruitment and randomization). *Communications in Statistics - Theory and Methods* 40(19–20): 3684–3699.

Anisimov V (2011b) Predictive event modeling in multicenter clinical trials with waiting time to response. *Pharmaceutical Statistics* 10(6): 517–522.

Anisimov V (2011c) Effects of unstratified and centre-stratified randomization in multicenter clinical trials. *Pharmaceutical Statistics* 10 (1): 50–59.

Anisimov V (2016a) Predictive hierarchic modeling of operational characteristics in clinical trials. *Communications in Statistics - Simulation and Computation* 45, 05, 1477–1488.

Anisimov V (2016b) Discussion on the paper "Real-time prediction of clinical trial enrollment and event counts: a review", by DF Heitjan et al, *Contemporary Clinical Trials* 46: 7–10.

Anisimov V, Yeung W, Coad S (2017) Imbalance properties of centre-stratified permuted-block and complete randomisation for several treatments in a clinical trial. *Statistics in Medicine*, 36 (8): 1302–1318.

Bakhshi A, Senn S, Phillips A (2013) Some issues in predicting patient recruitment in multi-center clinical trials. *Statistics in Medicine* 32(30): 5458–5468.

Barnard KD, Dent L, Cook A (2010) A systematic review of models to predict recruitment to multicenter clinical trials. *BMC Medical Research Methodology* 10: 63.

Bates GE, Neyman J. (1952) Contributions to the theory of accident proneness. *University of California Publications in Statistics* 1(9): 215–254.

Bernardo JM, Smith AFM (2004) *Bayesian Theory*, John Wiley & Sons, Inc., Hoboken, NJ, USA.

Carter RE, Sonne SC, Brady KT (2005) Practical considerations for estimating clinical trial accrual periods: Application to a multi-center effectiveness study. *BMC Medical Research Methodology* 5:11–15.

Cox DR, Isham V (1980) *Point Processes*, London: Chapman & Hall.

Deng Y, Zhang X, Long O (2014) Bayesian modeling and prediction of accrual in multi-regional clinical trials. *Statistical Methods in Medical Research* 26, 2: 752-765.

Gajewski BJ, Simon SD, Carlson SE (2008) Predicting accrual in clinical trials with Bayesian posterior predictive distributions. *Statistics in Medicine* 27:2328–2340.

Gajewski BJ, Simon SD, Carslon SE. (2012) On the existence of constant accrual rates in clinical trials and direction for future research. *International Journal of Statistics and Probability* 1:43–46.

Heitjan DF, Ge Z, Ying GS (2015) Real-time prediction of clinical trial enrollment and event counts: a review. *Contemporary Clinical Trials* 45, part A: 26-33

Johnson NL, Kotz S, Kemp AW (1993) *Univariate Discrete Distributions*. 2nd Ed., New York: John Wiley & Sons.

Johnson NL, Kotz S, Balakrishnan N (1994) *Continuous Univariate Distributions*, 2nd Ed. Vol. 1. New York: John Wiley & Sons.

Lachin JM (1988) Statistical properties of randomization in clinical trials. *Controlled Clinical Trials* 9: 289–311.

Lai D, Moy LA, Davis BR, Brown LE, Sacks FM (2001) Brownian motion and long-term clinical trial recruitment. *J. Stat. Plan. Inference* 93: 239–246.

Mijoule G, Savy S, Savy N (2012) Models for patients' recruitment in clinical trials and sensitivity analysis. *Statistics in Medicine* 31(16): 1655–1674.

Minois NN, Lauwers-Cances V, Savy S, Attal M, Andrieua S, Anisimov V, Savy N (2017) Using Poisson-gamma model to evaluate the duration of recruitment process when historical trials are available. *Statistics in Medicine*, 36(23): 3605-3620.

Rosenberger WF, Lachin JM (2013) *Randomization in clinical trials*, John Wiley & Sons, New York, USA.

Senn S. (1997) *Statistical Issues in Drug Development*. Chichester: John Wiley & Sons.

Senn S. (1998) Some controversies in planning and analysis multi-center trials. *Statistics in Medicine,* 17:1753–1756.

Senn S, Anisimov V, Fedorov V (2010) Comparisons of minimization and Atkinson's algorithm. *Statistics in Medicine* 29 (7/8): 721-730.

Snyder DL, Miller MI (2012) *Random Point Processes in Time and Space*. Springer.

Tang G, Kong Y, Chang CCH, Kong L, Costantino JP (2012) Prediction of accrual closure date in multi-center clinical trials with discrete-time Poisson process models. *Pharmaceutical Statistics,* 11: 351–356.

Williford WO, Bingham SF, Weiss DG, Collins JF, Rains KT, Krol WF (1987) The "constant intake rate" assumption in interim recruitment goal methodology for multicenter clinical trials. *J. Chronic Diseases*, 40: 297–307.

Zhang Q, Lai D (2011) Fractional Brownian motion and long-term clinical trial recruitment. *J. Statistical Planning Inference,* 141: 1783–1788.

Chapter 9
Better Together: Examples of Biostatisticians Collaborating in Drug Development

Russell Reeve, Seth Berry, and Brandon Swift

9.1 Introduction

A man was sitting near a table, when his supervisor approached him. The supervisor pointed to the table and told the man to clean it. The man looked puzzled and said he could not clean it. Usually the employee was very hard working, so this was unusual. "What do you mean you cannot clean it?" asked the supervisor. The employee replied "I do not know what you want to do with it. If you want to use the table for potting flowers, I am just going to dust off the dirt, and have a nice flat spot for the work. If you want to have a picnic on the table, then I may wash it off with water, and maybe scrub it clean. If you want to have a nice dinner, I'll put on a table cloth, maybe with a flower centerpiece. If you want to do surgery, I will clean with disinfectant, and also disinfect the walls, the floor, the doors, and any equipment in the room. Unless I know how you want to use the table, I cannot clean it properly."

This parable from quality guru Ed Deming illustrates (Walton 1986, Deming 2016) several important points that are important for biostatisticians in the drug development industry. Two points that are particularly relevant to this chapter are (1) the need for context in our work and (2) the critical importance of collaboration. These points are well-illustrated in this parable.

We cannot do our work without appropriate context. This is true of the table cleaner and is equally true of the biostatistician. The statistical analysis, the study design, the data collection plan, assay development and validation, manufacturing process development and quality control, formulation development, regulatory strategy, and almost every aspect of the job of a biostatistician needs to be governed

R. Reeve (✉) · S. Berry
IQVIA, Durham, NC, USA
e-mail: russell.reeve@iquia.com

B. Swift
Metvant Sciences, Durham, NC, USA

© Springer Nature Switzerland AG 2020
O. V. Marchenko, N. V. Katenka (eds.), *Quantitative Methods in Pharmaceutical Research and Development*, https://doi.org/10.1007/978-3-030-48555-9_9

by the context. The biostatistician needs to know how the study fits into the larger program and the objectives of the program, how the data analysis supports the trial, and how the development activity relates to the design and analysis. Examples of this will be discussed in each of the sections below. Understanding the context is key for making both the clinical and nonclinical work effective and without understanding the context important gaps in the outputs can derail trials and programs. And the context needs to go beyond the program itself, to also incorporate knowledge of the organizational objectives, tempered by the market. To understand the context, the biostatistician will need to collaborate with other disciplines. To design a trial, the biostatistician will need to talk with the medical expert, the pharmacokineticist, the data manager, the project manager, and the commercial team, whose thoughts are expressed through the target product profile. Since all of these individuals will provide key information and context that will need to be utilized, the biostatistician will also need to collaborate with all of these individuals. Hence, to understand the context, we also need constructive collaboration.

Biostatisticians within the pharmaceutical industry collaborate with a wide variety of scientists and experts in other disciplines. Statisticians collaborate in areas of drug design, assay development and validation, toxicology, manufacturing process development and quality control, pharmacokinetics, formulation development, clinical developers, data management, regulatory strategy, and commercial. No single method of collaboration will apply in all of these varied circumstances, though some common principles will apply. We will explore some of those principles in this chapter and give examples of successful and not so successful collaborative experiences.

Collaboration has certainly been an area of intense interest within statistical communities in the past. For example, Peck et al. (1998) consists entirely of industry/academic collaborations. While there have been many examples of industry/academic collaboration that has produced innovative statistics, there is still a need for additional collaboration with subject matter experts (e.g., Lee (2000)). Biostatistics, being motivated by applied problems, has a long history of collaboration. We only need to think of the foundations of statistics as a separate academic discipline with the agricultural field experiments of Fisher and the development of the t-test to solve specific industrial problems. Many foundational properties—such as the central limit theorem developed to solve insurance problems, split plot designs to solve agricultural research problems, and the sequential likelihood ratio test originally designed collaboratively with quality control engineers to solve manufacturing process monitoring problems—are now commonly employed in the practice of statistics.

In this chapter, we will discuss some case studies of fruitful collaboration. The themes are the importance of understanding the context of the work and the benefits of collaboration. These are chiefly case studies of various types, with data being masked to protect confidentiality. We start with clinical research, which has a never-ending list of problems for biostatistician involvement. Within clinical, we discuss the issues of biosimilar sample size, dose-response testing, adaptive design, trial design, and operational planning. We should note that sample size calculations may seem like a lone biostatistician task, but a successful sample size estimation is truly a collaborative exercise. We also discuss nonclinical collaboration, which is a very interesting area of application for biostatisticians. Areas in nonclinical statistics that we will present are in analytical similarity—of keen interest in biosimilar development—followed by assay development, formulation development, assay acceptance criteria, and software device application development, an area of growing interest among pharmaceutical companies.

9.2 Clinical

9.2.1 Biosimilar Sample Size for Equivalence Studies

Biosimilar products are compounds developed to be similar to a previously licensed biological therapy, and intended to be licensed for the same indications, or a subset of those indications. The biosimilar compounds are developed to mimic as closely as possible the structure of the predecessor compound, but the compounds are very large and are produced via biological systems, and hence may not be identical to the existing compound. Recent examples of products that have been approved for marketing of a biosimilar include Lapelga and Pegex for pegfilgrastim; Bevacirel and Cizumab for bevacizumab; and Amjevita and Amgevita for adalimumab. Most of the biosimilars under development are monoclonal antibodies or derivatives thereof. A ribbon diagram of a generic antibody is shown in Fig. 9.1.

Biological compounds revolutionized many areas of medical care. Biologics have been shown to have an improved benefit/risk profile compared to non-biologic treatments and are often the treatment of last resort in severe illnesses; see, e.g., Duffy (2013); Griffin and Morley (2013); Mosak and Furie (2013); Ahluwalia (2012); Ferrante et al. (2009); Scheinberg and Kay (2012); and Horton and Emery (2012). However, the downside to biologicals is that the compounds are very expensive. In fact, the average costs can be as much as 25 times higher than for a small-molecule drug (Thomson Reuters BioWorld). Hence, there is a need for cheaper alternatives to these costly but highly effective therapies, hence the interest in biosimilar products.

Until recently, there has not been any avenue for licensing these biological compounds in the United States even when the predecessor compound lost patent protection. For small molecule generics, the licensing is straightforward by using the abbreviated new drug application (ANDA) pathway. This is easier since the compound is identical to the reference compound, with the only difference being the formulation. For a biosimilar, the formulation may be similar, but the biologic compound itself may have amino acid sequences that differ from the reference biologic, hence the name "biosimilar."

Biosimilar development follows a stepwise approach, progressing from preclinical, to early phase clinical (often denoted as Phase I), and then to late stage clinical (often denoted as Phase III). The biosimilar must be shown to be analytically similar

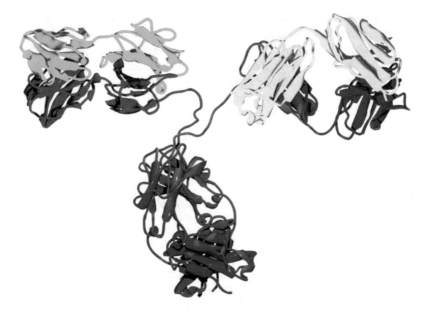

Fig. 9.1 A ribbon diagram of a monoclonal antibody. The molecular formula for trastuzumab is $C_{6470}H_{10012}N_{1726}O_{2013}S_{42}$, with a molecular weight of 145,531.5 g/mol. In contrast, aspirin has a molecular weight of 180.157 g/mol

to the licensed biologic compound. The objectives at each stage vary and build on the prior stages. Do not let the phase notations confuse the situation, as they do not directly correspond to the stages of a new molecular entity. In biosimilar development, Phase I is a confirmatory study, not an exploratory study, and can be more important (*cf.* FDA 2015: 18) than the efficacy study in patients (Phase III).

In this section, we will discuss the early phase clinical development. The objective is to show that the biosimilar is pharmacokinetically similar to the predecessor or reference product. Similarity is usually assessed via a bioequivalence study and appropriate statistical analysis following the FDA bioequivalence guidance. These bioequivalence studies tend to be run as parallel arms due to the long half-life, often in patients, and of fairly large size, ranging up to 180 patients, though some studies may be crossover. An important aspect that guides the decision between crossover and parallel design is the half-life (Table 9.1). Products with longer half-lives are better suited for parallel designs, even at the cost of additional patients.

Finally, the marketing strategy of the sponsor organization must be accounted for early in the development. If the sponsor is seeking a biosimilar marketing authorization only for a single region (e.g., United States (US)), then the sponsor will require only a two-arm study. However, if the sponsor seeks marketing authorization in both the US and European Union (EU) regions, a three-arm study will be required since regulators will require a reference product from each source region, and in this case multiplicity will need to be accounted for.

Table 9.1 Half-lives of selected biological agents with active biosimilar development

Compound	Half-life range	Half-life (weeks)	6 half-lives (weeks)
Pegfilgrastim	15–18 h	0.1	0.6
Etanercept	70 (7–300) h	0.4	2.5
Rituximab	22 (6.1–52) days	3.1	18.9
Bevacizumab	20 (11–50) days	2.9	17.1
Adalimumab	10–20 days	2.1	12.9
Tocilizumab	4 days	0.6	3.4
Panitumumab	7.5 (3.6–10.9) days	1.1	6.4

For example, a sponsor is designing a study to show PK comparability. In general, the regulatory authorities are looking for the sponsor to show that the biosimilar product shows comparable characteristics in the most sensitive population or the population where potential differences would most easily be observed. Several questions that need to be answered that will affect study design include:

- **Study population.** Healthy volunteers or patients? If patients, what disease and severity of disease?
- **Dose of product.** If the reference product has a dose-response relationship, then the dose should not be at the top of the dose-response relationship, but in the middle, since any performance differences at the top of the dose-response curve would be unlikely to be observed.
- **Study design.** Compounds with short half-lives (typically less than 5 days) would be better studied with a crossover design, since the comparisons between compounds will be based on intra-patient differences, eliminating inter-patient variability in the statistical comparisons. However, for longer half-life products (see, e.g., Table 9.1), a parallel design is preferable.
- **Endpoints.** Endpoints need to be selected and appropriate for the study design and population. The PK endpoints are often a version of area under the concentration-versus-time curve (AUC) and the observed maximum concentration (Cmax). Pharmacodynamic endpoints may also be studied if appropriate to the disease area and study design.
- **Variability.** Variability in the endpoints will determine the sample size, and this varies with study design, drug presentation, and possibly disease area. Crossover studies generally have lower variability than parallel since the inter-patient component is eliminated. Intravenous (IV) delivery generally has less variability than subcutaneous (SC), though in some cases variability as a result of SC administration can be reduced when hyaluronidase is used in the formulation. Furthermore, PK variability may differ between healthy volunteers and patients.
- **Multiplicity and power.** The marketing strategy will determine the number of treatment arms and hence whether multiple comparisons among the treatment arms are necessary. If the intended strategy is to seek licensing in EMA and FDA regulatory regions, then a three-arm study will be needed; if the strategy is the seek licensing in only one regulatory region, then a two-arm study will suffice. The power calculations must be consistent with the objectives of the study.

Table 9.2 Bevacizumab coefficients of variation (CV) for C_{max} and AUC

Study	n	Dose (mg/kg)	CV C_{max} (%)	AUC (%)
Study 1	15	10	51.0	
Study 2	25	7.5	67.2	36.8
Study 2	31	15	66.2	30.8
Study 3	30	5		32.5
Study 3	32	10		26.3

CV coefficient of variation, *n* clinical study sample size. PK parameters determine using standard non-compartmental analysis (NCA). Note that some papers reported only one of the two parameters of interest

For this study design, the compound being studies is bevacizumab. With a half-life of 2.9 weeks, a parallel study is indicated. In this example, we will assume a two-arm study, hence no need to adjust power for multiplicity of comparisons. The process will be to establish the variability of the PK endpoints based on prior literature. Based on the variability, then the sample size can be calculated.

Let us consider the variability. Often, the data reported in the literature is of fairly small sample size (n = ~30), with often different point estimates in each of the publically reported studies. For example, in a literature review of bevacizumab, the coefficient of variation for maximum observed concentration (C_{max}) was reported between 51 and 66% based on sample sizes of between 15 and 31, and for area under the concentration-time curve (AUC), the variability ranged between 26 and 36% (see Table 9.2). Even though the analysis of the data will be based on standard non-compartmental analyses (NCA) of the exposure parameters (e.g., AUC and C_{max}), a population PK model can help derive better estimates of the variability for the following reasons. Population PK models are often based upon a meta-analysis of data incorporating results from Phase I, II, and III studies, thus reflecting a much larger sample size. Furthermore PK data may often be collected using a sparse sampling (n = 2–3 samples per subject) which make calculations of AUC or C_{max} parameters unreliable or infeasible, but with a population PK modeling approach can be more accurately estimated.

In this example, a biostatistician worked with a pharmacokineticist, using population PK models reported in the literature, to simulate PK concentrations for virtual subjects. To achieve this goal, in silico patients were simulated as analytical methods will yield poor estimates of the actual variability due to the nonlinearity inherent in the PK model. To estimate the variability, a three-step process was implemented:

1. Using the population PK model, generate drug concentrations for K in silico patients from some large K (say 10,000).
2. Using the simulated drug concentrations, calculate the post hoc PK parameters, just as if these were concentrations from actual patients.
3. Calculate the variability, and use that to power the study.

Continuing with the case study of bevacizumab, a population PK model was developed by Lu et al. (2008), consisted of a two-compartment model with covariates on the parameters. The model was developed on Phase I through Phase III data in the original development of the compound and included data from 491 patients with a total of 4629 bevacizumab concentrations. Equations for the covariate models for clearance (CL) and volume of central compartment (V_c) are listed below. Further details and parameter estimates can be found in Lu et al. (2008).

$$
\begin{aligned}
\log CL = {} & \log \theta_1 + \log (1 + \theta_5 GDR) + \theta_6 \log (WT/74) \\
& + \theta_7 \log (ALBU/37) + \theta_8 \log (ALK/102) \\
& + \theta_{10} \log (SGOT/26)
\end{aligned}
\tag{9.1}
$$

$$
\begin{aligned}
\log Vc = {} & \log \theta_2 + \log (1 + \theta_{11} GDR) + \theta_{12} \log (WT/74) \\
& + \theta_{13} \log (ALBU/37)
\end{aligned}
\tag{9.2}
$$

In the model, the between subject variability for PK parameters assumes a log-normal distribution and is expressed using an exponential model

$$
P_j = \theta \cdot \exp \left(\eta_j \right)
\tag{9.3}
$$

where P is the parameter of interest, j is the jth individual, θ is the estimate of the population mean, and η_j is the deviation from the population mean for the jth individual, under the assumption that

$$
\eta \tilde{N} \left(0, \omega_\theta^2 \right).
\tag{9.4}
$$

with mean 0 and variance ω^2. The residual variability was characterized by an additive-proportional error model of the form:

$$
Y_{ij} = C_{ij} \cdot \left(1 + \vec{\varepsilon}_{ij} \right) + \varepsilon_{2ij}
\tag{9.5}
$$

where Y_{ij} is the observed concentration for the jth individual's i^{th} concentration, C_{ij} is the predicted concentration, and ε_{ij} is the residual proportional error term under the assumption

$$
\varepsilon \tilde{N} \left(0, \sigma_\varepsilon^2 \right).
\tag{9.6}
$$

with mean 0 and variance σ^2.

The pharmacokinetics expert implemented the model and used it to simulate concentrations for 10,000 in silico patients. Since the PK parameters are dependent on the covariates, the PK sampling scheme, and dose designated in the protocol, we simulated individual concentration-time profiles that reflect the planned study design and protocol. The results were based on 500 bootstraps with 200 subjects in each

Table 9.3 Summary statistics of non-compartmental analysis parameters calculated from 500 bootstrap data files with 200 in silico patients dosed at 2 mg/kg

Parameter	Mean	SD	%CV
$AUC_{0\text{-inf}}$ (μg·day/mL)	12,900	3720	28.8%
$AUC_{0\text{-tlast}}$ (μg·day/mL)	12,700	3510	27.6%
C_{max} (μg/mL)	1360	294.5	21.7%

replicate. PK parameters were calculated using an NCA approach using both the area under the concentration-time profile from time zero to infinity ($AUC_{0\text{-}\infty}$) and from time zero to the last sampling time ($AUC_{0\text{-tlast}}$). The parameters were summarized to calculate the mean, standard deviation, and CV, which could then be used to calculated sample size by the biostatistician. The summary statistics are shown in Table 9.3, where we see that the CV for AUC is approximately 28% and that for C_{max} is approximately 22%. In this case, we would expect AUC to dominate the sample size calculation. It is interesting that Knight et al. (2016) found CV of approximately 15–16% for AUC and 14–15% for C_{max}, using a 5 mg/kg dose, which is much lower than the results reported in Table 9.1.

Using this approach, several options are now available to help understand the design's operating characteristics and to optimize the trial design. We can look at the effect of the multiplicity of endpoints on power ($AUC_{0\text{-}\infty}$ and C_{max}, for instance) and to understand the effect of different covariate patterns in the current study relative to the originator study. In what can be an iterative optimization process, the pharmacokinetics can alter the sampling times based on this model to yield studies with the highest power, incorporating dropout timing, inclusion/exclusion criteria, quantification limits of the assays, population uncertainty, and other factors as needed, so the statistician can calculate the power or sample size based on the results. Working together, this optimization process can be made more efficient and will yield better trial designs than if the pharmacokineticist and biostatistician worked alone on their separate pieces.

The multiplicity between AUC and C_{max} may be an issue, since the correlation is relatively weak; see Fig. 9.2 for a plot of $AUC_{0\text{-}\infty}$ versus C_{max}. The pre-determined equivalence hypotheses for each parameter are calculated separately, but the trial will be a success only if both hypotheses succeed. To answer this question, the pharmacokineticist and the biostatistician used the population PK model to investigate the correlation between the primary endpoints and the effect this has on the power of the trial. The power under both the null and alternative hypotheses are shown in Table 9.4 under the assumption of a two-arm study, each with 60 patients and no dropouts. It was found that the Type I error rate of the joint hypothesis for both $AUC_{0\text{-}\infty}$ and C_{max} is very low, <0.01.

Combining the skillsets of a pharmacokineticist and a biostatistician allows for a better overall design. The pharmacokineticist provides expertise in the appropriate endpoints, PK modeling, blood sample timing, and effects of covariates on the blood concentrations, and the statistician provides the summarization and implications for trial results. Additionally, working together allows for a solution to be found more efficiently since less duplicated effort was required.

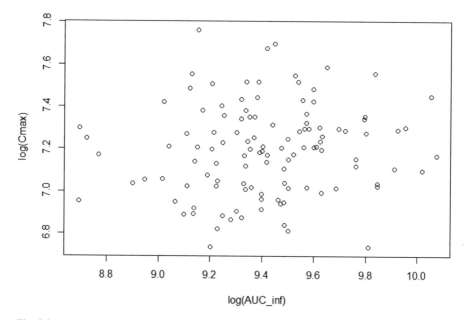

Fig. 9.2 Correlation between $AUC_{0-\infty}$ and C_{max} for n = 60 bevacizumab subjects simulated as a single virtual clinical trial using the population PK model published by Lu et al. (2008)

Table 9.4 Power calculations for bevacizumab for n = 60 under both null and alternative hypotheses, denoted by H

P{Reject H0|H}	$AUC_{0-\infty}$	C_{max}	$AUC_{0-\infty}$ and C_{max}
H = H0	0.049	0.045	0.006
H = HA	0.984	1	0.984

9.2.2   Trial Design via Simulation

Clinical trial design methods greatly enhance the opportunities for collaboration among many members of the trial design community, including the biostatistician, pharmacokineticist, physician, and operational team members. In fact, just pushing different members of the team to discuss the assumptions of the trial in preparation of a clinical trial simulation can be a useful and to make the study as rigorous as possible based on literature data. Many times what is considered to be true is in fact false, just by examining the literature in more detail. The following is one such example where the pharmacokinetic model is used as the basis for constructing pharmacokinetic-pharmacodynamic (PK-PD) relationships to then define the operational characteristics of the trial.

Using Phase I data, the pharmacokineticist developed a nonlinear mixed-effect population pharmacokinetic model. A two-compartment model with first-order absorption and elimination adequately fit the data, with body weight as a covariate on clearance. Because of large between subject variability in exposure, overlapping

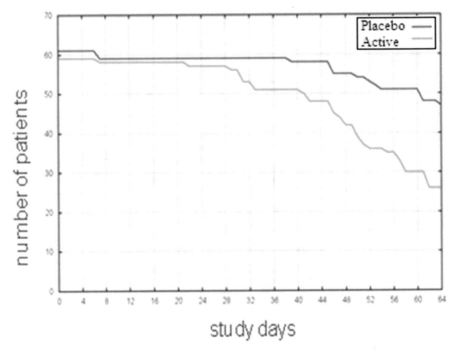

Fig. 9.3 Dropout rate of patients by treatment

exposure distributions could be expected among the proposed dose cohorts, making dose-response relationships more difficult to discern. A more robust study design could have been a randomized concentration-controlled trial, which would yield study cohorts with better separation in exposures, helping to clarify the dose-response relationship (see, e.g., Reeve and Hale 1994; Hale and Reeve 1994; Hale et al. 1998; Endrenyi and Zha 1994); however this approach was not considered.

Adverse events (AEs) observed in the multiple dose-ascending Phase I trial in patients were modeled as a function of dose. Using an unsupervised data analysis technique, a data-mining expert found that the level of adverse events increased for the first 4 weeks, then stabilized. However, it was clear that the actively treated patients had higher adverse event levels than the placebo patients. One advantage of this modeling approach is predictive scores are calculated for each patient based on their baseline characteristics. In this case, since adverse events are predominantly due to tolerability and are positively correlated with dropout probability (see Fig. 9.3), excluding patients that are more likely to not tolerate the drug could improve study performance by eliminating participants who are unlikely to benefit from the compound. One should be aware that this may not be appropriate in all cases: Oncology patients may not drop out of the trial due to tolerability, but rather only for lack of response or dose limiting toxicity, and in other indications one may not want to reduce the pool of potential patients due to a host of reasons, including

Fig. 9.4 Concentration-
adverse event relationship.
The solid line is the
predicted probability, and
the dashed lines are the 95%
confidence interval

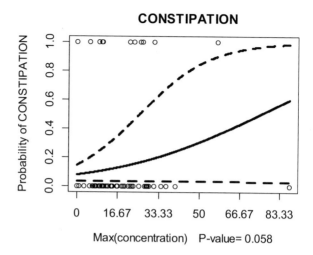

CONSTIPATION

desire to maintain a broad marketing authorization, lack of generalizability to a broader population based on a more narrow population, and recruiting.

Adverse event modeling is a critical and often overlooked component in trial simulation. In this case, modeling of AEs was critically important in the simulation process because of its effect on the dropout rate. Because we are often looking for unexpected safety signals, data mining methodologies can be useful in being able to detect safety concerns early in drug development. Based on experience within the drug development community, such as that with the Cox-2 inhibitors such as Vioxx which was found to have increased risk of cardiovascular events (Krumholz et al. 2007), safety modeling and data mining is critical to developing drugs and finding appropriate dosing regimens.

To further explore concentration-adverse event relationships, seven of the most commonly observed adverse events, as measured by incidence rate, were further modeled using logistic regression. The explanatory variable was chosen among the candidates C_{max}, AUC or average observed concentration (C_{avg}). Results of this modeling were fairly consistent among these three variables, as would be expected from a drug with linear kinetics. For several adverse events, including nausea and vomiting, statistically significant relationships were observed. The models indicated higher concentrations had significantly lower tolerability. See Fig. 9.4 for an example of an exposure-safety relationship or for a more thorough look; see, e.g., Tompson et al. (2013).

Since no efficacy data were available from the Phase I trial in healthy volunteers, a dose-response curve was not available for planning the study. Hence, it was decided that the best design would bracket the dose range covered in the Phase 1 study. From a PK-PD perspective, the design should be constructed to estimate the dose-response curve with sufficient precision that Phase III doses can be chosen. The endpoint and timing were selected in consultation with the medical expert on the program. Two design options were available: (1) a fixed dose-ranging design and

(2) an adaptive dose-ranging design. An adaptive design has the advantage of efficiently estimating the dose-response curve (cf. Reeve and Turner 2013). However, adaptive designs can be more complicated than fixed designs to plan and execute, and hence the benefits cannot automatically be assumed. In practice, adaptive designs require a fair amount of advanced planning, require statistical expertise versed in the issued of adaptive designs, and need careful wording in the protocol to ensure that the statistical properties of the trial are controlled and understood. Since the modeling from Phase I indicated linearity between doses and exposures, dose was used as a surrogate for drug exposure in designing the trial.

The fixed design is straightforward to simulate once the PK-PD model is settled. For the adaptive design, recruitment needed to be modeled in order to assure time during study execution for interim analysis and planned changes. The operations team was consulted on the rate of recruitment of this indication, and it was determined that the recruitment rate was expected to be slow relative to the 3-month time point at which the clinical efficacy endpoint would be observed. We should note that patient recruitment can be modeled as a mixture of Poisson processes, and this will be needed to adequately investigate the effect of any adaptive design. Other chapters of this book explore this process more thoroughly, so we will not here.

A Bayesian design was chosen, where arms would drop for futility if specific criteria were fulfilled. The upper bound on the number of subjects is denoted N. For this trial two values were compared: $N = 50$ and $N = 100$. If this design were fixed, $N/4$ subjects would be randomized to each trial arm. In the adaptive design, the trial would act as a fixed design trial until a fraction (f) of the total subjects have been randomized; the subjects in this fraction f were called the "run-in" group. After that point, the adaptive algorithm would adjust the probabilities of being assigned to each of the four treatment groups based on the accumulated data. The frequency of updating could be adjusted, from many interim analyses to only one. This model was constructed to perform the interim analysis at a fixed frequency in time, which yields a varying frequency in number of subjects analyzed, and hence the number of interim analyses varied among the studies simulated.

For this design, doses of 0, 5, 10, and 15 mg were chosen for study, the same as for the fixed design. The model chosen was the normal dynamic linear model (cf. Petris et al. 2009). Let μ_k, $0 \leq k \leq 3$ represent the mean of dose level k, where $k = 0$ represents the placebo group. Then the means are modeled by the relationship

$$\mu_k = \mu_{k-1} + \Delta_{k-1}, \tag{9.7}$$

where Δ_{k-1} is distributed as a Gaussian $N(0, \tau^2)$ and the variability parameter τ, which has the inverse gamma distribution $IG(\tau_0, \tau_0\tau_n/n)$, acting as a shrinkage parameter to reduce random variability in the mean estimates of each dose level. Each of the prior parameters in the prior can be adjusted to tune the performance of the adaptive algorithm so that the algorithm performs well over a set of dose-response curves. From prior studies, the standard deviation of the observations was estimated to be 10 units. Three dose-response curves were simulated, and the best design would perform well on all three scenarios: (1) null hypothesis case of no

Table 9.5 Simulation design parameters to optimize the adaptive trial

Standard deviation of differences among means (τ_0)	Maximum sample size	First futility sample size (fraction f)
5	50	15 (30%)
	50	25 (50%)
	50	35 (70%)
	100	30 (30%)
	100	50 (50%)
	100	70 (70%)
10	50	15 (30%)
	50	25 (50%)
	50	35 (70%)
	100	30 (30%)
	100	50 (50%)
	100	70 (70%)

response; (2) S-shaped function dose response (denoted as expected); and (3) U-shaped function dose response. The study would stop for futility if P(Success in Phase III) < 0.2. The study would be declared successful if the P(Success in Phase III) > 0.7 by the end of the study.

A factorial design (Table 9.5) on the study design parameters was performed in order to optimize those parameter values. Operating characteristics were proportion of subjects saved (due to stopping early for futility), maximum probability (across doses) that each non-placebo dose is better than placebo, and probability of success in Phase III trial, under the assumption of 300 subjects in the Phase III, where the best dose is taken forward.

Each parameter affected different operating characteristics. Effect of changing the fraction f on the probability of futility is shown in Fig. 9.5 (for the null hypothesis) and Fig. 9.6 (for an alternative hypothesis).

Results show that the value of τ_0 has an impact on the performance, but only for extreme values. For values greater than 1, τ_0 has minimal impact; see Figs. 9.7 and 9.8. Similarly, τ_n was also looked at. The inverse gamma parameter τ_n is an indicator of how much information is available on the variability of the treatment means; performance was robust once τ_n was greater than 1; see Fig. 9.7.

In this adaptive design, doses would be dropped if the predictive probability of superior relative to placebo dropped below 0.1. The trial was characterized a success if the dose with the highest probability of achieving success in a Phase III trial (assuming $N = 300$ in the Phase III trial) was greater than 0.7 and was considered a failure if this probability <0.3 at the end; intermediate values yielded an inconclusive trial. Measures of interest were the expected sample size savings from a fixed trial, probability of success, and predictive probability of success in the Phase III trial. Three scenarios were investigated: (1) null hypothesis of a flat dose-response curve; (2) expected dose-response curve with a significant improvement at the highest dose, and intermediate improvements at intermediate doses; and

Fig. 9.5 Effect of varying
fraction f on the probability
of futility under the null
hypothesis

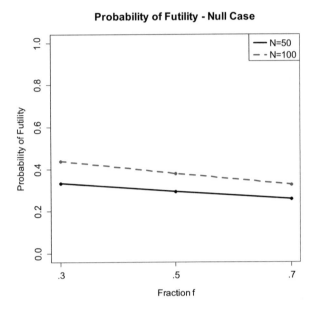

Probability of Futility - Null Case

Fig. 9.6 Effect of varying
fraction f on the probability
of futility under the
alternative hypothesis

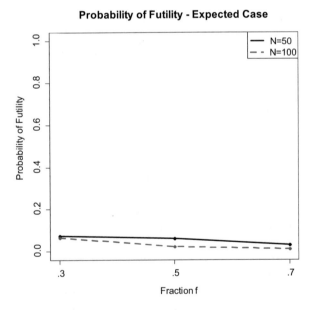

Probability of Futility - Expected Case

(3) U-shaped dose response where the maximum response occurs at an intermediate point and the maximum dose has an intermediate but still positive response.

A Bayesian adaptive design using four dose levels had high probability of success in scenarios 2 and 3 and lower probability of success in the scenario 1 versus a design with more dose levels. One concern was the priors on the parameters in a

Fig. 9.7 The effect of varying the expected value of τ, τ_0, for the null hypothesis

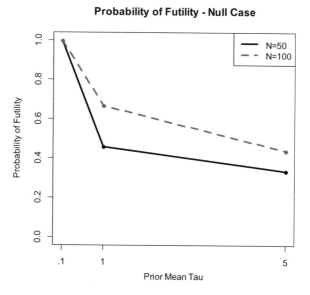

Fig. 9.8 The effect of varying the expected value of τ, τ_0, for the alternative hypothesis

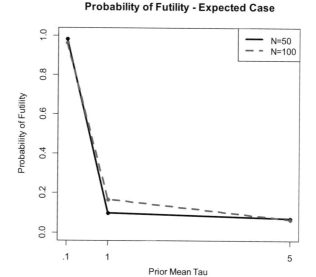

Bayesian framework might have a deleterious effect on study performance. However, our analysis indicated that within reasonable ranges, trial performance was fairly robust against variation in priors. Using an adaptive design would have saved on average between 10 and 20% of the cost of the trial, and so would have benefited the program with cost savings. Additionally, the adaptive design would have stopped the trial early for futility in this case, thereby providing supportive evidence to discontinue product development.

Decisions affecting the development of the compound and trial designs within that development were improved by the interaction among the different subject-matter expertise: clinical, pharmacokinetic, and biostatistics. Each expert contributed to the decision processes, by agreeing on which metrics should be employed, what endpoints were most valuable at each stage of development, and whether an innovative trial design could be used. Adaptive trials themselves require a degree of collaboration more stringent than the traditional designs, since the operational (e.g., blinding, drug supply, results communication with the sites, etc.), statistical, and clinical aspects (e.g., power of study, doses to be studied, endpoints used) are all closely linked.

9.3 Nonclinical Research and Chemistry, Manufacturing, and Controls (CMC)

9.3.1 Bioanalytical Assay Development

An assay is a procedure for detecting or quantifying an analyte. An analyte is that species of chemical, endogenous or exogenous, that is being analyzed, which typically resides in a biological sample; this sample is referred to as the matrix. For this example, an organization was developing an immunoassay, which uses immunological complexes to quantify the analyte, which in this case is a protein. For instance, consider an assay for interleukin-6 (IL-6), which is a large protein secreted by T cells and macrophages to stimulate immune response. A possible assay for quantifying IL-6 in blood would be an enzyme-linked immunosorbent assay (ELISA).

A sandwich ELISA consists of several steps, as shown in Fig. 9.9. Antibodies are used since they tend to be highly specific and have strong attachments. At each step, there are several parameters the analyst could adjust: concentration of the reagent, pH, and incubation time. The assay is performed in a rectangular 96-well (8 × 12 grid) PVC plate, with each plate well containing different concentrations of analyte. The steps of the assay are shown in Fig. 9.10.

The task for the biochemist is to (a) find which parameters (variables) have significant effect on assay performance, as measured by bias and variability, and (b) find optimal values for those significant parameters. In this case, it was chiefly concentrations of reagents and incubation times. After talking about the parameters with the biochemist, the variables of primary interest in the screening study were selected and are shown in Table 9.6. Since this was a screening study, a main effects model would be most appropriate (cf. Myers et al. 2016). A Plackett-Burman design is good for this sort of study, even with only seven factors. One could do a fractional factorial design with only 8 runs, but each run requires only 1 plate, and so 12 plates would not be excessive. Furthermore, Placket-Burman designs reduce the deleterious effects of confounding possible interactions with main effects by spreading the

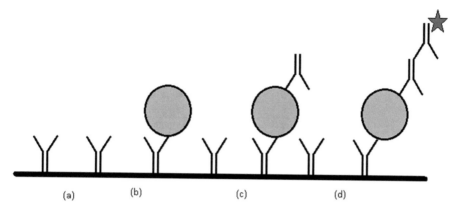

Fig. 9.9 Diagram of the steps to perform a sandwich ELISA. ELISA consists of several steps: (a) anti-antigens, called capture antibodies, are coated to the plate surface of each well; (b) antigen containing matrix is allowed to incubate in well, and antigen is captured/bound by the capture antibody; (c) detecting antibody (targeting another site on the analyte) are incubated and attach to the antigen forming the "sandwich" of capture antibody to antigen to detecting antibody; (d) anti-antibodies with marker attached (e.g., biotin) are incubated, and these anti-antibodies attach to the detecting antibodies; not pictured, a substrate is added, which interacts with the marker to form a color, with intensity being assumed proportional to the number of molecules of the antigen

---

Coat with Capture antibody
1. Coat the wells of plate with 1-10 µg/mL in carbonate buffer (pH 9.6)
2. Incubate overnight at 4°C

Blocking and Adding Samples
3. Add 200 µL blocking buffer
4. Incubate 1-2 hours at room temperature
5. Add 100 µL of diluted samples to each well (would normally have a dilution sequence down or across the plate to generate a curve)
6. Incubate 90 min at 37°C
7. Remove samples and wash plate twice with 200 µL phosphate buffered saline (PBS)

Detection Antibody
8. Add 100 µL of diluted detection antibody (normally constant to saturation)
9. Incubate 2 hours at room temperature
10. Wash plate 4 times with PBS
11. Add 100 µL of secondary antibody conjugated, diluted at the optimal concentration
12. Incubate 1-2 hours at room temperature
13. Wash plate 4 times with PBS

Fig. 9.10 Sandwich ELISA protocol as defined by Abcam (abcam.com)

Table 9.6 Key variables for screening study (step number from Fig. 9.10 in parentheses)

Variable number	Variable evaluated
1	Carbonate concentration
2	Incubation 2 (4)
3	Incubation 3 (6)
4	Detection antibody concentration (8)
5	Incubation 4 (9)
6	Conjugated antibody concentration (11)
7	Incubation 5 (12)

Table 9.7 Values of variables in Plackett-Burman design, along with sum of incubation times for each plate

Run	Var 1 (μg/mL)	Var 2 (hr)	Var 3 (hr)	Var 4 (μg/mL)	Var 5 (hr)	Var 6 (conc)	Var 7 (hr)	Total incubation time (hr)
1	10	2	2	High	3	High	2	9
2	1	2	1.5	High	3	High	1	7.5
3	1	1	2	Low	3	High	2	8
4	10	1	1.5	High	2	High	2	6.5
5	1	2	1.5	Low	3	Low	2	8.5
6	1	1	2	Low	2	High	1	6
7	1	1	1.5	High	2	Low	2	6.5
8	10	1	1.5	Low	3	Low	1	6.5
9	10	2	1.5	Low	2	High	1	6.5
10	10	2	2	Low	2	Low	2	8
11	1	2	2	High	2	Low	1	7
12	10	1	2	High	3	Low	1	7

The total incubation time is a key variable for the analyst

Var variable listed in Table 9.6, *conc* concentration, *hr* hours

interactions out among several different main effects, whereas a fractional factorial design would completely confound main effects with interactions. This design is shown in Table 9.7.

In talking over this design with the biochemist, our conversation turned to runs 1 and 5. The time to execute these runs was too long, making this experiment into a very long day. We had to cut off the corner, making the times shorter. Reducing all of the incubation times appropriately had very little effect on the statistical properties of the design, since all main effects were still estimable with approximately the same properties. Fortunately, Plackett-Burman designs are a type of D-optimal design, and experience indicates these tend to be fairly robust against departures from optimal. But the biochemist was able to organize the day in a reasonable period of time. Working with the biochemist, the runs were organized where the timing of each incubation start and stop allowed for the whole process to be completed by two technicians.

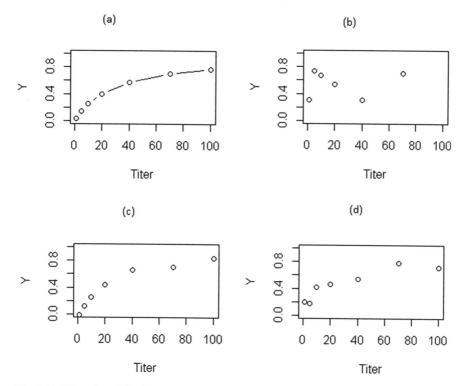

Fig. 9.11 Examples of titration curves resulting from a screening study; (**a**) perfect curve with no variability, presented for reference; (**b**) bad titration curve, given a low score; (**c**) excellent titration curve, given high score; (**d**) mediocre titration curve, given medium score

This whole process was made much easier by a couple of key factors: The statistician had engaged in assay work in the laboratory, learned the details of the processes, had a working knowledge of the biochemistry, and had gained the trust of the laboratory team by working with them on other projects, a partnership between biochemist and statistician. Hence, the statistician also knew that some shortcuts would be necessary: Run order was not randomized as would be normally the practice, but were ordered to accommodate laboratory processes. This allowed for some statistical risk, but was necessary given the practicalities of the problem. Additionally, since the statistician learned the language of biochemistry, they could easily communicate in the natural language of the problem.

The planned data was to calculate the mean and standard deviation of quality control (QC) samples, which had known concentrations of IL-6. Calculations are based on relative potencies calculated by comparing the horizontal distances between two Michaelis-Menten curves. Some of the data are presented in Fig. 9.11. Many of the runs failed to produce a titration curve that could reasonably be fit with a Michaelis-Menten curve. For example, in Fig. 9.11b the data appear as a random collection of values, and not as a curve. Looking at the curves together, the biochemist and statistician came on a different plan to analyze the results of the experiment. Plots of the curves were made and pinned to the walls of the laboratory for grading. The curves were graded according to their quality, with both the statistician and biochemist categorizing the results, with a score of 1 for a very poor curve and 5 for a very good curve. These scores were then analyzed using a linear regression model to estimate the factors that had the largest effect. The results were more difficult to analyze than expected since many of the curves were of lower quality than anticipated; while this posed difficulties, the collaborative nature of the work allowed for an alternative analysis plan and development strategy. It is difficult to imagine this experiment succeeding without the trust and the collaboration between both biochemist and biostatistician, who brought their own perspective to the problem, but could understand each other's problems and approach.

The result of this exercise was the identification of several key variables and the direction for improvement. At this point, the assay was run using operating parameters chosen from the curve quality analysis of the screening design. Based on the results of these confirmation runs (not shown here), the biochemist and statistician jointly decided that the quality of the assay was sufficient to move to the next phase: assay validation.

9.3.2 Bioanalytical Assay Acceptance Criteria

Measurement systems need to be developed and validated prior to use in studies following good clinical practice (GCP) guidelines. The validation process generates significant amounts of data that need to be analyzed and interpreted, and decisions about acceptability of the measurement system need to be pre-specified in standard operating procedures. Interactions between analytical chemists and statisticians are very productive in this area.

Consider the case of validation of an assay for amount of drug in a tablet. A common methodology is high-performance liquid chromatography (HPLC). In an HPLC, the compound of interest (analyte) is injected into an effluent that is under high pressure (often up to 1500 psi), and this mixture is pushed through a solid phase column to separate the analyte of interest from the other compounds in the effluent. The effluent is monitored at the end by a form of detector (ultra-violet visible light spectrophotometer, radiochemical, etc.) and measures the analyte over time (see step 7 in Fig. 9.12). The area of the peak in the chromatogram at a specific time is used to determine the amount of analyte exiting the column.

The peak areas (example units can be mV s) need to be calibrated to known standards. Reeve and Giesbrecht (1998) provide some data for a calibration curve. Given a standard with known quantity of drug, denoted x, then the peak area (denoted y) can be expressed by the simple linear equation

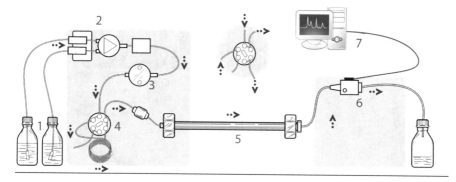

Fig. 9.12 Diagram of HPLC system. (1) Solvent, (2) gradient valve, (3) high-pressure pump, (4) sample injection loop, (5) analytical column, (6) detector, and (7) computer. Source: Download for free at http://cnx.org/contents/8419f350-7091-4f8f-bb0b-b777c5e97d96@4

$$y = a + bx + e, \tag{9.8}$$

where a and b are parameters to be estimated and e (with mean 0 and variance σ^2) represents assay variability. HPLC usually uses a linear calibration curve, though the variability is often proportional to the mean. Three approaches to the heteroscedasticity issue can be investigated:

- Weighted regression, with weights proportional to $1/x^2$
- Box-Cox transformation
- Log-log transformation

Teeter-Totter Model of Regression

A good example for regression leverage that gives non-statisticians an intuitive understanding is a teeter-totter. The angular force (leverage) on a teeter-totter is proportional to the square of the distance from the fulcrum times the force acting at that point; in a regression problem, the fulcrum is always $\bar{x}$, and the force is the distance between the fitted value and the observed value. Hence, a point farther from the fulcrum (x = 1000 in the example, since $\bar{x}$ = 180) has greater influence than does a point closer to the fulcrum (x = 0). This effect can be seen, e.g., in Fig. 10.14, where the deviation from the fitted line is most pronounced at the lower end of the calibration curve.

It is helpful to explain regression as a series of springs attached to a linear board, with a fulcrum at the means of the independent and dependent variables. Seen in this light, one clearly wants the springs attached to the board so that the attachment points are uniformly spread out, which is what happens in the log-log regression. In the weighted regression, the springs are attached in a cluster just below the fulcrum, with one spring attached to the top end: The

(continued)

springs do not alter the behavior of the angular forces on the board imparted by
the springs, but only the relative spring constants.

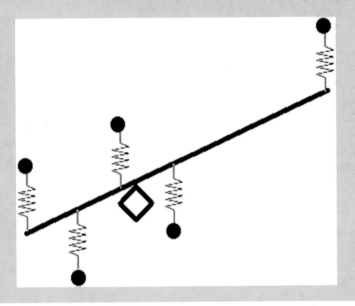

The weighted regression approach is often preferred by the scientists, since much
of the software developed and shipped for free with the equipment uses this
approach. If we assume e is normally distributed, then this approach is compatible
with the distributional assumptions. The weighting by $1/x^2$ is due to the fact that
$a \approx 0$ and hence x is approximately proportional to the mean of y. But the properties
of this approach are not necessarily well-understood by the scientists, and it is the
responsibility of the statistician to explain the issues. One critical issue is the
influence of the extreme observations on fit. This may not be a big issue in the
case of manufacturing quality control samples since the range of concentrations is
fairly limited, clustering around 100% of the label strength (%LS). For bioanalytical
assays, the range of concentrations (multiple orders of magnitude) can be large, and
in those cases the standards tend to be placed in a geometric progression (e.g., 0, 1,
3, 10, 30, 100, 300, 1000). Even with appropriate weighting, this generates large
relative errors at the bottom end of calibration range, since most of the influence will
be in the top sample. The leverage of a point is defined as how much the prediction
moves as the observation moves or the change in the predicted value $\widehat{y}$ as a function
of the change in the observation y at the same point. Mathematically, this is given by

$$\frac{d\widehat{y}}{dy} = \frac{1}{n} + \frac{(x - \bar{x})^2}{\sum_{j=1}^{n}(x_j - \bar{x})^2} \qquad (9.9)$$

The influence of a point is the product of the leverage and the "pull" of the data, which is proportional to the difference between the observation and the predicted value. See the Teeter-totter Model of Regression box for an explanation based on a physical process, the teeter-totter. Often the physical analogies are helpful to give subject-matter experts an intuitive grasp of statistical properties.

Re-expressing the data to a more appropriate scale is an excellent method for improving calibrating performance and is underappreciated by most analytical scientists. In statistical jargon, this process of re-expressing on a different scale is called a transformation. In this application, a transformation that stabilizes the variance across the calibration curve will be the preferred scale. The Box-Cox family of variance stabilizing transformations has been shown to work well in many calibration applications. The family consists of the transformation indexed by a parameter λ given the expression

$$y \rightarrow \left(y^\lambda - 1\right)/\lambda. \tag{9.10}$$

The limit of this transformation as $\lambda \rightarrow 0$ is the log transformation, and hence the log-log transformation is actually a special case of the Box-Cox family. The family tends to give reasonably similar results across a wide range of values for the parameter λ, and hence using a value for λ other than the optimal value typically yields similar benefits. Therefore practitioners will often use a set of parameters that should be tried first, such as $\lambda \in \{0, 0.25, 0.5, 0.75, 1\}$.

Consider the calibration data shown in Table 9.8 (Dolan 2009). The data are plotted in Fig. 9.13 along with four different prediction lines. Included also are the prediction lines for each of three different weighting schemes and also for a log-log

Table 9.8 Example calibration data for an HPLC assay

Concentration	Peak area ratio
5	0.0632
5	0.0725
10	0.1126
10	0.1344
50	0.6078
50	0.583
100	1.0714
100	1.1227
500	5.129
500	5.4232
1000	10.3892
1000	10.5105
5000	46.7262
5000	51.1182

Concentration represents known standards of a given concentration, and peak area ratio represents areas of an analyte of interest relative to that of another compound, known as an internal standard.

Fig. 9.13 Plot of calibration data. The four regression lines are also superimposed for the three weighting schemes plus the log regression approach. Ratio (y-axis) represents area of an analyte of interest relative to that of the area of the internal standard. conc (x-axis) represents known standards of a given nominal concentration

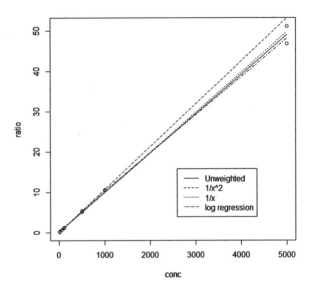

regression. The mean of the concentration is 952, and hence the fulcrum of the teeter-totter sits at about the 1000 concentration. The effect of the weighting is not as large as one would expect, but it appears the $1/x^2$ weighting produces a counterintuitive result, where the calibration curve is higher than either of the points at a concentration of 5000. A log-log plot gives some insight into the differences between the fits; see Fig. 9.14. On this plot, it is clear that the unweighted and the $1/x$ weighting schemes produces predictions too high at the lower end of the calibration range, and these would yield unreliable results. The $1/x^2$ weighting and the log-log regression yield similar results. The residual plots of both the $1/x^2$ weighting scheme and the log-log regression, however, paint different stories, and it is clear than the log-log regression is a better fit to the data (Fig. 9.15). The reason for this is not the heteroscedasticity, since both methods appropriately account for that, but rather the placement of the fulcrum and the springs.

The key question of interest is whether the assay is precise and accurate enough. The role of the statistician is to answer this question in a manner that is scientifically useful and statistically meaningful, but also understandable to the biochemist. This will be answered in the context of the metric known as percent recovered or the predicted concentration of a known sample that is treated as an unknown divided by the actual amount in the sample. If the calibration curve fits the calibration data, then the recovery should equal 100%, and this is true regardless of shape of the curve, assuming strict monotonicity. To see this, let the response y be modeled as a function of the concentrations x by the function

$$y = f(x) + e,$$ (9.11)

Fig. 9.14 Plot of calibration data on the log-log scale. From this perspective, all weight schemes produce similar results on the upper half of the curve, but vary wildly on the lower half. Ratio (y-axis) represents area of an analyte of interest relative to that of the area of the internal standard. conc (x-axis) represents known standards of a given nominal concentration

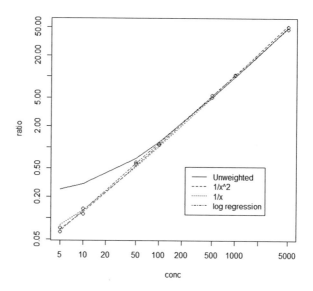

Fig. 9.15 Residual plots of $1/x^2$ weighting scheme and the log-log regression

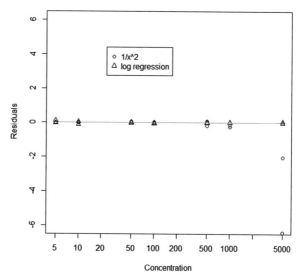

for a differentiable, invertible function f and error $e \sim N(0, \sigma^2)$. The predicted concentration x_p is then calculated as

$$x_p = f^{-1}(y - e) = f^{-1}(f(x) - e) \approx x + ue, \qquad (9.12)$$

for some constant u. The approximation at the end becomes an equal if f is linear. In this case, we have the relative recovery, denoted R, given by the expression

$$R \equiv x_p/x = 1 + ue/x. \qquad (9.13)$$

To develop the best statistical approach to accepting or rejecting the method, the statistician and the scientist will need to work together. A couple of approaches that have been found useful is to test the hypothesis

$$H_{01} : E\{R\} = 1 \text{ versus } H_{A1} : E\{R\} \neq 1. \qquad (9.14)$$

This hypothesis tests for a difference between actual and desired recovery; i.e., do we see a difference from the preferred recovery? H_{01} implies that there is no difference, and H_{A1} implies that there is a difference. This works well in the case of an assay with a relatively defined variance structure, and it is uncertain as to how large a difference is important. For release testing, another test may be more appropriate based on an equivalence hypothesis of the form

$$H_{02} : E\{R\} \leq 1 - \delta \text{ or } E\{R\} \geq 1 + \delta \text{ versus } H_{A2} : 1 - \delta < E\{R\} \\ < 1 + \delta, \qquad (9.15)$$

where δ is predefined constant. In many release testing cases, $\delta = 0.06$.

Let us contrast the pairs of hypotheses being considered here. For the hypothesis pair H_{01} and H_{A1}, the objective is not to reject the null hypothesis, since that would indicate that the assay is flawed in some way: It provides evidence that the recovery is not 100%. The equivalence hypothesis pair of H_{02} and H_{A2} provides a statement on the acceptable nearness to 100% recovery, and the objective is to reject the hypothesis H_{02} that the recovery differs from 100% by more than the acceptable difference. In terms of motivation, the biochemist will prefer to not reject H_{01}, but will want to reject H_{02}. However, the value of the acceptable deviation from 100%, δ, is a critical parameter in the equivalence hypothesis, one that should be discussed between the biochemist and the statistician. Each can provide useful information to provide insight on a value that would be useful. This discussion is critical to have and can only be accomplished in the context of a collaborative effort.

In general, the equivalence hypothesis H_{02} would be a better choice than the testing of the point null hypothesis H_{01} because it provides evidence that the mean recovery is acceptably close to the desired value. One consequence of setting up the problem this way is that it rewards better development: The difference hypothesis H_{01} would be rejected less often if less data are collected, and H_{01} would be rejected more often for an assay with very little variability. In contrast, the power to reject equivalence hypothesis H_{02} would be increased with a larger sample size, and also H_{02} would be rejected more often if the assay has very little variability. Hence, the difference hypotheses reward poor assay performance and poor validation procedures, whereas the equivalence approach rewards good assay performance and careful validation procedures. Let $P\{A \mid \theta\}$ denote the probability of accepting the method when $E\{R\} = 1 + \theta$. In the case of H_{01}, we accept the method if we fail to reject the null hypothesis; in the case of H_{02}, we accept the assay if we reject the null hypothesis. Then we have the following two properties:

- $P\{A \mid \theta\}$ increases as the sample size increases under H_{02} for any $-\delta < \theta < \delta$, but decreases under H_{01} for any $\theta \neq 0$.
- $P\{A \mid \theta\}$ increases as the variability of the assay decreases under H_{02} for any $-\delta < \theta < \delta$, but increases under H_{01} for any $\theta \neq 0$.

9.3.3   Formulation Development

This case study will look at the development of a dry-compression tablet formulation. Most pharmaceutical products designed for oral administration are not amenable to direct compression into tablets and hence need additional ingredients to support tableting.

To understand the thinking of the formulation scientist, one needs to understand the manufacturing process of the tablets. Tablet manufacturing is made in a series of steps. The steps typically include the following:

1. Agglomeration:

   (a) Most often done with wet granulation, but some tablets use dry granulation

2. Mix the drugs and the excipients.
3. Preparation of binder solution.
4. Mix binder solution with dry mix to form wet mass.
5. Dry the moist granules.
6. Mix the dry granules with lubricants.
7. Press into tablets:

   (a) Without the lubricants, the mix will clog the system.
   (b) But with too much lubricant and not enough binder, the tablets will not hold together in the bottle.

8. Coat.

To hold the tablet together after the press, tablets contain binding agents. However, the tablet must also function once in the biological system, and specifically the tablet needs to dissolve efficiently in the appropriate organ (stomach versus small/large intestine), and not dissolve before then. Hence, tablets often have a disintegrant to allow the absorption of the drug.

When working with formulation scientists, the first question that arises is how many ingredients are being considered, and the second is how many different formulations one can afford to develop. This gives the boundaries in which to work. For developing a formulation, a response surface design was used and included discussions with the formulation scientists. The formulation scientist may or may not be familiar with designed experiments, so the statistician may need to provide some instruction on the benefits of a response surface design. This is primarily due to formulation scientist reliance upon the concept of one-factor-at-a-time (OFAT) experiments. OFAT designs are inefficient and can be misleading in the presence of interactions.

A degree of pragmatism is needed for the biostatistician as well, since the perfect D-optimal experiment may not be satisfactory for the experimental conditions. And the time it takes to develop the perfect experiment may be more effort than possible benefit. To illustrate this, while working with a pharmaceutical scientist developing a tablet formulation, six critical variables were identified that needed to be investigated:

- Amount of talc
- Amount of magnesium stearate
- Amount of cellulose
- Amount of water in the wet massing step
- Wet massing time
- Die pressure

Other variables may also affect tablet performance, but these were the ones that the pharmaceutical scientist wished to investigate at this point. Since no investigation into the product had commenced, it was decided a screening trial would be most useful. In a screening experiment, interaction terms are ignored, and a design only for the main effects is constructed. A typical main effects design is a 12-run Plackett-Burman design, which is shown in Table 9.9. In the display, a low value for a variable is coded as −1 and a high value as +1. The advantage of a Plackett-Burman design is that possible interactions are spread across three different variables, and not confounded with any specific variable. Hence, they are fairly robust in a setting where getting maximum information quickly is important, but interactions are likely

Table 9.9 Complete Plackett-Burman design for 12 runs

FID	X1	X2	X3	X4	X5	X6	X7	X8	X9	X10	X11
1	1	1	1	1	1	1	1	1	1	1	1
2	−1	1	−1	1	1	1	−1	−1	−1	1	−1
3	−1	−1	1	−1	1	1	1	−1	−1	−1	1
4	1	−1	−1	1	−1	1	1	1	−1	−1	−1
5	−1	1	−1	−1	1	−1	1	1	1	−1	−1
6	−1	−1	1	−1	−1	1	−1	1	1	1	−1
7	−1	−1	−1	1	−1	−1	1	−1	1	1	1
8	1	−1	−1	−1	1	−1	−1	1	−1	1	1
9	1	1	−1	−1	−1	1	−1	−1	1	−1	1
10	1	1	1	−1	−1	−1	1	−1	−1	1	−1
11	−1	1	1	1	−1	−1	−1	1	−1	−1	1
12	1	−1	1	1	1	−1	−1	−1	1	−1	−1

FID Formulation ID. Note can have up to 11 variables. Order of runs should be randomized. Variables are X1 through X11; −1 indicates a low setting for the variable, 1 indicates a high setting

Table 9.10 Factorial 2^{6-3} design

FID	X1	X2	X3	X4	X5	X6
1	−1	−1	−1	1	1	1
2	1	−1	−1	−1	−1	1
3	−1	1	−1	−1	1	−1
4	1	1	−1	1	−1	−1
5	−1	−1	1	1	−1	−1
6	1	−1	1	-1	1	-1
7	-1	1	1	-1	-1	1
8	1	1	1	1	1	1

FID Formulation ID

to exist. In this case, six of the columns were selected to use in the design, and the remaining five were ignored; if however, we decided later to add another factor, we could then use one of the remaining columns for that new factor.

The formulation scientist was grateful for the design, went off to think about it. A week later the formulation scientist returned, explained that this design would take too long to complete, and asked to reduce the size of the design. Another option would be a 2^{6-3} standard design, which is shown in Table 9.10. In this design, interactions would be directly confounded and hence was a more risky design than the 12-run Plackett-Burman design, but with the payoff of 33% fewer formulations to construct. Again, after explaining the benefits and risks with this design, the formulation scientist went off to plan the experiment.

Another week later the formulation scientist returned, once again explaining that this design was also too time-consuming, requesting another reduction in the size. While the design could be reduced to a seven run design, thereby dropping one variable, the biostatistician strongly recommended against that course of action due to the increased risk and advised an analysis of this design with fewer runs would not be possible. At this point, the biostatistician asked how long it would take to run all eight formulations. The answer was 2 or 3 days. This is a classic example of over-optimized designs, since we spent nearly 3 weeks to shave off 1 or 2 days of laboratory work. Cost otherwise was not an issue. The follow-up was that the design was executed on the eight-run format and the key variables were identified to move the program forward.

Trust between the formulation scientist and the biostatistician is important in process design and optimization problems, especially as the cost of the experiment increases. When prior data are available, scientists are reluctant to run new planned studies, but would prefer to analyze already collected data. This is not always the optimal plan, but this can usually be addressed only if the biostatistician is considered part of the team. For this reason, it is best if the biostatistician works with the pharmaceutical scientists repeatedly, instead of dropping in as a "rescue" expert. The reason that prior data may not answer the questions lies in the working of interactions, which are usually not well-understood. In another tablet manufacturing problem, friability was an issue. The culprit was thought to be in the wet massing step, which is critical for producing consistently high-quality tablets, but other steps could not be ruled out. Data on the past 50 lots was assembled, with the idea of analyzing the data to assess the effects of different variables.

A multivariable linear regression was assembled to fit the data. First variable selection using backward elimination, followed by stepwise regression, was used to narrow down the field of variables to study. This produced six variables of interest, but with relatively poor fitting results. To improve fitting, higher-order polynomial terms were added, to the point of adding up to quartic terms. Since the model generated predictions that were inconsistent with experience in the manufacturing of tablets, management concurred with the biostatistical team that this model was not an appropriate solution, and a more controlled line of attack must be attempted, hence a planned experiment.

A planned experiment in a full-scale manufacturing setting is no small undertaking, since the plant must be taken out of service to run the experiment and millions of dollars of active pharmaceutical ingredient (API) and excipients are involved. As we discussed elsewhere, large amounts of resources are at risk in these high-stakes experiments. Hence, a lengthy round of discussion involving the biostatistical team, formulation team, and manufacturing engineers, including the quality control team, were initiated.

In these cases, the biostatistical role is essential, but delicate. The biostatistician possesses the expertise and the technological know-how to develop a line of attack to efficiently answer the question. But one must be wholly committed to and considered part of the team; otherwise this process is likely to end in a sub-optimal solution, possibly even acrimony. Consider the viewpoint of the manufacturing engineer, someone who has extensive education and many years of experience running a tablet manufacturing facility. The engineer is facing a problem that he cannot solve in a timely manner. He is unlikely to appreciate an outsider, with no knowledge of manufacturing issues, telling the engineer that there is a better way of solving the problem. In these cases, consulting can be counterproductive. The biostatistician truly needs to collaborate with the subject-matter experts, and the easiest path to success is to be a valuable part of the team, with actual knowledge and experience in these problems. And the way to become part of the team is to get out of the office, into the plan, into the laboratories, involved in the QC decisions. In short, become an actual pharmaceutical scientist that takes full responsibility for the operations along with the technical and managerial team of the facility.

9.3.4 Software as a Medical Device (SaMD)

Many medical devices incorporate software; for example, home-based glucose monitoring devices have physical components, but the functionality of the device would be non-existent without the software built into them. Conversely, software can also be the device. These software devices can facilitate better dosing than would be available otherwise. Pharmacokineticists and biostatisticians play a key role in developing, evaluating, and gaining marketing approval for these types of precision dosing devices.

SaMD can be used to help personalize a dose for an individual patient, and this can be achieved in different ways. For example, one can have a target exposure level for a patient, and the dose or dosing interval can be altered to achieve a target exposure level or response. For example, aminoglycoside dosing in infectious disease, Factor VIII/Factor IX in hemophilia, or warfarin for anticoagulation, where the target is to achieve an international normalized ratio[1] (INR) between 2.0 and 3.0.

Developing SaMD tools to help determine an individualized dosing regimen to achieve a specific exposure level can be useful in several contexts, including:

- Patient care, where achieving a target exposure level helps to improve product performance (e.g., in renal, hepatic, or immune-impaired patients; special populations like pediatrics/geriatrics; transplant patients; addressing drug-drug interactions; and optimizing the usage of expensive medications)
- Clinical studies, where a randomized concentration-controlled trial will have advantages over more traditional randomized dose-controlled trials

For this example, the exposure parameters of interest were time above a target through concentration, clearance, and area under the concentration-versus-time curve (AUC). The SaMD aims to reduce the burden on the patients in terms of the number of blood draws used to adequately estimate these parameters. The goal was to use only two samples to estimate each parameter, instead of the full complement of eight or nine samples. This sample reduction is not a new concept; this was successfully performed for mycophenolate mofetil in a clinical trial in renal transplant patients in the early-1990s in order to properly dose patients in an RCCT (see, e.g., Hale et al. 1998; Reeve and Hale 1994; Hale and Reeve 1994; Reeve 1996). To construct this SaMD, we need:

1. A population PK model based on dense sampling.
2. An algorithm which produces Bayesian posterior estimates of the PK model parameters based on a small subsample of time points, using the population PK model parameters and variability estimates (e.g., standard deviation of the random effects in the population PK model) as the priors.
3. An implementation of the model in software with a simple delivery method to the point of use (e.g., a website or mobile interface).
4. A method for evaluation of the software device. This may involve development of a comparative trial, with corresponding sample size calculations to validate the software estimation and predictions.

---

[1]The INR is the ratio of prothrombin time between a test and normal tissue $(PT_{test}/PT_{normal})^{ISI}$, for some factor ISI which is a function of the particular normal (control) sample.

As can be seen, this requires the close collaboration of several different areas of expertise, including pharmacokinetics, regulatory, biostatistics, and software development.

In this case study, a population PK model was developed for the compound by the pharmacokineticist using a nonlinear mixed effects modeling software called NONMEM (*ICON* Development Solutions, Elliott City, Maryland), for use by a precision dosing software application. The population PK model consisted of a two-compartment structural IV model with between subject variability terms for both clearance (CL) and the central compartment volume of distribution (V_c) along with a proportional within subject variability (residual) error model. Weight and creatinine clearance were both identified as significant covariates for CL in a median normalized manner. Weight was also identified as a significant covariate on the V_c in a median normalized manner. For model validation, the population PK model demonstrated suitable model stability after evaluation of the condition number (e.g., condition number less than 20 Mould and Upton (2013)) and non-parametric bootstrapped confidence intervals (e.g., confidence interval endpoints within 20% of the point estimate). Likewise, evaluation of numeric and visual predictive checks indicated that the model adequately predicted concentrations.

The device user interface collected the individual patient demographic, weight, and creatinine clearance values. In addition, the interface also collected the patient's current dosing regimen and PK sample collection activities with the date and times of each. These data were then fed into the Bayesian estimation algorithm, originally implemented using the post hoc random effects prediction built into the NONMEM system. However, to achieve faster reporting speeds on the device to be used in the clinic, the model was re-coded into C++ since NONMEM was found to run slowly in a mobile or web environment (other typical mobile or web interface computer languages include Java and Perl). The individual parameter estimates along with graphical representation of the model fits were presented within the interface. Finally, the individual parameter estimates could then be used to predict exposure levels of potential new dosing regimens for selection to optimize the exposure levels (see Fig. 9.16).

The clinical trials used for validation of the medical device was relatively simple to design in terms of implementation using intra-patient comparisons of the dosing regimen AUC values produced by the software device (based upon the minimal sampling scheme) with AUC obtained by NCA methods using the full profile. The criteria for success were that 95% of all patients have device AUCs within $\pm 15\%$ of the NCA AUCs and that 99% are within $\pm 20\%$. We also summarized the results using the root mean squared error (RMSE $= [\Delta^2 + v^2]^{1/2}$ where Δ is the mean difference and v is the standard deviation of the within-subject differences) of the difference in predicted and actual AUC within the same subject.

Data to support the sample size calculation came from two sources: (1) historical data from completed clinical studies and (2) simulated data. Historical data are data from subjects that have already been analyzed within other trials of the clinical program. Simulated data were constructed by creating virtual patients with realistic covariate relationships and simulated concentration levels based upon the population

Fig. 9.16 Screenshot of a precision dosing software application mobile user interface

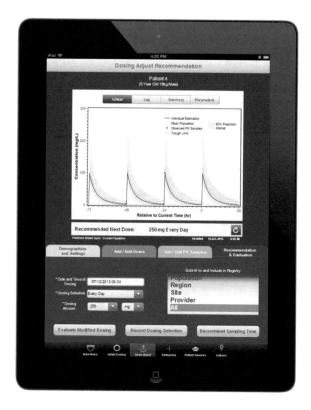

PK model developed from the clinical studies (historical data). The simulations were useful since the sample size in the historical data is fairly limited, and the variability estimate would have a large inherent uncertainty. The simulated results can be thought of as a bootstrapping approach to better estimate the uncertainty in the variability (Fig. 9.17).

As noted, the device estimate of AUC is derived from a Bayesian calculation based on the population PK model using just a few optimal samples. Two and three sample options were looked at with regard to the choice of the sparse sample times used to estimate the predicted AUC. The mean, standard deviation, and root mean squared error were estimated for both the historical and the simulated data.

Given the variability and the proportion of success estimated from both the historical and simulated data, the sample size can be calculated for both the proportion and the RMSE endpoints. For the proportion, the point estimate of the proportion needs to be larger than 95%, and hence power will be defined as the probability that the estimate of the proportion within ±15% is at least 95%.

The power, denoted π, on the proportion can be calculated as

$$\pi = 1 - \text{Bin}(\lfloor 0.95n \rfloor, n \mid p = 0.97) \tag{9.16}$$

Fig. 9.17 Schematic of the clinical trial, and the comparisons needed. The standard method is the traditional PK data analysis which involves the estimation of individual pharmacokinetic parameters through nonlinear regression using an individual's dense concentration-time data. A second stage then calculates descriptive summary statistics such as mean parameters estimates, variance, and covariance of the individual parameter estimates obtained during the first stage

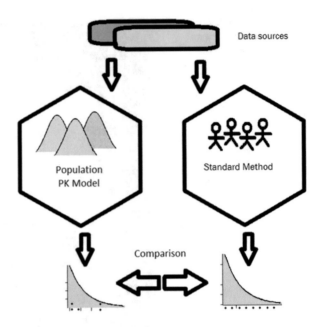

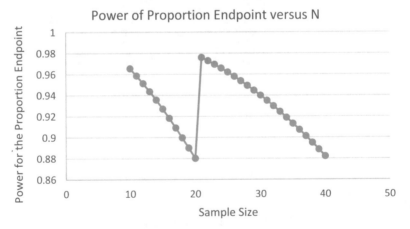

Fig. 9.18 Probability of observed proportion within 15% being greater than 95% given the estimate of 97% based on historical variability

where $\lfloor x \rfloor$ is the greatest integer less than x and Bin(k, n | p) = P{X ≤ k | n, p} is the cumulative distribution function for a binomial random variable. The power function is shown in Fig. 9.18. We note immediately that increasing sample size does not increase the power necessarily, but may in fact reduce it. This behavior often comes as a surprise to both biostatisticians and pharmacokineticists alike and will need to be discussed with the trial team to ensure adequate trial power. The minimum power occurs on multiples of 20, and this is due to the discreteness of the binomial distribution.

This project requires close collaborations between the pharmacokineticist, biostatistician, and software developers to succeed. The pharmacokineticist brings expert knowledge of the PK model and the possibilities for dose adjustment, along with practical knowledge of behavior in the clinic. Physicians also can be involved to support what dose time point would be acceptable to patients, how the device should function for ease of interpretation by the clinical customers, and knowledge of which patients to include in the clinical study. Likewise, the software developer needs to work with the team very closely to implement the model in a native device language, ensure that the device's user interface works well on the platforms being used, and can provide necessary outputs. And the biostatistician needs to provide power calculations, device testing data and scenarios, and work closely with the pharmacokineticist as the models are optimized to achieve good parameter estimation.

9.4   Conclusion

Collaboration within the pharmaceutical industry between biostatisticians and subject-matter experts is very productive. Collaboration allows for solutions to problems that would be difficult without the collaboration and allows the solutions to be developed much more efficiently than without the collaboration. Biostatistical input is valuable in many areas of clinical development, including clinical trial design, nonclinical areas such as assay development, manufacturing process development and control, and formulation development, and in newer areas such as personalized precision dosing. Collaboration is also very rewarding for the biostatistician, since working with our colleagues in other areas of expertise allows the biostatistician to contribute to the solutions of difficult, important problems facing the drug development organization.

Collaboration of biostatisticians across the organization can also contribute to cost savings. Consider the case of model-based drug development (MBDD), which requires a close collaboration between biostatisticians, pharmacokineticists, and clinicians. MBDD is the process of using predictive models, based on statistical and pharmacokinetics-pharmacodynamics modeling, including exposure-response models. Based on an analysis of Lalonde et al. (2007), the cost savings within one organization was $75 million for 2006 and $100 million for 2007. Savings accrued chiefly through two benefits:

- Smaller dose-response studies instead of the traditional Phase II studies
- Fewer late phase studies, since the information used in drug development is improved under the MBDD paradigm

The experience of the authors with MBDD is that it improves decision-making within drug development through two mechanisms:

- Better quantitative decisions; using a learn and confirm approach to the drug development process is more efficient than traditional development methodologies.
- Forces active collaboration among different experts.

MBDD itself is a collaborative method, whereby biostatisticians, pharmacokineticists, and clinicians develop models that describe the input/output systems (i.e., dose-exposure-response models). This process requires input from each of the different areas of expertise, and the model is the language that everyone can use to describe the biological and clinical trial process.

References

The E.D. Deming Institute (2016) https://www.deming.org/theman/theories/fourteenpoints, accessed 4 July 2016.

Walton, Mary (1986) *The Deming Management Method, Perigee Books*, New York, NY

Peck, R., Haugh, L. D., & Goodman, A. (1998). *Statistical Case Studies: A Collaboration Between Academe and Industry (Instructor Edition)* (Vol. 3). Siam.

Lee Y (2000) The Sustainability of University-Industry Research Collaboration: An Empirical Assessment, *The Journal of Technology Transfer*, Volume 25, Issue 2: 111-133

Dolan J (2009). Calibration curves, Part V: Curve weighting. *LCGC North America*, Vol 27, Issue 7, pp 534-540.

Krumholz HM, Hines Junior HH, Ross JS, Presler AH, and Egilman DS. 2007. BMJ. Jan 20; 334 (7585): 120–123. doi: https://doi.org/10.1136/bmj.39024.487720.68

Tompson D, Crean C, Reeve R, Berry N. S. (2013). Efficacy and Tolerability Exposure–Response Relationship of Retigabine (Ezogabine) Immediate-Release Tablets in Patients With Partial-Onset Seizures, *Clinical Therapeutics*, Volume 35, Issue 8, 1174 - 1185.

Endrenyi, Laszlo, and Jiuhong Zha (1994) Coparative efficiencies of randomized concentration- and dose-controlled clinical trials, Clin Pharmaco Ther, 56, pp. 331-338.

Hale, Michael D., Nicholls, Andrew J., Bullingham, Roy E.S., Hené, Ronald, Hoitsma, A., Squifflet, Jean-Paul, Weimar, W., Vanrenterghem, Yves, Van de Woude, Fokko J. and Verpooten, Gert A.(1998) The pharmacokinetic-pharmacodynamic relationship for mycophenolate mofetil in renal transplantation, *Clinical Trial and Therapeutics*, **64**, pp 672-683.

Hale H and R Reeve (1994) Planning a randomized concentration controlled trial with a binary response, *Proceedings of the Biopharmaceutical Section of the ASA* 1994.

Reeve, R and M Hale (1994) Results and efficiency of Bayesian dose adjustment in a clinical trial with a binary endpoint, *Proceedings of the Biopharmaceutical Section of the ASA* 1994.

Reeve, R (1996) Efficiency of randomized concentration-controlled clinical trial *Communications in Statistics*, Vol 25, No 9, pp 2169-2188.

Reeve, R, and Turner R (2013) Pharmacodynamic models: Parameterizing the Hill equation, Michaelis-Menten, and the logistic curve, and relationships among these models, *Journal of Biopharmaceutical Statistics.*

Lu, J. F., Bruno, R., Eppler, S., Novotny, W., Lum, B., and Gaudreault, J. (2008). Clinical pharmacokinetics of bevacizumab in patients with solid tumors. *Cancer chemotherapy and pharmacology*, 62(5), 779-786.

Lalonde, RL et al. "Model-based Drug Development." Clinical Pharmacology & Therapeutics. Vol. 82(1); pgs 21-32. July 2007.

FDA (2015) Scientific Considerations in Demonstrating Biosimilarity to a Reference Product. Guidance for Industry

Knight B, Rassam D, Liao S, Ewesuedo LR. (2016) A phase I pharmacokinetics study comparing PF-06439535 (a potential biosimilar) with bevacizumab in healthy male volunteers. *Cancer Chemotherapy and Pharmacology*. Volume 77, Issue 4: 839–846

G. Petris et al. (2009) *Dynamic Linear Models with R*, Use R, DOI: https://doi.org/10.1007/b135794_2, Springer Science.

Myers R, Montgomery D, Anderson-Cook C (2016). Response Surface Methodology: Process and Product Optimization Using Design Experiments. John Wiley & Sons. Hoboken, NJ, USA.

Mould D, and Upton R N (2013) Basic concepts in population modeling and model-based drug development—Part 2: Introduction to pharmacokinetic modeling methods. CPT Pharmacometrics Systems Pharmacology. Vol 2, No. 4: e38. doi: https://doi.org/10.1038/psp.2013.14.

Duffy MJ, (2013) Tumor Markers in Clinical Practice: A Review Focusing on Common Solid Cancers. Medical Principles and Practice 22 (1):4–11

Griffin MM, Nick Morley, (2013) Rituximab in the treatment of non-Hodgkin's lymphoma – a critical evaluation of randomized controlled trials. Expert Opinion on Biological Therapy 13 (5):803-811.

Jatinder P. Ahluwalia, (2012) Immunotherapy in Inflammatory Bowel Disease. Medical Clinics of North America 96 (3):525-544.

Ferrante M, D'Haens G, Rutgeerts P, Vermeire S, Van Assche G, (2009) Optimizing biologic therapies for inflammatory bowel disease (ulcerative colitis and crohn's disease). Current Gastroenterology Reports 11 (6):504-508.

Horton SC, Emery P, (2012) Biological therapy for rheumatoid arthritis: where are we now?. British Journal of Hospital Medicine 73 (1):12-18.

Reeve, R and Giesbrecht, F (1998) In (ed). Peck, R, Haugh, L, and Goodman, A Statistical Case Studies, Chemical assay validation, pp 7–14.

J Mosak, R Furie, (2013) Breaking the ice in systemic lupus erythematosus: belimumab, a promising new therapy. Lupus 22 (4):361–371.

Scheinberg MA, Kay J, (2012) The advent of biosimilar therapies in rheumatology—"O Brave New World". Nature Reviews Rheumatology 8 (7):430-436.

Printed in the United States
by Baker & Taylor Publisher Services